LACTATION SPECIALIST SELF-STUDY SERIES

Module 4
The Management
of Breastfeeding

Rebecca F. Black, MS, RD/LD, IBCLC

Dietitian, Lactation Consultant, Researcher
President, Augusta Nutrition Consultants
Augusta, Georgia

Leasa Jarman, MS

Education Consultant
Augusta, Georgia

Jan B. Simpson, RN, BSN, IBCLC

Nurse, Lactation Consultant
Tuscaloosa, Alabama

JONES AND BARTLETT PUBLISHERS

BOS

World Headquarters
Jones and Bartlett Publishers
40 Tall Pine Drive
Sudbury, MA 01776
978 443-5000
info@jbpub.com
www.jbpub.com

Jones and Bartlett Publishers Canada
P.O. Box 19020
Toronto, ON M5S 1X1
CANADA

Jones and Bartlett Publishers International
Barb House, Barb Mews
London W6 7PA
UK

Cover illustration is a woodcut print by Russell Wray, Gull Rock Pottery,
325 East Side Road, Hancock, ME 04640.

Acknowledgment: Supported in part through funds from the Georgia WIC Program, Maternal and Child Health Branch, Division of Public Health, Georgia
Department of Human Resources.

Library of Congress Cataloging-in-Publication Data
The management of breastfeeding / edited by Rebecca F. Black, Leasa Jarman,
   Jan B. Simpson.
         p.   cm.—(Lactation specialist self-study series : module 4)
         Includes bibliographical references.
         ISBN 0-7637-0193-9 (alk. paper)
         1. Breast feeding—Study and teaching.   I. Black, Rebecca F.
   II. Jarman, Leasa.   III. Simpson, Jan B.   IV. Series.
   RJ216.S885   1997
   613.2'69--dc21   97-25569
                                                                                      CIP

Sponsoring Editor: Karen McClure
Production Editor: Joan M. Flaherty
Editorial/Production Service: Ocean Publication Services
Design/Typesetting: Ruth Maassen
Cover Design: Hannus Design Associates
Cover Illustration: Russell Wray
Cover Printing: Malloy Lithographing
Printing and Binding: Malloy Lithographing

Printed in the United States of America
02   01   00   99   98   10   9   8   7   6   5   4   3   2   1

Contents

Preface

Lactation consultants number in the thousands; they represent the varied disciplines of counseling, education, nursing, nutrition, occupational therapy, pharmacy, physical therapy, psychology, and medicine. The differing backgrounds of lactation consultants and the lack of a widespread educational program of study for lactation consulting results in professionals with strengths in particular areas of lactation. As we enter the next millenium, and possibly more control of healthcare resources by managed care and less choice by the consumer, it is imperative that those in lactation consulting share a base knowledge from many disciplines to compete and survive. As resources shrink, health-care professionals must expand their clinical skills to improve their marketability. Because boundaries separating prenatal, hospital, and postpartum services are becoming less defined, organizations and hospitals strive to compete for services outside their traditional roles.

The Lactation Specialist Self-Study Series draws extensively from the literature of all related disciplines. It is designed in four separate modules to present a systematic overview of the profession (support, process, science, and management of breastfeeding), emphasizing and reviewing areas for study usually lacking in the academic preparation of nurses and nutritionists.

The Management of Breastfeeding, Module 4 of *The Lactation Specialist Self-Study Series,* explores the developmental stages of infancy and the importance of viewing feeding assessment in the context of the expected physiologic state of the infant during the postpartum transitional period through late infancy. Discussion of sensory capabilities, as well as newborn reflexes, and how to incorporate the knowledge into assisting the breastfeeding infant are reviewed.

Issues of prolonged lactation, such as attachment, sleep, crying, and starting solids, are presented in Chapter 1. The nutritional needs of the infant and toddler are also discussed in Chapter 1 of this module, because nutrition is an integral component of the management of lactation as an infant develops. The section on nutrition for the breastfed infant in this module builds on the nutrition information provided in the section on breastfeeding assessment in *The Process of Breastfeeding,* Module 2, and in the section on the biochemistry of human milk found in *The Science of Breastfeeding,* Module 3 of *The Lactation Specialist Self-Study Series.*

Chapter 2 of this module presents information on the impact of maternal and infant health issues to lactation management. The influence of maternal metabolic diseases, viral infections, contraceptive choices, and medication use are carefully explored.

Thermal regulation, hypoglycemia, hyperbilirubinemia, infections, growth deficits, iron-deficiency anemia, and oral infant health care comprise the selected topics discussed in the section on infant health issues.

Chapter 3 includes information about breastfeeding infants who are premature; are neurologically impaired; have Down syndrome; have cleft lip and/or palate; or have functional variations of the palate, tongue, and jaw. This chapter, Special Lactation Circumstances, also covers guidelines for breastfeeding while pregnant, tandem nursing, breastfeeding multiples, adolescents who breastfeed, the maintenance of lactation during mother and infant separation, and relactation and induced lactation.

The format of the module is designed to be reader-friendly, with pre- and post-test questions for each section, extensive reference lists, and a useful index. There are 320 multiple-choice questions in *The Management of Breastfeeding*—the pre- and post-test format helps the learner gauge his or her knowledge about the content covered prior to and after completion of a section. The format easily lends itself to use in a formal learning environment, such as an undergraduate or graduate curriculum, or for the student or clinician looking for a systematic way to prepare for the profession or obtain informal continuing education credits.

Acknowledgments

In 1992, the state of Georgia public health nutrition section identified the need to update the knowledge and skills of practicing nurses and nutritionists in the field of lactation. The *Lactation Specialist Self-Study Series* was first developed as an eleven-volume set of modules and was supported in part through funds from the Georgia WIC Program, Maternal and Child Health Branch, Division of Public Health, Georgia Department of Human Resources. Many individuals were instrumental in the early development of the series. I wish to thank Carol McGowan for her vision of the project and the faith that the project would finally come to fruition, Gwen Gustavson for her pilot teaching of the curricula to nutritionists in two health districts in Georgia, and Irene Frei and Frances Wilkinson for their support of the project by providing the necessary resources.

Many other individuals have helped this series become a reality: Tracy Howie and Jerry Smith were invaluable for their technical computer expertise; Debi Bocar, Martha Brower, and Julie Stock reviewed all four modules and provided excellent suggestions about them for continuing education applications as well as feedback for improvement; Jatinder Bhatia and Elizabeth Williams also provided valuable constructive feedback from the medical community about selected modules.

I would be remiss if I failed to thank the behind-the-scene supportive individuals who kept my business running for what, at times, must have seemed like forever. Emily Kitchens, my business manager, is invaluable to me and without her organizational abilities, tireless energy, and loyalty, Augusta Nutrition Consultants, Inc., would fold. The lactation consultants and peer counselors on staff filled in for me in many situations and provided valuable insight for the series. Many dietetic interns enrolled in the Augusta Area Dietetic Internship combed the library in search of articles, as did Donna Wilson. The librarians at the Medical College of Georgia never wearied of my requests for reprints and seemingly daily presence on the Medline. Thanks also go to the nutrition and pediatric professors at the Medical College of Georgia School of Medicine and Graduate School for their willingness to answer questions and interpret literature.

Jan Simpson, one of the editors, was very instrumental in the *Lactation Specialist Self-Study Series*. Not only did she write several of the chapters but she also helped in the development of the content of the modules as well as the completion of the applications for nursing continuing education credits. Jan and her family worked many hours to get the series finished. Leasa Jarman, another editor, provided expertise on test construction and evaluated each module for completeness of the objectives and each test for accurate measurement of the objectives. Thanks also go to the individual contributors who are too numerous to mention here but are all named on the Contributors' list.

I wish to thank my family—Tony, Helen, and Marie—who gave so willingly of Mom and accompanied me on several trips to educational workshops. Many evening hours and weekends were lost to the *Series* and their support was essential to its successful completion. Finally, I wish to acknowledge the presence and guidance of the Lord Jesus Christ who gives me the strength to press on to the prize of eternal life through Him.

Rebecca Black

List of Contributors to and Reviewers of Module 4

Contributors

Rebecca F. Black, MS, RD/LD, IBCLC
President, Augusta Nutrition Consultants, Inc.
Augusta, Georgia

Donna Calhoun, BS, IBCLC
Lactation Consultant
Breast Expressions
Augusta, Georgia

Bryn Hamilton, RD/LD, IBCLC
Neonatal/Pediatric Dietitian in Private Practice
Augusta, Georgia

Leasa Jarman, MS
Education Consultant
Augusta, Georgia

Robin McRoberts, MS, RD/LD
Public Health Nutritionist
Augusta, Georgia

Jan B. Simpson, RN, BSN, IBCLC
Lactation Consultant in Private Practice
Tuscaloosa, Alabama

Richard A. Simpson
Pediatric Dentist
Tuscaloosa, Alabama

Reviewers

Debi Leslie Bocar, RN, MEd, MS, IBCLC
Oklahoma City, Oklahoma

Martha K. Grodrian, RD/LD, IBCLC
Dayton, Ohio

Pamela D. Hill, PhD, RN
Chicago, Illinois

Kathleen E. Huggins, RN, MS
San Luis Obispo, California

Karen Sanders Moore, RNC, MSN, IBCLC
Saint Louis, Missouri

Julie Stock, MA, IBCLC
Chicago, Illinois

CHAPTER 1

Developmental Stages and Implications for Lactation Management During Infancy

SECTION A

Postpartum Transitional Period

Donna Calhoun, BS, IBCLC
Rebecca F. Black, MS, RD/LD, IBCLC

LEARNING OBJECTIVES

At the completion of this section, the learner will be able to do the following:

1. Identify the sensory reactions and reflex behaviors of the newborn.
2. Recognize the importance of mother–baby interdependence during the postpartum period.
3. Discuss average, quiet, and active babies' responses during the newborn period in relation to breastfeeding.
4. Describe the four stages of maternal role acquisition and appropriate counseling strategies for each stage.

OUTLINE

I. Introduction

II. Bonding and Breastfeeding

    A. Physical adjustments

    B. Psychological adjustments

    C. Neuromotor reflexes of the newborn
        1. Rooting
        2. Sucking and swallowing
        3. Babkins palmomental response
        4. Startle (Moro) reflex
        5. Asymmetrical tonic neck reflex
        6. Stepping reflex
        7. Extension or tonic labyrinthine reflex

D. Inborn teat order behavior
E. Sensory capabilities of newborns
   1. Visual senses
   2. Auditory senses
   3. Flavor characteristics
F. Case report

III. Behavioral Assessment and Breastfeeding

A. Quiet babies

B. Average babies

C. Active babies

D. Case report

IV. Development of Parenting Behavior

A. Maternal role acquisition

B. Paternal issues

PRE-TEST

For questions 1 to 6, choose the best answer.

1. Cutaneous stimulation and breastfeeding augment newborn physiological adjustments after birth. Which of the following is not part of this process?
   A. Respiration and blood circulation
   B. Sucking activity
   C. Hair growth
   D. Attachment behavior patterns
   E. Digestive stimulation

2. Allowing the newborn to suck at the breast immediately after birth protects the mother from
   A. neglect.
   B. hemorrhaging.
   C. pituitary malfunction.
   D. thyroid disease.

3. Postpartum hormonal surges affect the emotional state of the mother and intensify her
   A. nesting instinct.
   B. motherly behavior.
   C. psychosis.
   D. fatigue.

4. Which of the following is not a factor influencing mother–baby interaction?
   A. Odor
   B. Crying
   C. Touch
   D. Clothing color
   E. Eye-to-eye contact

5. Knowledge of newborn neuromotor reflexes is instrumental for
    A. teaching nonprimitive behavior.
    B. managing appropriate positions for the baby during breastfeeding.
    C. establishing feeding duration and frequency.
    D. all of the above.

6. Based on neuromotor behaviors, humans are categorized as
    A. nesting mammals.
    B. rooting mammals.
    C. aquatic mammals.
    D. mother-clinging mammals.

For questions 7 to 10, choose the best answer from the following key:
    A. Tonic labyrinthine reflex
    B. Babkin palmomental response
    C. Rooting reflex
    D. Inversion prone response

7. This response is not an example of infant primitive reflexes.

8. This response is often misinterpreted as maternal rejection.

9. This response will intensify sucking activity when stimulated during breast-feeding.

10. This response is recognizable by the hand in the mouth.

For questions 11 to 13, choose the best answer.

11. Breastfeeding may be especially important for the high-risk infant because it
    A. improves respiratory functions.
    B. increases bradycardia and decreases body temperature.
    C. optimizes blood oxygenation.
    D. decreases body temperature.
    E. improves respiratory functions and optimizes blood oxygenation.

12. Newborn sucking triggers the releases of prolactin and
    A. estrogen.
    B. progesterone.
    C. oxytocin.
    D. epinephrine.

13. SMYLI is an acronym that stands for
    A. self-regulating, mother, youth, lateral, interaction.
    B. self-regulating, mother, young, lateral, interaction.
    C. self-regulating, mother, young, longitudinal, interaction.
    D. self-regulating, mammal, youth, longitudinal, increase.

For questions 14 to 17, choose the best answer from the following key:
    A. The quiet baby
    B. The average baby
    C. The active baby

14. Increases the possibility of stimulation deprivation.

15. Communicates actively through eye contact, attentive listening, and entrainment.

16. Changes in environment may disrupt the cyclic organization of these infants.

17. May have erratic sleep and wake patterns and/or feeding habits.

For questions 18 to 20, select the best answer from the following key:
   A. **True**
   B. **False**

18. Human infants develop close relationships adequately without bonding to one caregiver.

19. Sucking is an infantile behavior necessitating restriction for proper maturation of the child.

20. Bottle feeding offers a baby the same quality stimulation as breastfeeding.

Introduction

Breastfeeding as a continuum in the reproductive process is more than a method of providing nutrition to the young. It offers an exo-uterine domain that perpetuates and enhances the infant's development into childhood. The material herein reflects many years of scientific observation and evaluation of mental and physical responses between mother and child. The fact that Homo sapiens have survived for many years is validation that the human reproductive process is precisely designed to the smallest detail.

Zoologists realize the necessity to duplicate the natural environment and recognize the impact that unsuitable surroundings have on the ability of females to conceive, birth safely, and nurture their young. Likewise, accumulating statistics press our medical professionals and educators to reevaluate current procedures and practices, which, on improvement, will present a more accommodating environment for birthing and raising human children.

The main focus of this section is the mother and infant pair. This does not imply that other relationships, such as father, siblings, and extended family members, are not crucial to the nursing couple. Rather, the point is to emphasize the importance of the core relationship. Each detail of this interdependent relationship has a stabilizing principle, leading to ever-increasing lines of development for the mother and infant dyad. Recognition of the whole picture will aid us in the support of the breastfeeding couple and deepen our understanding and appreciation of the role of breastfeeding in human development.

Bonding and Breastfeeding

The *transitional newborn*, as described by Gene C. Anderson, is: "any just delivered newborn who is undergoing the process of physiological, and perhaps psychologic, adaptation from intrauterine to extrauterine life" (Anderson, 1988). Much like the marsupial that is born extremely immature, the human infant is dependent on environmental support and stimulation for growth. Like the marsupial, the umbilical cord and placenta are replaced with the breast and nipple to continue providing nutrition and numerous impulses to facilitate the infant's bodily functions.

Enticed by his newness, the mother lifts her baby to her breast, touches him or her, and feels a sense of wonderment. Attractive characteristics of the newborn elicit behavioral responses from the mother and, as the baby begins to suckle at the breast, this signals to the body that the birth is complete.

PHYSICAL ADJUSTMENTS

During the period following birth, the newborn has many physiological adjustments to make beyond the comfort of the mother's womb. Breathing, maintaining body temperature, feeling unrestricted body movement, feeling sensations on the skin, bowel activity, and circulatory moderations all require regulation. Research with kangaroo care (Anderson & Vidyasagar, 1979) has shown that keeping the high-risk infant in contact with the mother's body has a tremendous benefit for babies having difficulty during the transitional period (see Chapter 3 of this module). As noted by Montegue (1971):

The cutaneous stimulation the baby receives from the mother's caressing, from the contact with her body, its warmth, and especially the peroral stimulations—that is, the stimulations received during the suckling about the face, lips, nose, tongue and mouth—are important in improving the respiratory functions and through this means the oxygenation of the blood.

The colostrum from the breast primes the digestive tract, emptying the meconium and leaving a coating of immunizing properties.

Neurologically, the baby's senses are stimulated through the skin, encouraging him or her to open the eyes, recognize the mother's scent, taste her skin and milk, feel her warmth, hear her voice, and develop a sense of time or being. By allowing the newborn to stay with the mother, he or she is able to bridge the transformation from a fetus to a neonate.

For the mother, the physical changes are pertinent to her survival and well-being just as much, and breastfeeding augments the progress of the third stage of labor. The sucking of the newborn triggers the release of two hormones in the mother, prolactin and oxytocin. Oxytocin contracts the uterus, reducing uterine bleeding and prompting the expulsion of the placenta. Once the placenta has been expelled, there is a marked increase in the level of prolactin. Prolactin affects the functions of the breast and signals the beginning of lactation. The sucking newborn protects the mother from hemorrhaging and intensifies her mothering feelings, which in turn guarantees the infant's survival.

Reciprocal interactions affect every system—sensory, hormonal, immunological, and behavioral—in the mother's and baby's body (Kennell & Klaus, 1987); the interactions can occur simultaneously during the first days of life (see Figure 1A–1). The long-term ramifications to the child, parental interaction, and social structure by interrupting the progression of these steps is not known.

PSYCHOLOGICAL ADJUSTMENTS

Dr. D. W. Winnicott, in his talk "The Ordinary Devoted Mother," sums up the importance of the status of mothering (Lebenthal, 1985):

> We must be able to apportion etiological significance (not blame), and that is that in no other way can we recognize the positive value of the ordinary devoted mother factor—the vital necessity for every baby that someone should facilitate the earliest stages of the processes of psychological growth, or psychosomatic growth, or shall I say the growth of the most immature and absolutely dependent human personality.

S   self-regulatory

M   mother

Y   young

L   longitudinal (uninterrupted by birth)

I   interaction

As soon after birth as circumstances allow, early interaction is strongly encouraged. Ideally, mother and baby would be in a setting that facilitates close proximity at all times. For high-risk infants, the mother would be included in as much of the child's care as reasonably possible. Anderson labeled this kind of supportive environment with the acronym SMYLI (smile).

Examples of this would be kangaroo care (Anderson, 1989) and rooming-in arrangements. During kangaroo care, the mother simply holds her diaper-dressed baby under her blouse, with the baby in an upright, prone position between her breasts, allowing self-regulated breastfeeding. For term infants, most hospitals permit rooming-in—the baby remains in the mother's room during the postpartum stay. SMYLI arrangements permit the nursing pair to experience reciprocal interactions to facilitate strong attachment behaviors and assist the newborn to adapt to extrauterine life.

During the first few days following delivery, but particularly during the first few minutes and hours, the mother and her newborn share a physiologic need for generalized peristalsis. Inherent in self-regulatory mother–young interaction is generalized sensory contact, self-regulatory sucking and swallowing to satiety, and perhaps the dynamic action of ingested colostrum. These phenomena promote a parasympathetically governed (i.e., cholinergically governed) organic set in which

Figure 1A–1

Mother-to-infant and infant-to-mother interactions.

Source: Adapted from Kennell, JH, and Klaus, PH (1995). *Bonding: Building the Foundations of Secure Attachment and Independence*, p. 79. Reading, MA: Addison Wesley. Used with permission of authors.

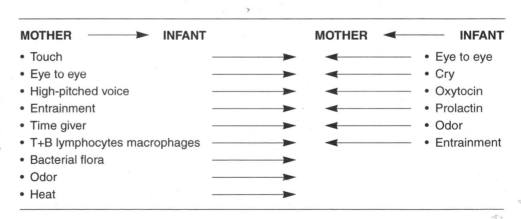

MOTHER ⟶ INFANT		MOTHER ⟵ INFANT
• Touch	⟶ ⟵	• Eye to eye
• Eye to eye	⟶ ⟵	• Cry
• High-pitched voice	⟶ ⟵	• Oxytocin
• Entrainment	⟶ ⟵	• Prolactin
• Time giver	⟶ ⟵	• Odor
• T+B lymphocytes macrophages	⟶ ⟵	• Entrainment
• Bacterial flora	⟶	
• Odor	⟶	
• Heat	⟶	

generalized peristalsis results in vascular perfusion, glandular secretion, and optimal body function (Neely, 1979; O'Doherty, 1986). Thus, optimal postpartum and extrauterine physiologic adaptation is facilitated. This mutual need, which is best and most naturally met by breastfeeding, causes the mother and her newborn to be initially dependent on each other for mutual caregiving-comfort, which can be achieved in association with each other.

Such pleasant associations, occurring over and over again, not only facilitate bonding but also mean more energy and contentment to share with the father. The mother and her newborn need to be free to interact with each other in a self-regulatory fashion from the moment of birth. Any lessened opportunity to interact constitutes some degree of deprivation (Anderson, 1989). Klaus and associates (1995) discuss physical and physiological interactions that help to build parent–child relationships in their book *Bonding: Building of Foundations of Secure Attachment and Independence.*

NEUROMOTOR REFLEXES OF THE NEWBORN

For the clinician working with infants, knowledge of normal reflex behavior will facilitate handling of the newborn, provide assessment criteria for recognizing disturbances, and, later, assist in positioning for breastfeeding.

In three million years, the evolution of newborn behavior and capability has not changed (Sugarman, 1988). The infant of today has the same needs and neurological functions as were present in prehistoric newborns. These abilities are basically for survival and many resemble primate behavior in which the young are carried constantly on a furry body. Humans are categorized as "mother-clinging" mammals. Our most rudimentary skills are grasping and turning the head to clear the airway. *Reflexes* are predictable movements in response to various stimuli. *Primitive reflexes* are those that occur automatically during intrauterine life. The following are the neuromotor reflexes of the newborn:

- Rooting
- Sucking
- Swallowing
- Babkins palmomental response
- Startle (Moro) reflex
- Asymmetrical tonic neck reflex (ATNR)
- Stepping reflex
- Extension or tonic labyrinthine reflex

Newborn babies are usually alert and active in the sensitive period following birth. A wakeful period of generally an hour or so in which active eye contact and vigorous sucking or licking at the breast occurs will ensue if not impeded by maternal medications or routines that separate mother and infant (Righard & Alade, 1990).

Rooting

Brushing the baby's cheeks with a breast or any material causes the baby to turn his or her head in that direction. This elicits a searching action with the lips and tongue. When breastfeeding, the baby will search for the nipple. A touch on the center of the lower lip causes sublaxation of the lower jaw. The mother can utilize this reflex to facilitate latch-on by lifting her breast and moving the nipple lightly over the center of the lower lip. The baby's response to the stimulus of touch varies depending on whether the baby is hungry or whether external circumstances, such as medications given during labor, have temporarily altered the baby's response.

Sucking and Swallowing

The baby draws a nipple or finger into the mouth, forms a seal of negative pressure around it with the lips, and uses peristaltic (wavelike massage) movements of the tongue against the object in an attempt to ingest it. Sucking in itself is a complex sensory-motor response because of sensitive pressure points located in the mouth. Rooting or grasping for the breast and moving the tongue appropriately are innate while how wide to open the mouth must be learned by the baby as he or she adapts to the mother's body. Swallowing normally accompanies sucking.

Prenatally, infants have the ability to suck; infants can be seen by ultrasound sucking their thumbs. The suck reflex is evident by 24 weeks (Herbst, 1981). The fetus can swallow by 11 weeks (Miller, 1982), and sucking and swallowing is established by 32 weeks (Amiel-Tison, 1968; Bu'Lock et al., 1990). By 37 weeks, the combination of sucking, swallowing, and breathing is well coordinated (Bu'Lock et al., 1990).

Babkins Palmomental Response

The head and mouth are linked neurologically. If the mouth or cheek is stroked, the hand on the same side will form a fist and the infant will open his or her mouth and bring the fist to the mouth. This is an effective tool for the newborn to use in calming, comforting, and finally controlling reactions (Brazelton, 1992a). According to O'Doherty (1986), this reflex is:

[A] legacy from our more hairy days; the hairy ape has the palmomental reflex that makes him cling to the mother when he is put to the breast, leaving the mother's hands free. . . . The palmomental reflex persists in quite a strong form . . . [and] bidirectional-grasp promotes sucking. Just as suck promotes grasping . . . the grasp may be induced if sucking is weak.

This may prove to be a beneficial technique to incorporate when developing treatment plans for breastfeeding difficulties.

Startle (Moro) Reflex

When the baby senses a loss of support or balance, he or she responds by throwing the arms wide with the hands open, then the arms begin to close together again and hands close. When the baby feels supported again, he or she resumes a neutral position—hands centered over chest, head symmetrical, legs flexed against abdomen.

Asymmetrical Tonic Neck Reflex

Head rotation to either side produces chin/extension and occiput/flexion; the infant assumes a fencing position. This posture is often misinterpreted as maternal rejection when, actually, it is only a fleeting response to a stimulus.

Stepping Reflex

The stepping reflex is involuntary. Parents mistakenly confuse this activity with the later development of walking. This reflex lasts only two to three months. To stimulate this movement, hold the baby upright, lightly touch the tibia against a surface, and the newborn will automatically step up, alternating each foot.

Extension or Tonic Labyrinthine Reflex

In this posture the head is thrust backward, producing shoulder retraction, arching back, and lower limbs extended straight. Babies with low muscle tone (hypotonic) slump forward when held prone. Hypertonic babies manage to arch upward. Babies who tend to hyperextend have difficulty with positioning for breastfeeding. Tonic flexation of the head and neck reduces mobility of the jaw, tongue, and throat, causing difficulty with latch-on and sucking.

As part of the neurodevelopmental examination of infants, these reflexes should be elicited. Their presence or absence, or the degree, need to be considered along with motor findings as part of the overall diagnostic picture. The following factors influence muscle tone:

1. Medications (barbiturates, analgesics, anesthesia and epidurals) given during labor and delivery
2. Neurological disturbances
3. Delay resulting from prematurity or low birth weight

For the breastfed infant who exhibits deviant reflex behavior, clinical assessment by a professional trained in this field will be necessary to coordinate corrective intervention techniques with the lactation consultant. Particularly long sessions of working to put an infant to the breast can overwhelm newborns. How babies cope, react, and interact during breastfeeding sessions gives signals about how to best interact with a particular baby to health-care workers. Babies can express being overwhelmed by crying or shutting down. Newborns are controlled by their reflexes and may need help in combining rooting and sucking to breastfeed effectively. See Table 1A–1 for a summary of newborn reflexes and positioning (Tully & Overfield, 1996).

In his Neonatal Behavioral Assessment Scale, Brazelton describes several techniques that utilize the neuromotor reflexes for assessing individual variations in babies (Brazelton, 1973, 1984). A description of how to use the scale is available on videotape and can be ordered from the Brazelton Institute (Children's Hospital, Boston, MA). In difficult breastfeeding situations, the tool may be helpful to assist counselors with understanding how to interpret an individual baby's behavior.

INBORN TEAT ORDER BEHAVIOR

Inborn teat order has been observed in other mammals. Work by Australian researchers measuring milk synthesis using a computer-image method also revealed human infant nipple preferences (Daly et al., 1993). Mothers have known this for years, as have experienced lactation consultants, but this is the first study to lend support to the idea that infants may prefer one breast over the other.

Table 1A-1   Newborn Reflexes and Breastfeeding

I. The complete rooting reflex involves turning toward a stimulus which touches the area of the mouth, opening the mouth, thrusting the tongue out and pulling in what ever is presented. The sucking reflex is stimulated by anything that touches the back of the hard palate or the back of the tongue.

    A. The tongue must thrust out over the lower gum and cup under the breast, pulling the nipple to the palate.

    B. For effective feeding, the breast must be far enough in the mouth for the tongue to compress the lactiferous sinuses against the roof of the mouth, allowing milk to flow freely through the nipple.

II. To facilitate correct latch-on, positioning the baby and mother comfortably is important.

    A. Place the baby with his whole body facing the breast. The ear, shoulder, and hip will be in a straight line and the hips will be flexed.

    B. Have the mother's arm well supported under the baby's head so that as she relaxes during the feeding, the baby does not feel as if his head is falling and bite reflexively.

    C. Rotate the baby's shoulders forward, placing one arm on either side of the breast, as if hugging it.

    D. Avoid touching any part of the face except the lips to elicit a simple rooting reflex. Do not confuse the baby with several messages at the same time.

    E. If necessary, stroke the tip of the baby's tongue with the nipple (or a finger) to elicit thrusting and to get the tongue out over the lower gum.

    F. Support the breast near the lower lip so it does not slip out of the mouth when the baby pauses between bursts of sucking.

    G. Pull the baby close to the breast so the nipple can go as far back in the mouth as possible. If necessary, adjust the baby's body position slightly to free the nose.

    H. To remove the breast from the baby's mouth, it is important to remember the biting reflex and put a finger between the baby's gums so he can bite on the mother's finger instead of on her nipple as his head is moved.

III. There is a wide range of normal reflexive responses that can be easily misinterpreted.

    A. Most newborns can only attend to one stimulus at a time and will close their eyes while feeding. This is not sleep but an attempt to concentrate.

    B. Babies may breastfeed in bursts of 10 to 20 suck/swallows and a pause, just as adults pause while eating.

    C. A baby who begins to feed and then stops sucking and appears to be in a deep sleep may be shutting down because he cannot manage to pull the nipple far enough back in his mouth to trigger the sucking reflex.

    D. A baby who arches his back as he is brought to the breast or who bobs his head back and forth at the breast but never latches onto the nipple is not rejecting the breast. In the uterus, it was effective to arch the head back because that stretched the wall of the uterus close to the face and held the baby's hand still at the mouth. A baby who is bobbing his head back and forth is making repeated attempts to grasp the nipple at the right angle. Usually, careful positioning of the baby while holding the breast can prevent arching and bobbing.

IV. There are several markers of a good feeding, which can be assessed and taught to the mother.

    A. The baby should be satisfied after feeding long enough to soften the first breast and contentedly releasing the second (usually, about 15 minutes on each breast) and remain fairly content for $1\frac{1}{2}$ to 2 hours.

    B. The mother's breasts should get softer and lighter through the feeding.

    C. After losing weight for a few days (up to 7% of birth weight), the baby should begin to gain weight.

    D. The baby should be having at least 6 wet diapers and 2 bowel movements every 24 hours by the time the baby is 4 days old.

    E. The mother's nipple should pull into a molded form to fit the baby's mouth during the feeding. The mother can look at it as the baby releases it. The nipple should resemble an orthodontic bottle nipple.

    F. If the mother's nipple has a raw and/or bloody line either vertically or horizontally at the tip, the baby is probably abrading the tongue against it. This incorrect suck usually prevents emptying of the breast because the baby is pinching the nipple shut and preventing milk flow.

    G. When the baby begins breastfeeding, his shoulders, arms, and hands should relax. He should not continue to struggle to get his hands in his mouth. He should feed in long bursts of suck/swallows. If he continues struggling as he is sucking, try:

        1. Gently pulling down on the lower jaw to position the tongue correctly, while the breast is lifted and pushed further into the mouth.

        2. Pushing in on the baby's back between the shoulder blades to straighten his neck and body, thus relaxing the jaw and allowing freer breathing and swallowing.

Source: Mary Rose Tully and Mary L. Overfield (1996). Lactation Consultants of North Carolina, Raleigh. Reprinted with permission.

SENSORY CAPABILITIES OF NEWBORNS

The visual, auditory, tactile, vestibular, olfactory, and gustatory senses are very important during the first year of cognitive, physical, and emotional development. Auditory senses can be stimulated by talking slowly; exaggerating letters, vowels, and words; and using the infant's name often. Singing, humming, music, the sound of the ocean, and a heartbeat or the dryer all are noticed by the infant and serve to develop the cognitive function of hearing.

Another cognitive function is sight, and mobiles, crib bumpers, blankets with contrasting patterns, black-and-white cards, and the faces of caregivers are easy tools to use to develop this sense. Skin-to-skin contact, water play, soothing baths with a caregiver, and massage are just a few ways to explore the physical sense of touch. Rocking, swinging, carrying, riding in a carriage or car, and supervised play in a waterbed introduce the physical sense of movement. Body odors and cooking odors can evoke emotional responses in adults, and infants have been shown to recognize the smell of mother's milk.

Visual Senses

Retinal structures and the optic nerve are not complete at birth. Breastmilk is particularly suited to further development of these structures because of its high concentration of docosahexanoic acid—a long-chain polyunsaturated Ω-3 fatty acid. See Module 3, *The Science of Breastfeeding,* Chapter 2, for further discussion of this topic.

Neonates focus best at a range of 8 to 12 inches—a distance approximated when the infant is feeding at the breast. Moving objects are preferred to stationary ones, and neonates are able to track objects as they move (Kessen et al., 1970). The human face holds the neonate's attention longer than other visual patterns (Frantz, 1965; Kagan, 1966; Lewis, 1969). Sharp contrasts, such as between black and white, are known to visually stimulate neonates but are recommended to be used for only brief periods. New parents need to be made aware of the newborn's incredible visual responsiveness.

Klaus and Kennell demonstrated that eye-to-eye contact is an early and important way for parents to accept that the baby is theirs. When newborns "fix" on their parents' faces, their eyes brighten and communication begins (Klaus & Kennell, 1970, 1976, 1982). Brazelton (1992b) describes an alert, three-day-old infant who imitated him by sticking out her tongue in response to his sticking out his tongue. The mother of the infant was so surprised by what her infant could do that she made a profound statement—"I'll treat her like a her rather than an it"—in response to Dr. Brazelton's question of what observing this behavior meant to her. This lends support to lactation consultants who often say the word "open" and demonstrate the requested behavior to the baby by opening their own mouths when working with babies who do not open their mouths wide for feeding.

Auditory Senses

Hearing is developed by the gestation age of seven months, with the fetus showing signs of responding to internal and external sounds. Differences in pitch elicit varying reactions in neonates with shrill, low sounds disturbing and alarming the infant and soft, high-pitched sounds calming the infant (Levanthal & Lipsitt, 1964; Weir, 1976). Newborns also can differentiate familiar voices from those of strangers. The mother can use talking to the infant as an effective way to reorganize a fretful infant prior to feeding. Even when an infant is in deep sleep, a slight stir may be observed when one quietly speaks near his or her ear. Other changes observed include changes in breathing patterns and a slight opening of the eyes. The sound of soft voices close to the infant assists the infant to gradually stir and wake up. Exceptions to this would be after a feeding or play period, or trauma, when the infant is in an exhausted sleep period (Brazelton, 1992b).

Flavor Characteristics

The sense of taste develops in the early weeks of gestation. Taste cells appear in the fetus by 7 to 8 weeks and are mature by about 14 weeks gestation (Bradley, 1972; Bradley & Stern, 1967). The fetus is first exposed to different tastes by swallowing amniotic fluid, which includes glucose, lactic acid, and urea (Liley, 1972; Pritchard, 1965). Studies show that there is a preference for sweet substances over bitter ones (Liley, 1972).

Newborns will consume more of a sugar solution than a plain-water solution (Deson et al., 1973). This preference continues as long as sweetened solution is offered and preference at age two is significantly correlated to the amount of solution consumed at six months of age (Chiva, 1979). If sweetened water is not offered after birth, there seems to be a diminished acceptability to it (Beauchamp et al., 1991). Different facial expressions in newborns can be elicited with sweet, sour, and bitter, but not salt, solutions (Rosenstein & Oster, 1990).

To understand the development of human taste perception and preference during gestation, Maone and associates (1990) developed a method to study taste perception in preterm infants without the delivery of fluids. A nipple-shaped gelatin medium was embedded with the taste substance to be studied, and infants born preterm (>33 weeks) were allowed to suck or mouth the medium. When the medium was sweetened with sucrose, the infants produced more frequent, stronger sucking responses than when offered a latex nipple.

This is interesting in light of the findings that sucking on a pacifier enhances growth efficiency (Bernbaum et al., 1983; Field et al., 1982), which has come into question based on the work of Ernst et al. (1989). These authors found a lack of improved growth outcome related to nonnutritive sucking in premature infants with very low birth weight who were fed a controlled nutrient intake. Is the intensity and the frequency of the suck important to the enhanced growth found in the other studies and would increasing the carbohydrate concentration in the form of simple sugars increase the intensity and/or frequency of the suck?

Infants do not appear to have a preference for salt, and it is presumed this taste is learned (Beauchamp & Cowart, 1990; Dahl, 1958). As a child ages, there is a preference for higher salt concentrations. Infants four to five months of age and five and one-half to six and one-half months of age drank more saline water than plain water (Beauchamp et al., 1986). Preschool children prefer highly salted foods more than adults do and prefer salted foods to salted water (Beauchamp & Cowart, 1990).

Sour and bitter tastes seem to be rejected by infants (Vasquez et al., 1982). Malnourished infants preferred a casein derivative in soup while well-nourished infants rejected it. This may show that protein-depleted infants have a specific taste for which there is a physiologic need (Vasquez et al., 1982).

Foods and various drinks in the maternal diet, such as garlic and alcohol, can affect the flavor of the breastmilk. Breastfed infants breastfeed less after mothers consume alcoholic beverages. Infants of mothers who drank orange juice with a small dose of ethanol versus the infants of mothers who drank orange juice without ethanol consumed less breastmilk during a three-hour testing session (Mennella & Beauchamp, 1991).

Another test of 11 breastfeeding mothers and their infants was conducted on two days separated by one week to examine the effect on infant intake for four hours following post-beverage consumption of a 0.3-g/kg dose of alcoholic beer on one day versus an equal volume of nonalcoholic beer on the other day. The infants consumed significantly less milk during the testing session in which their mothers drank the alcoholic beer (Mennella & Beauchamp, 1993). Mothers often did not recognize nursing sessions were cut short, but did feel that their breasts were not completely empty. An altered taste may have been responsible.

Little is known how foods in the maternal diet affect the sensory qualities of the milk. It is known that the flavor of the milk from lactating cows and rats is altered by the flavor of certain foods (Babcock, 1938; Galef & Clark, 1972; Galef & Sherry, 1973; Shipe et al., 1978). It is not unreasonable to assume that flavors from food do contribute to flavors in human milk since maternal dietary factors have been shown to influence breath (Kostelc et al., 1981; Sastry et al., 1980), urine and fecal matter (Moore et al., 1984), and hand odor (Wallace, 1977). In fact, a recent study indicates that breastfed infants accept vegetables better than formula-fed infants (Sullivan et al., 1994); and it is speculated that the breastfed infant has been experiencing a variety of flavors from the mother's milk and, as a result, is more open to acceptance of vegetables. Further research is needed to determine how maternal dietary differences affect human milk flavor and ultimately growth and development in the infant.

The fetus develops its olfactory system between six- and nine-weeks gestational age (Bossey, 1980). The amniotic fluid develops odors originating from the maternal diet (Hauser et al, 1985) and disease states, which may be present in the fetus (Martuis et al, 1988). Newborn infants have a good sense of smell and can detect a wide range of odors (Engen et al., 1963; Self et al., 1972).

A breastfed infant can separate the odors of his mother's breast and underarm odors from other body odors. Bottlefed infants cannot do this, so it is believed the skin-to-skin contact and proximity of the infant's nostril aid this development (Cernoch & Porter, 1985). Bottlefed infants have also been reported to prefer the breast odors of lactating women (Makin, 1987). There are similarities in the volatile substances present in human milk and amniotic fluid (Schaal, 1988; Stafford et al., 1976), and the normal fetus has open airway passages that are bathed in amniotic fluid (Schaffer, 1910). Animal studies have found that exposure to odors during gestation affects odor preferences postnatally (Hepper, 1987).

Mothers who are breastfeeding find that introducing a bottle after a few weeks is more successful if done by the father or another caregiver because the infant preferentially turns toward the smell of her breast. By seven days after birth, infants can differentiate their own mother's breast pad from that of another mother (MacFarlane, 1975).

BONDING AND BREASTFEEDING CASE REPORT

Sarah gave birth to an eight-lb., two-oz. (4198 g) baby girl by emergency cesarean section. The baby was diagnosed with esophageal atresia requiring surgical repair in two days and was placed on intravenous fluids in the neonatal intensive care unit (NICU) with medications to prevent infection. Sarah used a hospital breast pump every three hours to stimulate milk supply. Two weeks after the surgery, Sarah was allowed to begin breastfeeding the baby.

Initially, the baby would not root or cooperate with any stimulation to her mouth. She would close her eyes, become limp, and purse her lips tightly together. Sarah was discouraged by her baby's behavior and considered weaning. Knowing the contribution that human milk can give to a baby's health motivated Sarah not to give up.

Four days after the first attempt, Sarah brought the baby home. Feeding the baby required much time spent pumping her breastmilk, cleaning the pump equipment, washing and sterilizing bottles, and preparing bottles to feed. Sarah knew that breastfeeding the baby would be simpler and would increase the opportunities for rest.

Sarah contacted a lactation consultant (LC). During the first consult, the baby repeated the same behaviors. Sarah was worried that her baby was damaged or not healthy enough for the work of breastfeeding. The LC observed that Sarah did not cuddle her baby or hold her close, but kept the baby held at a distance on the edge of her lap or up high on her shoulder. When the baby was laid in the crib, she would hyperextend. When cradled in the hands of the LC, she would extend her legs straight out and brace her feet on the LC's chest with eyes shut and mouth pursed.

The lactation consultant recommended that Sarah and her baby spend a lot of time together in skin-to-skin contact to recreate the initial steps of interaction that were missed after the birth. The baby had experienced many traumas and unpleasant sensations during the stay in the NICU and, as a result, developed defense mechanisms to block out pain or forced procedures. Sarah, too, was disappointed in her baby. Instead of a round, chubby baby, healthy and eager to nurse, her baby was skinny, had a shaved head, and was unresponsive.

Sarah began to take her baby to bed with her and to carry her around most of the day. The baby was given massages with emphasis to the face and mouth. Sarah bathed the baby with her in warm water, holding her close throughout. Sarah continued feeding with the bottle at regular intervals, but would offer the breast whenever the baby cued a need to suck. Within several days, the baby began to breastfeed and bottle feeding was abandoned.

Behavioral Assessment and Breastfeeding

Within the broad range of normal behavior, infant temperament is generally divided into three categories:

1. Quiet
2. Average
3. Active

Each type involves a different approach to breastfeeding management. Sucking patterns, sleep cycles, levels of irritability, feeding duration and frequency, and neuromotor activity are all factors affected by the temperament of the baby. Behavioral assessment evaluates the intensity of a given attribute, and how to best interact with that attribute. Appropriate response on the part of the mother is important to the survival and stability of the infant. Therefore, caregivers should participate in helping the mother to recognize her baby's individual communication cues, and how to accommodate those needs.

During the transitional period after birth, mothers in a SMYLI setting learn to interpret and interact with their infants' behavior earlier than mothers who are routinely separated from the baby (Anderson, 1989). Breastfeeding in a SMYLI environment is self-regulated and requires little management by caregivers other than assessing the latch-on efficiency. Consequently, parents are able to develop parenting skills appropriate to the temperament of their infant.

QUIET BABIES

Infants who are labeled as quiet usually earn this title because of the low incidence of crying. During periods of hunger or discomfort, these infants are subtle in their modes of communication. They may not outwardly react to changes in their environment, such as being moved about from room to room. These "good babies" generally sleep four to five hours, feed briefly, then return to sleep. Mothers need to observe the nonverbal cues of these infants in order to adequately meet their needs. Good babies are at risk of missed feeds, stimulation deprivation, and missed experiences of bonding because they are left sleeping for prolonged periods; mothers indicate a hesitancy to awaken the babies. Infrequent breastfeeding increases the possibility of neonatal jaundice, poor milk supply in the mother, and the potential for latch-on problems.

Nonverbal cues indicating needs in the quiet baby include sucking motions with the mouth, flexed arms and fists while asleep, shifting positions or squirming, changes in breathing patterns and facial expressions, mouth opening without crying, rooting, sucking on fingers, and eye contact. Sometimes it may be up to the mother to initiate care and attention to regulate "cyclic organization" for the baby (Neely, 1979). Mothers of extremely quiet infants need encouragement to stimulate the babies—to pick them up, talk to them, and elicit responses.

During breastfeeding, quiet infants may have loose muscle tone, requiring sufficient support from the mother and extra pillows to maintain effective latch-on and to keep the mother comfortable during long breastfeeding sessions. Falling asleep, or sucking at intermittent rates, necessitates frequent, short feeds. Switching breasts when the sucking rate slows is one method to stimulate the baby to nurse longer and to keep the milk supply up but it requires careful monitoring of weight gain to ensure sufficient intake of the higher-fat hindmilk. Also, being held skin-to-skin, carried about, and hearing mother's voice arouses the baby to a more aware state even though the eyes are closed and baby appears to be sleeping. Offering the quiet infant time for leisurely sucking at the breast increases the infant's visual attentiveness and eye movement, and provides more interaction with the environment (Neely, 1979).

AVERAGE BABIES

Average babies respond to their environment with a wide variety of communication cues. Average levels of activity encompass a wide area, overlapping some quiet behavior and active behavior, yet the infant does not demonstrate those attributes consistently, only sometimes. Average sleep and wake cycles range in length from 2- to 3-hour intervals, with periods of quiet alertness without crying for 10 to 20 minutes. Neuromotor activity is flowing and varied, with firm muscle tone. Babies adjust to handling and being moved about with crying for brief periods, then calm when held and talked to. The average baby communicates actively through eye contact, attentive listening, and entrainment and cries when nonverbal cues are not answered.

Depending on the sleep and wake cycle, average infants feed every 2 to 3 hours. Sucking rates will vary from 3 to greater than 10 sucking bursts with pauses of equal length. They may nurse once during a 2-hour period or feed off and on during a 2-hour period.

ACTIVE BABIES

Active babies are sometimes labeled "fussy" babies, or high-need babies or colicky, because of their frequent and sometimes lengthy crying periods. Their sleep and wake patterns may be erratic, as well as their feeding habits. These infants require prompt attention to avoid hysterical crying. When hunger or discomfort cues are given, these infants become impatient and are difficult to calm. Changes in environment may disrupt the cyclic organization of these infants and their sleep and wake patterns vary from day to day without regulation by the mother. These types of children thrive on dependable activity routines in their environment.

During feeds, they may breastfeed vigorously for 5 to 10 minutes and be satisfied, or they may breastfeed vigorously then spend long lengths of time in leisurely suckling. Allowing these infants to breastfeed at one breast per feeding will increase the leisurely sucking periods. Active babies often have strong sucking urges and may fill themselves to the point of discomfort when nursing from two breasts. For these infants, increased opportunities for nonnutritive sucking helps them to regulate their cyclic organization. Some mothers find using a pacifier helpful because the baby wants to have sucking pleasure but does not need more milk. Neely (1979) found that nonnutritive sucking increased regular sleep patterns, decreased episodes of irritability, and increased quiet, alert states. Crying and irritability reduces the opportunities for the infant to have positive stimulation from his or her mother.

Mothers with active babies need encouragement and emotional support. Well-meaning friends and relatives may blame the mother for her child's behavior, telling her she's spoiling the baby or that her milk is not sufficient for his or her needs. Active babies need a lot of attention to help them gain control, stay calm, and learn to interact with their environment.

In summary, all behavioral types of infants benefit from continuous contact with the mother and breastfeeding. Newborns and mothers are considered "mutual caregivers" (Anderson, 1988). Mother–infant separation after birth has far-reaching implications that affect psychological and physical adaptation to extrauterine life. According to Anderson (1988):

The maternal milieu offers the ideal micro-environment wherein a mix of salient stimuli can be made available to the newborn in optimal fashion . . . for the exercise of amazing abilities which the newborn is now known to possess, and which can be demonstrated under the proper condition.

Psychologically, mothers are adapting to a new role in their lives. They must have optimum conditions to help them to develop strong attachments to their young, to guarantee growth, and to nurture their infants' balanced behavior. Separation after birth predisposes the mother to feelings of separation toward her baby. Developing attachment is the core of this intricately woven relationship—breastfeeding ties them together physically and emotionally.

BEHAVIORAL ASSESSMENT AND BREASTFEEDING CASE REPORT

Tina gave birth to twin boys by a normal vaginal delivery with no complications. Breastfeeding was initiated two hours after birth. Rooming-in was practiced for the 32 hours they spent in the hospital. Tina had several relatives who had successfully breastfed for extended periods of time. There was much help around home and encouragement for Tina's challenge of breastfeeding twins.

During the hospital stay, both babies were breastfed simultaneously for every feed. Both babies slept at the same time and the larger one would awaken first with the smaller following suit within a minute or two. At home the larger baby (baby A) began to sleep for longer periods and remain in a quiet, alert state for several minutes before signaling hunger with crying, then breastfeeding for only 10 to 15 minutes. The smaller baby (baby B) slept for shorter periods and would wake up screaming and would breastfeed for nearly an hour. Tina worried that baby B was not receiving adequate milk and baby A was losing interest too soon. Her mother suggested Tina get a consultant to evaluate the breastfeeding performance of each baby to rule out any problems.

During the consult, the lactation consultant observed that both babies latched on well and were sucking as expected. After evaluating the breastfeeding history, the mother and LC surmised that this was a case of individual temperaments and breastfeeding patterns. The consultant suggested that Tina closely watch for the waking activity of baby B to avoid the abrupt wake-up crying and to respond to the hand-to-mouth activity of baby A rather than waiting for him to cry.

By the next day, baby B was less frantic during breastfeeding sessions when Tina would put him to breast before he was fully awake. However, he continued to have hour-long nursing sessions. Baby A nursed longer when Tina put him to breast when he began to stir from sleep and began rooting on his hand; however, his quiet, self-contained behavior continued. Weight gain for both babies was normal even though baby A gained more rapidly than baby B. The pediatrician attributed this to their different temperaments and metabolism.

Tina began to attend a support group for mothers of twins. Three of the mothers there had breastfed twins and had experienced a situation similar to Tina's. This knowledge and support motivated Tina to continue breastfeeding. She realized that it was not a problem to correct, rather it was a condition requiring her adaptation. As the twins grew older, their temperaments were more distinctive. Baby B was a high-need infant requiring frequent breastfeeding and nonnutritive sucking to remain calm and attentive. Baby A was usually content to sit and play on the floor or in the crib. Tina was grateful for the extended family in her home. She felt that baby A would not have received enough attention from her alone because of the amount of time spent soothing baby B.

Development of Parenting Behavior

MATERNAL ROLE ACQUISITION

Mothering requires skill and patience. The replacement of extended families and close community ties by small nuclear families has left many women in Western cultures without appropriate role models. Bocar and Moore (1987) describe maternal role acquisition as a four-stage process—anticipatory, formal, informal, and personal. They draw from the work of Thornton who defined an expansion of the role acquisition process from one stage to four (Thornton, 1975).

Bocar and Moore (1987) also offer an explanation for the behavior observed in the antepartum and postpartum periods by mothers, complete with counseling strategies for the lactation consultants (see Table 1A–2). In the anticipatory stage the mother collects information about what mothers "should" do beginning with her own experience in her family. Colman and Colman (1971) describe *quickening*, or the first movements of the fetus experienced by the mother, as the first perception of the baby as a separate being.

Galinsky (1981) describes the image-making stage of parenthood in which parents draw on memories and fantasies of parenthood. Expectations are formed in the anticipatory stage and are helpful only if realistic (Thornton & Nardi, 1975). Loss of expectations by the mother of the preterm infant may need to be addressed by the LC. She has lost not only the anticipated experiences of bonding, breastfeeding immediately after delivery, taking the baby home soon after delivery, and so on but also has lost the expectation of a beautiful, plump, cooing baby.

In the formal stage, the mother sees her role as fulfilling "must" behaviors (Berlo, 1960). These include the day-to-day duties of feeding, holding, diapering, and so on to be done one specific way, which is often determined by the surrounding culture. In this stage of role acquisition, the mother responds best to consistent information and few choices regarding how to care for her baby. Mothers are particularly vulnerable and aware of negative or contradictory comments from individuals they perceive as experts in baby care (Mercer, 1981; Rubin, 1961, 1967a). In this stage, the *doula*, the person who mothers the mother, is of benefit in nurturing and supporting the new mother (Brown & Hurlock, 1977; Raphael, 1973). Lactation consultants may be drawn into this role in the absence of close family members.

The birth of a new baby is a developmental milestone in the evolution of the family and often causes added stress. Encouraging a venting of emotions and offering suggestions for developing a relationship with the new baby can be helpful (Bocar & Moore, 1987). The LC can help the mother view her baby as a separate being or partner, which is crucial to the attachment process (Klaus & Kennell, 1982; Mahler, 1967; Sarbin, 1954).

Enhancement of the mother's self-confidence during the formal stages, through the mastery of child-care duties, leads to enjoyment of the new baby (Coopersmith, 1967; Kitzinger, 1980) and a progression to the next stage of role acquisition. During the informal stage, mothers begin to move from the "must do" to "may do" stage (see Table 1A–3). During this stage, mothers look to peers as role models (Rubin, 1967a) and accept that there is more than one way to "parent" the baby. A

Table 1A-2   Major Counseling Strategies for the Four Maternal Role-Acquisition Stages

Stage	Descriptive Comment
1. Anticipatory	Promote realistic expectations
2. Formal	Provide simple, consistent suggestions in easily mastered segments
	Provide specific, positive feedback regarding maternal behavior
3. Informal	Introduce alternatives in a nonthreatening environment
4. Personal	Encourage positive self-assessment and the sharing of infant-care techniques with other mothers

Source: Bocar, D, Moore, K (1987). *Acquiring the Parental Role: A Theoretical Perspective.* In Auerbach, K (Ed.), *Lactation Consultant Series.* Schaumburg, IL: La Leche League International. Reprinted with permission.

Table 1A-3   Mother's Descriptions of Behavior Associated with the Four Maternal Role-Acquisition Stages

Stage	Descriptive Comment
1. Anticipatory	"Mothers should do . . ."
2. Formal	"Mothers must do . . ."
3. Informal	"Mothers may do . . ."
4. Personal	"I do . . ."

Source: Bocar, D, Moore, K (1987). *Acquiring the Parental Role: A Theoretical Perspective.* In Auerbach, K (Ed.), *Lactation Consultant Series.* Schaumburg, IL: La Leche League International. Reprinted with permission.

mother must find her comfort level as she explores the mothering alternatives she observes around her (Bocar & Moore, 1987).

The next stage Bocar and Moore describe is the personal stage in which the mother's behavior evolves, having replaced the "perfect-mother" fantasy with more realistic expectations of her style (Bocar & Moore, 1987; Heffner, 1978). Maternal role acquisition is thus achieved as mothers become comfortable with their past mothering experiences and choice of future direction (Erikson, 1956). In this stage, when describing maternal behavior, mothers abandon "should do," "must do," and "may do" phrases for the present tense "I do" (Bocar & Moore, 1987; Rubin, 1967b).

PATERNAL ISSUES

The immediate postpartum period may be the first time the father recognizes the baby as separate from the mother. His view of the family as a unit as opposed to a couple begins to take shape as he experiences the baby when holding, diapering, and bathing. Often he may be unsure about the new infant and experience feelings of ambivalence. The father's desire for involvement may be high or low as reflected in his attendance at childbirth or breastfeeding classes, participation as a labor partner, and behavior after the birth (Cronenwett, 1982; May & Solid, 1984; Peterson et al., 1979).

Jordan and Wall have studied the male's perspective of "fathering" and provide valuable insights for supporting the father during breastfeeding (Jordan, 1986, 1990, 1991; Jordan & Wall, 1990, 1993). They describe feelings of jealousy, resentfulness, and being left out as common. They contend that anticipatory guidance, by an experienced father of a breastfed infant, about breastfeeding with an emphasis on sharing and suggestions for supporting the couple's relationship and enhancing the father–infant relationship can be very beneficial as a new father acquires the "fathering" role (Jordan & Wall, 1993).

The father's role should not be overlooked because studies have shown the father to be important in the infant-feeding decision and the duration of breastfeeding (Baranowski et al., 1983; Beske & Garvis, 1982; Bevan et al., 1984; Black, 1990; deChateau et al., 1977; Morse, 1987). See Module 1, *The Support of Breastfeeding*, Chapter 1, for further discussion of the father's role in breastfeeding initiation and duration.

POST-TEST

For questions 1 to 6, choose the best answer.

1. Which of the following is not an example of infant primitive reflexes?

    A. Rooting
    B. Startle reflex
    C. Babkin palmomental response
    D. Tonic labyrinthine reflex
    E. Inversion prone response

2. The _____ is often misinterpreted as maternal rejection.

    A. stepping reflex
    B. startle reflex
    C. tonic labyrinthine reflex
    D. Babkin palmomental response

3. The _____ will intensify sucking activity when stimulated during breast-feeding.

    A. startle reflex
    B. Babkin palmomental response
    C. asymmetrical tonic neck reflex
    D. stepping reflex

4. The _____ will inhibit tongue and jaw mobility when the newborn is placed in a supine position to breastfeed.

    A. startle reflex
    B. Babkin palmomental response
    C. tonic labyrinthine reflex and asymmetrical tonic neck reflex
    D. asymmetrical tonic neck reflex and startle reflex

5. Factor(s) that do not influence muscle tone and primitive reflexes are

    A. analgesics and anesthesia.
    B. neurological disturbances.
    C. prematurity.
    D. swaddling.

6. Infant characteristics that trigger "motherly responses" include all of the following except

    A. eye-to-eye contact.
    B. crying.
    C. odor.
    D. low birth weight.

For questions 7 to 11, choose the best answer from the following key:

A. True   B. False

7. Using the breast as a pacifier has no benefit for mother or baby.

8. Early postpartum mother–baby interaction is essential to the development of a reciprocal relationship.

9. Mothers participating in rooming-in with their newborns develop appropriate parenting skills earlier than mothers who do not.

10. Infants labeled as "good babies," who are content to be left alone for long periods, are at risk of sensory deprivation.

11. Prompt gratification of an infant's distress signal builds trust in his or her caregivers.

For questions 12 to 16, choose the best answer.

12. Infant communication cues are designed to
    A. mimic animal behavior.
    B. control and manipulate adults.
    C. stabilize nervous behavior.
    D. keep mother close.

13. SMYLI is an acronym for describing support environments post-birth such as would be found in
    A. kangaroo care.
    B. central nursery care.
    C. rooming-in.
    D. separation of mother and infant.
    E. kangaroo care and rooming-in.

14. Physical, sensory, hormonal, and behavioral communication from mother-to-infant and infant-to-mother is best described by which term?
    A. Reciprocal interactions
    B. Bonding cycle
    C. Kangaroo care
    D. Postpartum transitional period

15. Humans are categorized as
    A. nesting mammals.
    B. mother-clinging mammals.
    C. rooting mammals.
    D. aquatic mammals.

16. Neurologically, the infant is stimulated by
    A. touch, smell, taste.
    B. increases in prolactin and oxytocin.
    C. colostrum.
    D. passage of meconium.

For questions 17 to 20, choose the best answer from the following key:
    A. The quiet baby
    B. The average baby
    C. The active baby

17. May require mother to intervene and regulate cyclic organization.

18. May need to switch breasts when sucking rate slows.

19. Needs varied neuromotor activity and firm muscle tone to assist the baby in adjusting to handling by caregivers.

20. Needs leisurely sucking at the breast and nonnutritive sucking to help this infant to regulate cyclic organization.

SECTION B

Growing Up Breastfed

Donna Calhoun, BS, IBCLC
Rebecca F. Black, MS, RD/LD, IBCLC

LEARNING OBJECTIVES

At the completion of this section, the learner will be able to do the following:

1. Recognize the importance of stimulation to emotional growth of mother and baby, and the contributions of breastfeeding to this growth.
2. Describe developmental milestones in normal child development and their effect on the breastfeeding relationship.
3. Discuss normal sleep patterns of breastfed infants.
4. Describe benefits to the infant from prolonged lactation.

OUTLINE

    D. Six to twelve months

    E. Case study

IV. Prolonged Lactation Issues

    A. Infant sleep patterns

    B. Infant fussiness and/or crying

    C. Other issues

PRE-TEST

For questions 1 to 7, choose the best answer.

1. Successful breastfeeding provides the optimum milieu for mother and baby to develop
    A. separation anxiety.
    B. similar personalities.
    C. deep attachments.
    D. identity conflicts.

2. Attachment behavior patterns prepare the infant for
    A. basic intuitive abilities.
    B. future relationships with others.
    C. insecurities.
    D. psychopathic treatment.

3. The increased prolactin levels produced when breastfeeding has a direct effect on maternal
    A. pancreatic activity.
    B. ovarian activity.
    C. breathing activity.
    D. mucosal dryness.

4. Prolonged breastfeeding promotes
    A. overfeeding.
    B. dental caries.
    C. normal growth.
    D. obesity.

5. An infant's system is developmentally not ready for starches before four to six months because
    A. all of the infant cereals have sugar.
    B. infants' gastric acid secretions are high.
    C. pancreatic amylases are not available in duodenal fluids.
    D. infants have low secretion of salivary amylase.

6. An infant signals readiness for solid foods when she or he
    A. refuses to breastfeed.
    B. is able to sit up, chew, and swallow without gagging and reach for food.
    C. begins to drool and has teeth.
    D. is able to sit unsupported for long periods of time.

7. Between the ages of four to six months, changes in the infant's behavior are often misinterpreted as signals to begin weaning because the infant
    A. nurses for shorter periods and less frequently.
    B. is easily distracted by activity in the environment.
    C. plays with toys.
    D. is active with gross-motor skill development.

For questions 8 to 12, choose the best answer from the following key:
    A. Low-risk signs of infant attachment
    B. High-risk signs of infant attachment

8. A weak crying response from the infant.

9. Moderate touching and body sculpturing elicits positive responses from the infant.

10. The infant cries to signal unmet needs

11. Rageful crying (without tears) by the infant.

12. Weak contact in eye-following response by the infant.

For questions 13 to 17, choose the best answer.

13. The infant is most alert in the first 24 hours during the
    A. 3rd to 20th hour post-birth.
    B. first 6 hours post-birth.
    C. first 2 hours post-birth.
    D. last 6 hours of the first 24 hours post-birth.

14. Cluster feedings are described as
    A. 6 to 7 feedings in a 3- to 4-hour period.
    B. 2 to 3 feedings every 3 hours for 24 hours.
    C. bottle feedings given by caregivers other than the mother.
    D. feedings from only one breast clustered together in a 2- to 3-hour period.

15. Training infants to sleep for long periods at night
    A. cannot be achieved for infants under 8 weeks of age.
    B. may be detrimental to SIDS-prone infants.
    C. helps infants develop trust.
    D. is believed to foster the development of shame and doubt.

16. Breastfed infants have been found to be _____ irritable and display _____ arousal than bottle-fed infants when under stress.
    A. more; less
    B. less; more
    C. more; more
    D. less; less

17. Breastfeeding toddlers between the ages of 12 to 18 months consume
    A. 25% less energy than nonbreastfed toddlers.
    B. 25% more energy than nonbreastfed toddlers.
    C. less minerals than nonbreastfed infants.
    D. less vitamins than nonbreastfed infants.

For questions 18 to 20, choose the best answer from the following key:
   A. **Low-risk parenting**
   B. **High-risk parenting**

18. Parent seeks medical assistance only when a crisis occurs.

19. Parent uses frequent face-to-face positioning with eye contact and appropriate smiles.

20. Parent touches, strokes, or talks to baby minimally and in an emotionless state.

Introduction

Although healthy attachment to our young is possible without breastfeeding, it is believed by many that the degree of attachment is deepened and enhanced with the inherent qualities of breastfeeding. This discussion of attachment in the context of breastfeeding is meant to illustrate the continuum process that has so long been a part of human experience. "We have conspired to baffle this long-standing knowledge so utterly that we now employ researchers full time to puzzle out how we should behave toward children, one another and ourselves" (Liedloff, 1977).

Attachment can form as early as two weeks of life, when an infant can differentiate a familiar person from a stranger, when the infant signals for his or her mother and prefers her presence. The common practice of separating mother and baby after birth interrupts the process of bonding and both may begin to show symptoms of detachment, which is a defense mechanism of separation (Magid & McKelvey, 1987). As we shall see, such interruption may lead to child abuse or emotional disturbances for the mother and/or the infant. Even in situations in which separation is unavoidable, such as prematurity or illness, the attachment process can be repaired as much as possible by understanding the bonding cycle (see Figure 1B–1). Assisting parents to learn this process, hopefully, will help them heal emotional wounds. Breastfeeding, especially in unavoidable situations, offers the mother and infant a chance to have some sense of normalcy.

Figure 1B–1

First Year of Life Cycle

Source: From McKelvey, CA, Magid, K. *High Risk: Children Without a Conscience*, p. 74. Copyright © 1987 by Dr. Ken Magid and Carole A. McKelvey. Used by permission of Bantam Books, a division of Bantam Doubleday Dell Publishing Group, Inc.

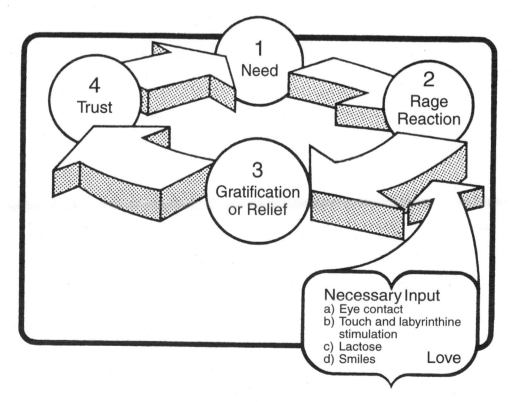

Long-Term Effects of Breastfeeding on Emotional Growth

All of a baby's communication cues are designed to keep mother close. Her presence ensures security, warmth, and source of food, in addition to exposing a baby to the rhythms and habits of her lifestyle. Her arms become the seat of learning, her breasts a comfort zone. As Liedloff (1977) describes it:

The human continuum can also be defined as the sequence of experience which corresponds to the expectations and tendencies of the human species in an environment consistent with that in which those expectations and tendencies were formed.

During gestation, the human infant experiences close physical containment, and when he or she is born, expects an environment that conforms to what the baby has come to know is right. Mother, as we have seen earlier, is the ideal milieu for the newborn and young infant. This attachment is the foundation for all other attachments in life. According to Magid and McKelvey (1987):

The bond that a child develops to the person who cares for him in his early years is the foundation for his future psychological development and for his future relationships with others.

During the postpartum period while mother and baby are learning to interact with each other, synchronizing sleep/wake patterns, and so on, the foundation of trust is developing. Without trust in the caregiver, the bonds of attachment are weakened, so to safeguard this process, recognition of how trust forms is necessary. Erikson (1963) describes the period of birth to one year of age as the period when trust or mistrust develops. To develop trust, the basic needs of food, warmth, and comfort must be met, as well as the need for mutual giving and getting between the infant and caregivers.

ATTACHMENT PARENTING

For the health-care professional involved with mother–baby pairs, it is crucial to recognize healthy and unhealthy attachment patterns of behavior. Breastfeeding success depends on communication and interaction. Mothers having difficulty with the mechanics or emotional adjustment of learning to breastfeed should be referred to a lactation consultant and a social support system before discharge. For the mothers of sick or premature infants, social support should be part of the care to be provided.

For the average breastfeeding couple, many of these concerns do not come into play. Breastfeeding itself enhances a mother's ability to attune herself to her infant. Many mothers claim a boost to their self-confidence as a result of successfully breastfeeding, especially when the birth did not meet their expectations or there were complications with the baby. Increases in self-esteem also have been reported for educated, low-income minority women (Locklin & Naber, 1993). Tables 1B–1 and 1B–2 summarize low- and high-risk signs of infant attachment and parental behaviors.

Table 1B–1   Infant Attachment Behaviors

Low-Risk Signs	High-Risk Signs
Infant cries to signal unmet need and when gratified will gradually terminate crying.	Weak crying response or rageful crying (without tears) and/or constantly whining.
Infant may sometimes resist cuddling but with moderate touching, and body sculpturing, infant will positively respond to mother's positive nurturing.	Poor clinging and extreme resistance to cuddling and close holding (fights to get free). Arches back when picked up (after first six weeks of life) and seems "stiff as a board."
Baby can fixate on mother's eyes and develop good following response, especially when nursing or smiling.	Weak contact in eye-following response. Infant will highly resist close face-to-face eye contact and consistently avert gaze (even if cuddling is permitted).
Infant may have some nursing difficulty (mother's nursing difficulty, i.e., inverted nipples, etc.) but can adapt and quickly develop healthy response.	Baby has poor sucking response and does not motivate to approach mother for receiving nurturance. Can also be due to developmental difficulties, i.e., cleft palate.
Baby gurgles, chortles, and has smiling response, especially when primary caretaker smiles.	Infant resists smiles even when tickled or played with lovingly. No reciprocal smile response.
Infant sparkles with life and a varied combination of emotions from sad to mad to glad. He looks and feels "right."	Infant is extremely passive and lifeless and seems to be in another world with no positive response to humans. Not attached to anything. Later this passivity will give way to rage. Baby looks and feels "like something is wrong."

Source: From McKelvey, CA, Magid, K. *High Risk: Children Without a Conscience*, p. 248. Copyright © 1987 by Dr. Ken Magid and Carole A. McKelvey. Used by permission of Bantam Books, a division of Bantam Doubleday Dell Publishing Group, Inc.

ATTACHMENT PARENTING CASE STUDY

Becky gave birth, by vaginal delivery, to a seven-lb. (3178 g) baby girl at a military base hospital in Wisconsin during the winter. Baby was kept in a central nursery except for 30-minute feeding times every four hours. Becky's husband was overseas and there were no family members within traveling distance. Her upbringing was in a two-parent family with four siblings; her father and mother were harsh disciplinarians, withholding affectionate responses for special occasions.

Becky firmly believed in the merits of breastfeeding, but felt that infants must be taught proper habits and behaviors. Baby was fed on a strict four-hour schedule and diapers were changed only at those times; she was kept in the crib at all times other than to be fed. Becky scheduled playtimes—three times a day for 20 minutes—whether the baby was asleep or crying. If her baby persisted in crying, Becky would leave the room and shut the door.

The six-week check-up was missed due to heavy snow. When Baby was two months old, Becky took her to the clinic. The pediatrician noted that the baby was only 10 oz. (283 g) over birth weight. He questioned Becky about her breastfeeding management and strongly suggested she breastfeed the baby more frequently. When the doctor picked the baby up to play with her, she

Table 1B–2   Parental Behaviors

Low-Risk Parenting	High-Risk Parenting
Mother exhibits positive interest in baby at birth and is eager to interact.	Mother withdraws and assumes a negative psychological and physical posture regarding baby at birth.
Mother wants to hold, caress, and respond to infant's vocalization. Makes positive statements about baby—"She's adorable."	Minimal touching, stroking, or talking to or about baby unless in negative manner—"Be quiet." May hold infant tensely.
Happy mother is filled with radiance, even, at times, tears of joy.	Emotionless and flat affect or depressed and angry. Sometimes tears of sadness.
Mother is attuned with baby's need for a balance of stimulation and quiet time. They develop a healthy rhythm together of play and rest.	Mother overstimulates baby by too much talking and touching. Mother sometimes plays in inappropriate or hostile ways (cruelly teasing infant).
Mother frequently establishes face-to-face positioning with eye contact and appropriate smiles.	Mother doesn't establish eye contact except when angry and rarely smiles or does so inappropriately (when infant is in pain).
Plays with infant when awake (but doesn't overdo it) and places baby in stimulating area to observe and interact with others. Shows ability to comfort child and appears strongly attached.	Leaves infant, when awake, for long periods in isolation and doesn't show the ability to comfort the baby when needed. Handles baby roughly or in detached manner and may be abusive and neglectful.
Mother provides infant with proper and preventative medical assistance. Concern for diet, diaper changes, and health of baby.	Mother fails to provide basic supplies for well baby care and is angry at most baby behaviors. Mother doesn't seek medical assistance unless a crisis occurs.
Mother is basically happy and satisfied about being a mother and primary caretaker.	Mother is unhappy, frustrated, and angry at being a mother and the primary caretaker.

Source: From McKelvey, CA, Magid, K. *High Risk: Children Without a Conscience*, pp. 250–51. Copyright © 1987 by Dr. Ken Magid and Carole A. McKelvey. Used by permission of Bantam Books, a division of Bantam Doubleday Dell Publishing Group, Inc.

arched and stiffened her back and legs. As he handed the baby to Becky, he noticed that she did not look at her baby, but quickly placed her in the portable carseat. The doctor set an appointment date for follow-up in one month.

At the next visit, a behavior specialist observed the doctor's examination of the baby. Later, he concurred with the pediatrician that the baby and mother were exhibiting abnormal behavior. The pediatrician arranged for Becky to be sent an invitational letter announcing a mother–baby play group on base. For the first three sessions Becky was uncomfortable being with new people. She also felt self-conscious in front of women who held and kissed their infants. However, she looked forward to the meetings and continued to attend. Two of the mothers living in her apartment building were also without their husbands and they all began getting together to have dinner.

During the next several clinic visits, the doctor was pleased to see Baby and her mother beginning to respond to each other. When he would come into the exam room, the baby cried to be held by her mother and would cling tightly to mother's protecting arms.

Developmental Stages

THE NEONATAL PERIOD

Some of the important management issues during the neonatal period that impact on the establishment of breastfeeding include thermal regulation, metabolic adaptation, glucose control, and the presence of hyperbilirubinemia in the neonate. Chapter 2 of this module discusses glucose control and hyperbilirubinemia in more detail.

Thermal Regulation

Maintaining body heat in newborns is crucial. Methods vary with the institution but include knit caps and radiant warmers. Infants have a low-to-moderate ability for nonshivering thermogenesis (Cannon et al., 1988). Mothers help maintain temperature by holding the baby to use their body heat and prepare a nest (Christensson et al., 1992). When compared to infants placed on a cot, infants with skin-to-skin contact maintained body temperature better; this was measured by actual body temperatures. The pattern of temperature changes was also different and the skin-to-skin group showed a rapid increase followed by a slow steady rise. The infants on the cots had a rapid increase until 30 minutes when it leveled off. This may be due to vasoconstriction for heat conservation. Infants on the cots cried for a significantly longer period of time than those in the skin-to-skin group. The crying should have caused a temperature increase (Hammarlund et al., 1986; Riesenfeld et al., 1987), but did not (Christensson et al., 1992). See Chapter 2 for more on thermal regulation.

Metabolic Adaptation

A long-held view of breastfeeding infants as hyperactive, behaviorally disorganized infants has been supported by studies, which compared visual and auditory orientation items on the Neonatal Behavioral Assessment Scale (NBAS) (DiPietro et al., 1987), crying following handling (Bell, 1966), soothing (Korner & Thomas, 1972), feeding (Bernal, 1972), and other forms of stimulation of bottle- and breastfed infants. This view has been challenged by research utilizing spectrum analysis of long-term heart-rate variability as a method by which the behavioral organization of bottle- and breastfed infants can be evaluated. This technique measures the rhythmic changes in arousal that occur over time. These rhythmic heart-rate changes form patterns, which reflect several central and autonomic nervous system functions (Berg & Berg, 1987). In development, these rhythmic oscillations increase the complexity of heart-rate variability. It is believed that less complexity in the temporal organization of an infant's long-term heart-rate variability may be evidence for disrupted behavioral organization (Lester, 1984; Zeskind, 1981; Zeskind & Lester, 1981; Zeskind et al., 1991).

To test this theory, Zeskind et al. (1992) measured heart rates and behavioral states of 14 breastfed and 14 bottle-fed newborn infants every 30 seconds for two continuous hours. A greater number of reliable cycles in heart rate were observed in the breastfed infants. Also, lower overall mean heart rates and lower mean heart rates in quiet and active sleep states were observed in the breastfed infants. Bottle-fed infants had more periods of quiet sleep than breastfed newborns. Neonatal heart rate is used as a measure of energy utilization (Woodson et al., 1983).

Zeskind et al. (1992) conclude that breastfed newborns show more complex, yet energy-efficient, patterns of behavior during quiet rest. They further recommend asking how bottle feeding may diminish newborn behavioral organization rather than how breastfeeding enhances behavioral organization since sleep promotion by differing amino-acid concentrations of many infant formulas has been reported (Yogman & Zeisel, 1983). In addition, plasma amino-acid profiles have been found to respond to different types of feeding (human milk, casein-predominant formula, and whey-predominant formula) in the immediate neonatal period (Cho et al., 1990).

FOUR TO SIX WEEKS

At four weeks, the asymmetrical tonic neck reflex position predominates; his or her dominant neuromotor skills are still primitive reflexes and automatic. The head sags forward when in a sitting position. The infant will thrust his or her arms and legs when playing. If the baby is on his or her tummy, the head turns to clear the nose from the bed and he or she lifts the head briefly. The infant may be able to roll part way from back to side. Fine-motor characteristics of four weeks include fisted hands, which clench on contact. The infant can only see an object in his or her line of vision and follows it to the midline. Eye movements are well focused, and the baby may follow the movement of objects close by. Any toy put into the infant's hand will be dropped immediately.

Besides crying, the infant begins small throaty sounds and responds to a caregiver's voice. The infant stares indefinitely at the surroundings and reduces his or her activity to look at an observer's face; he or she may smile back at a face or voice. The baby fixes his or her eyes on the mother's face in response to her smile and makes eye-to-eye contact. The infant responds positively to satisfaction and comfort and negatively to pain. He or she adjusts his or her posture to the body of the person holding the infant and can root and suck at the breast well. He or she can recognize parents' voices. Most of the time, the four-week-old infant has a vague and impassive expression. Daily patterns of sleeping, crying, and eating are highly disorganized. He has 5 to 10 daytime feedings and 2 to 6 night feedings.

Normally, after the first six weeks postpartum, the daily routine for mother and baby gets easier to manage. Mother has learned her baby's cues and is able to respond easily; she may feel more relaxed and confident in her ability to make sufficient milk to satisfy him or her. The infant's cyclic organization is more stabile; sleeping patterns become more dependable as do feeding patterns. Assuming the bonding cycle is unbroken, the baby actively searches for his or her mother when hearing her voice or seeing her nearby. He or she displays pleasure with coos and active body movements or sucking motions of the mouth.

By six weeks of age, babies have a well-defined nursing style. Still needing to feed frequently, the six-week-old may breastfeed 8 to 12 times in a 24-hour period, and signals this need through rooting and grasping skin or clothing to pull his or her mouth close. At about six weeks of age, there is an increase in appetite; infants usually go through an appetite (growth) spurt and need the extra calories. It is important to reassure mothers that this is normal and nothing is wrong with their breastmilk. It's also important to stress increased breastfeeding sessions may be needed and that cereal should not be offered yet.

TWO TO SIX MONTHS

During this span of time, the baby develops rapidly physically and mentally. As the baby grows larger, his or her appetite increases accordingly. Infants will experience growth spurts around two months and four months of age. Again, it's important to stress to the mother that this is normal behavior. Take the time to reassure her that breastfeeding is the best food for her baby. This is why it is so important that the mother continue to let the baby lead the frequency and duration of feeds. Failure to do so compromises adequate milk supply and nutritional intake for the baby. Mother's milk at this age is still the mainstay of the infant's diet and meets all nutritional requirements. See Module 3, *The Science of Breastfeeding*, for more information on the nutrient and immunologic content of breastmilk and the infant's needs.

While breastfeeding, infants of this age begin to pay more attention to their immediate environment. Mothers find this stage very rewarding because of the increased interactions with their babies. As many of the primitive reflexes become suppressed, many gross-motor skills emerge. Reaching out, caressing, smiling, patting, laughing, and playful behavior make breastfeeding sessions more leisurely and interesting. Head shaking or bobbing, pushing backward with the arms and hands, jerking leg movements, and turning away to locate a noise across the room are all normal activities for the four- to six-month-old baby feeding at the breast. Unaware mothers may interpret this as disinterest on the part of the baby and initiate weaning unnecessarily.

At this age, infants are easily pacified by frequent breastfeedings. The infant will interrupt a feeding to turn to look at a familiar person coming into the room and/or to smile at mother. Frequent feedings at the breast continue to be enjoyed. Infants are developmentally ready for cereal when they can sit upright by themselves and can hold their heads steady. These behaviors are usually exhibited at about five to seven months of age. Also, at this time, the tongue thrust reflex is beginning to diminish. As solids begin to contribute calories in the diet, the infant may not breastfeed as long or drink as much formula.

Separation anxiety can begin as early as four months or younger. Infants cry when mother is out of sight and calm down only when picked up. Some babies of a sensitive nature request to be breastfed when stressed by new or unusual events, so breastfeeding continues to help babies adjust to life beyond the womb.

For the mother at this stage, breastfeeding is a source of enjoyment and gives her a feeling of satisfaction watching her baby mature and thrive. No longer an intensive process of manipulation, breastfeeding the baby has become second nature requiring minimal preparation. Around four to six months, some babies may begin teething, and mothers may become concerned about biting.

SIX TO TWELVE MONTHS

The average baby at this age is usually beginning to move beyond the boundaries of mother's arms. Sitting alone, crawling, playing with toys, standing, walking, and taking an avid interest in the world fill an infant's waking hours. Nursing at this age is brief, but the frequency is still individually based. Mobile infants can assume a variety of positions to feed in: standing, kneeling, propping a foot on mother's shoulder, and sometimes requesting to nurse by helping mother undo her clothing. Older babies often request to feed for other reasons besides hunger; breastfeeding is a source of comfort and closeness in a world full of new changes. Average infants sleep six to ten hours at night, whereas active infants may sleep less. Most infants take at least two naps during the day.

For mothers who have breastfed this long, questions about weaning usually are voiced by family members or friends. Extended breastfeeding is not common in Western cultures even though it has been the global norm for millions of years. Many women choose to continue to breastfeed beyond the first year for personal reasons and health reasons. Psychologically, sucking continues to be a need inherent in childhood behavior. According to Bumgarner (1990):

Sucking is a necessary leveler for rapidly growing little people—so much that most children who do not nurse seek an alternative—bottle, pacifier, thumb, fingers, hair, blanket-corner, etc. They show us through the persistence of such behaviors that young children need the calming and reassuring effects of sucking as much or more than some of us adults need our "pacifiers." . . . Sucking . . . will cease all by itself once it has done its job. The dependence upon less effective behaviors or upon objects may not go away nearly so easily or readily.

Several excellent resources are available to continue with in-depth reading about developmental stages. Brazelton has written two books—*On Becoming a Family: The Growth of Attachment Before and After Birth* (1992a) and *Touchpoints: Your Child's Emotional and Behavioral Development* (1992b)—which may be helpful to professionals and laypersons.

DEVELOPMENTAL STAGES CASE STUDY

Tina's twins were allowed to breastfeed until they weaned on their own during the toddler years. When the twins were three months old, baby B awakened two to three times a night to breastfeed, whereas baby A awakened only once. To help Tina get more rest, her husband suggested they sleep together with the twins in the family bed. Grandmother recommended giving baby B cereal before bedtime to help him sleep longer. After three nights of feeding baby B two tablespoons of rice cereal, the pediatrician was called because the infant was crying heavily. The doctor speculated that the baby was constipated, and suggested using a suppository to relieve it. The baby passed a large pasty stool and Tina abandoned the use of cereal as a sedative. Baby B resumed his usual night patterns and Tina adapted to his frequent feeds.

At six months old, baby A would breastfeed only in a quiet place free of strangers and noise. Even while out shopping for a few hours with his mother, baby A would wait to breastfeed in the car or at home. Baby B enjoyed lots of diversion. He would breastfeed in spurts, taking time to look across the room or follow the dog. He would practice leg jerking, putting his toes in Tina's face, giggling, and playing peek-a-boo under her shirt. While out shopping, he was most content in a back carrier rather than in the stroller, and would request a feeding when tired and sleepy.

By the time the boys were a year old, baby B was walking and climbing the furniture. Baby A was crawling and standing, content to rummage in drawers and cabinets. Both continued to breastfeed. Baby A breastfed only three or four times, with the bedtime feeding lasting the longest. Baby B breastfed frequently at odd times during the day, usually when he had a fall or fright or was tired. During the night, he would breastfeed at least one or two times. Baby B fed himself normal table meals that were cut into bite-size pieces. Baby A preferred to be spoon fed mashed vegetables and fruits. Neither infant had any interest in meats.

At two years, both boys ate a wide variety of meats, vegetables, fruits, and cereals. Both were nearly equal in motor development; however, baby B had a tendency to try more daring stunts and pedal a tricycle. Baby A spent more time looking at picture books and followed his grandfather doing household chores. Baby B would engage in games and wrestling with older cousins; baby A would sit on the sidelines cheering on the action. Baby A breastfed only to go to sleep; baby B would breastfeed for a few seconds only when hurt or distressed. Tina had difficulty remembering when baby B last breastfed, but deeply relished the bedtime breastfeeding with baby A.

Prolonged Lactation Issues

INFANT SLEEP PATTERNS

Newborns exhibit many states of awareness, varying from quite alert to deep sleep, on a continuum. Levels of arousal can be categorized into many states ranging from very quiet sleep to hard crying (Anderson, 1988). The extremely receptive, wakeful period following birth usually lasts for a couple of hours and is followed by a sleepy period, which may last as long as 20 hours, for both the mother and infant. Increasing wakefulness occurs at 20 to 24 hours of age with the infant showing readiness to feed cues every couple of hours. Often episodes of cluster feedings occur during the first few days in which as many as six or seven feedings will occur in a three- to four-hour period. Unfortunately, these cluster feedings may occur at night as the infant's nocturnal tendencies surface. These tendencies may be the result of maternal activity before birth. When the pregnant mother is active during the day, the movement lulls the baby to sleep and, then, when the mother sleeps, the fetus's activity increases. Pryor and Pryor (1991) refer to the baby as being on "uterine time" during the postpartum period before he or she adapts to the cues of light and dark.

Pinilla and Birch (1993) investigated environmental influences on sleep/wake cycles by studying whether exclusively breastfed infants could be taught to sleep from 12:00 AM to 5:00 AM without waking during the first eight weeks of life. Treatment groups used focal feeds (a breastfeed between 10:00 PM and midnight)—feeding interval lengthening by use of alternative caregiving behavior, and maximization of environmental differences between day and night—to elicit longer sleep episodes at night. The "treatment" was effective in lengthening the duration of nighttime sleep. These researchers contend that because frequent nighttime waking often results in early termination of lactation, the parents' ability to teach an infant to lengthen his or her nighttime sleep periods will make the continuation of breastfeeding easier for the mother (Pinilla & Birch, 1993). This view is not supported by many lactation consultants.

The push for infant independence is part of our (Western) cultural child-care patterns; thus, solitary sleeping of infants is considered normal. Yet parent co-sleeping is widespread and practiced by the majority of the world's people. The child-care pattern of infants sleeping for long periods in social isolation from parents has only recently been studied for its psychological or biological consequences (McKenna, 1993).

Parental sounds, smells, gases, heat, and movement during the night are stimuli the infant has experienced as a fetus; proximity to these is expected by the infant. Human infants are the least neurologically mature primates. Born with only 25% of its adult brain volume, the infant develops and adapts slowly. Pilot studies of the physiological effects of mothers and infants sleeping apart and together found sleep, breathing, and arousal patterns of co-sleeping mothers and infants to be entwined in important ways (McKenna et al., 1991). Mothers induce small transient arousals that theoretically may be important in preventing sudden infant death syndrome (SIDS)—for prone infants to resist a SIDS event (McKenna, 1986; McKenna et al., 1991). Infant sleep, heart rate, breathing, and arousal levels are affected by parental stirrings, especially breathing sounds and vocalizations (Chisholm, 1986). McKenna (1993) proposes co-sleeping be conceptualized as a continuum ranging from same-bed contact to elimination of infant–parent sensory exchanges such as when infants sleep alone in a distant room with the door closed.

Steinberg et al. (1992) hypothesize that plasma tryptophan concentrations (which are known to alter adults' sleep and working patterns) may influence infants' sleep latency. Formula-fed infants' plasma tryptophan concentrations are lower than those of human milk-fed infants, so an experiment was designed to look at whether formulas with varying tryptophan concentrations were of significance in altering plasma tryptophan and the ratios of plasma tryptophan to other large neutral amino acids (LNAA). The plasma tryptophan:LNAA ratios were predictive of a difference in infants' sleep latency. Significantly shorter sleep latencies were observed when tryptophan was added in an amount to obtain ratios similar to those of infants fed human milk over infants whose formula contained tryptophan in lower levels that did not approximate the ratios of those fed human milk.

INFANT FUSSINESS AND/OR CRYING

Infant fussiness is often reported by breastfeeding mothers as a persistent problem (Chapman et al., 1985; Graef et al., 1988; Humenick & Van Steenkist, 1983; Kearney et al., 1990). Normal infants, regardless of feeding method, are reported to gradually increase their amount of crying to a peak in irritability at about two months, with an average of two to two-and-one-half hours in a 24-hour period (Barr, 1990; Brazelton, 1962).

Associations between infant feeding and infant behavior have been difficult to find conclusively. Breastfed newborns have been shown to display more arousal than bottle-fed infants following an anthropometric examination (Bernal & Richards, 1970). In another study, breastfed infants were found to be more irritable during the first ten days of life (Bernal, 1972).

In a small group of infants, those who breastfed have been shown to have higher arousal level when under stress (heel prick and first immunization) than those fed formula (Worobey & Lewis, 1989). Failure to recognize a heightened infant awareness as a cause of fussiness of those who are breastfed may result in premature weaning. Counseling that focuses on the organizational function of crying and teaches viewing it as a developmentally expected occurrence may help alleviate mothers' fears.

General observations about crying made by Barr (1990) include:

- A progressive increase in crying, peaking during the second month and then gradually decreasing
- A diurnal phase, clustered in the evening hours, with peak crying during the second month of life
- A between-individual variability, which is most marked during crying peaks; a large degree of within-individual variability from day to day
- Early crying that is not modifiable by differences in caregiving style

Increased carrying (beyond typical Western society patterns) has been shown to reduce crying and fussiness by 43% at six weeks and by 54% during the evening in a randomized controlled trial (Hunziker & Barr, 1986). Higher levels of plasma lactic acid and blood glucose were associated with the crying of boys, aged 1 to 3. Although lactic acid builds up when adults exercise, it may be elevated in children through a stress response (Aono et al., 1993).

Fussiness can be caused by formula intolerance. In a study comparing formula change and its effects on fussiness, there was little change in hydrogen excretion with no difference in crying or fussiness with a reduced lactose formula. A change to a soy-based formula showed a significant reduction in hydrogen excretion and its related decrease in fussiness. This decrease continued with prolonged use and, by day eight, there was a 40% decline in fussiness (Barr et al., 1991). Crying also increased in newborn infants who had an extra water feeding but there was no difference in infants who received an extra formula or lactose-carbohydrate feeding (Oberlander et al., 1992). Infants with an atypical ponderal index (PI) have hyperphonated (usually high-pitched) cry sounds, poor performance on the NBAS (Neonatal Behavioral Assessment Score), and poor regulation of behavioral state, which are believed to be due to disrupted autonomic and behavioral organization (Lester, 1984; Zeskind, 1981; Zeskind & Lester, 1981).

Crying is often given as a reason for the early introduction of solids and a decrease in breastfeeding frequency. Mothers often view crying as an indication that feeds are inadequate and/or that the infant's nutritional needs are not being met.

Some of the prebirth causes of newborn babies' crying, fussiness, and/or irritability include anoxia (a deprivation of oxygen during prolonged labor); prematurity; maternal high blood pressure; maternal drug use such as heroin, phenobarbital and other barbiturates, or cocaine; cigarette smoking; and marijuana smoking (Jones, 1992). The result of these causes for an infant include excessive irritability, difficulty sleeping, superexcitability, fussiness with a shrill cry, sleep disruptions, trembling, and/or a baby that easily startles.

Colic is defined by the rule of threes—a baby cries for longer than three hours, for more than three days in a row, for three months. Colic is upsetting to all who are around the baby. According to Jones (1992), young infants show pain through their voice (whimpers, groans, high-pitched cries), facial expressions (grimaces, chin quivers, furrowed brow area), body movements (tense and rigid, fist clenching, pulling in of arms and legs, shallow rapid breathing), color changes (red face, purple lips, an unusually pale appearance), and changes in behavior (interrupted sleep, irritability, fussiness, extremely active or very sluggish and unresponsive). Medications, such as dicyclomine hydrochloride, are commonly given to older colicky babies but are generally not recommended for young infants.

The maternal diet is often blamed for colic symptoms but the only validated cause is from the overconsumption of milk products by lactating women (Jakobsson & Lindberg, 1983). A milk-free diet can be tried temporarily if the mother is found to be consuming excessive quantities (greater than four servings per day) of milk products. In the short term, it would certainly do no harm to the mother if she is desperate to try something—anything—to help the baby. If dairy products in the maternal diet is the problem, often the infant will experience green, frothy stools, gas, a rash, and/or a stuffy or runny nose.

OTHER ISSUES

Other management issues in prolonged lactation include the introduction of solids, maintaining an active lifestyle while breastfeeding, breastfeeding an older infant, tandem breastfeeding, contraception during breastfeeding, managing maternal or infant illness while breastfeeding, and when and how to begin weaning. These issues are discussed in Chapters 2 and 3 of this module.

POST-TEST

For questions 1 to 6, select the best answer.

1. Without _____, the development of healthy attachment will be damaged during early childhood.
   A. a father
   B. a stimulating environment
   C. strict upbringing
   D. trust

2. Healthy attachment signs in an infant include
   A. a weak crying response or rageful crying.
   B. resistance to cuddling.
   C. no reciprocal smile response.
   D. cries to signal need and stops crying when need is met.

3. Detached patterns of behavior are most likely to develop in
   A. children of high-risk parenting.
   B. infants with low-risk signs of attachment.
   C. premature infants.
   D. infants and parents who practice co-sleeping.

4. Factors that indicate an infant's readiness for solid foods include
   A. refusal to breastfeed.
   B. drooling and teething.
   C. sitting alone, chewing and swallowing, reaching for food.
   D. crawling and pulling up to a standing position.

5. When denied sucking stimulation at the breast, an older infant may
   A. seek an alternative such as hair, fingers, thumb, and so on.
   B. take a nap.
   C. eat excessively causing obesity.
   D. wean abruptly.

6. Ecological child spacing is intensified by breastfeeding when
   A. mother allows unrestricted sucking.
   B. birth control pills are taken in conjunction with breastfeeding.
   C. father sleeps in a separate room.
   D. thyroid and pituitary functions are hindered.

For questions 7 to 12, choose the best answer from the following key:
   A. High-risk parenting
   B. Low-risk parenting

7. Face-to-face positioning with eye contact.

8. Provides infant with preventive medical assistance.

9. Handles baby in detached manner with flat affect.

10. Balances baby stimulation with quiet time.

11. Minimal touching, stroking, or talking to baby.

12. Imbalance of stimulation and quiet time.

For questions 13 to 15, choose the best answer.

13. Extended breastfeeding promotes
    A. normal growth.
    B. more allergies.
    C. dental caries.
    D. undernutrition.

14. Determining when to begin solids should be based on
    A. developmental factors.
    B. physiological factors.
    C. both A and B.
    D. neither A nor B.

15. An optimal time for breastfeeding is when the infant is
    A. crying to be fed.
    B. in a light sleep.
    C. in a deep sleep.
    D. in a quiet, alert state.

For questions 16 to 20, choose the best answer from the following key:
    A. True
    B. False

16. Adding solid foods to the two-month-old infant's diet increases his or her nutritional intake.

17. Pancreatic maturation is a key factor for determining an infant's readiness for solid foods.

18. Weaning culmination requires the absence of breastfeeding and bottle use.

19. One-year-olds may have a psychological need to continue breastfeeding.

20. Breastfeeding promotes the development of a synchronized/symbiotic relationship between mother and baby.

SECTION C

Nutrition for the Breastfed Infant

Robin McRoberts, MS, RD/LD
Rebecca F. Black, MS, RD/LD, IBCLC
Richard A. Simpson, DMD

LEARNING OBJECTIVES

At the completion of this section, the learner will be able to do the following:

1. Give three indications of adequate feedings in breastfed infants.
2. Give developmental milestones that can guide the introduction and progression of solid foods into the infant's diet.
3. Explain the recommended sequence for the introduction of solid foods for the breastfed infant.
4. Cite three contributions of extended breastfeeding to the health and well-being of the toddler.
5. Cite recommendations for the supplementation of breastfed infants with vitamins and/or minerals.

OUTLINE

I. Introduction

II. Nutritional Needs of the Infant

    A. Macronutrient needs
       1. Energy
       2. Protein
       3. Fat
       4. Carbohydrates

    B. Selected micronutrient needs
      1. Zinc
      2. Calcium
      3. Sodium
    C. Intake and growth of the breastfed infant

III. Suggested Guidelines for Feeding the Breastfed Infant

    A. Assessing intake
    B. Progressing to solids
      1. Digestive maturation
      2. Introducing solids
    C. Nutritional needs of infants and children
    D. Extended lactation
    E. Weaning

IV. Nutrients of Specific Concern for the Breastfed Infant

    A. Vitamin D
    B. Fluoride
    C. Iron
    D. Vitamin K
    E. Mothers with marginal diets

PRE-TEST

For questions 1 to 4, choose the best answer.

1. The recommended caloric distribution for the infant is
    A. 40% to 50% fat, 7% to 11% carbohydrate, remainder is protein.
    B. 25% to 30% fat, 7% to 10% protein, remainder is carbohydrate.
    C. 40% to 50% fat, 7% to 11% protein, remainder is carbohydrate.
    D. 40% to 50% carbohydrate, 7% to 11% fat, remainder is protein.

2. The recommended progression of solids is
    A. cereals, fruits, vegetables, meats.
    B. fruits, vegetables, cereals, meats.
    C. cereals, fruits, meats, vegetables.
    D. cereals, vegetables, fruits, meats.

3. If an infant experiences fussiness, diarrhea, rash, or blood in the stool, a parent might suspect
    A. growth deficit.
    B. food allergy or intolerance.
    C. kwashiorkor.
    D. marasmus.

4. An example of a recommended nutrition practice in the first six months of infancy is
   A. cereal fed through an infant feeder.
   B. feeding mixed foods prior to plain foods.
   C. offering a new food daily for seven days.
   D. offering iron-fortified infant cereal between four and six months of age.

For questions 5 to 8, choose the best answer from the following key:

   A. Breastfed infants   B. Formula-fed infants

5. _____ consume more calories at four months of age.

6. _____ have higher skinfold measurements at 9 to 15 months of age.

7. Growth charts are based on _____.

8. _____ have lower weight for height at four months of age.

For questions 9 to 12, choose the best answer from the following key:

   A. If responses 1, 2, and 3 are correct   D. If response 4 is correct
   B. If responses 1 and 3 are correct   E. If all are correct
   C. If responses 2 and 4 are correct

9. Infant indicators of an adequate intake include
   1. frequent sleep episodes over four to five hours.
   2. increases in length, weight, and head circumference.
   3. feeding durations of one hour or more.
   4. evidence of milk transfer.

10. Good sources of iron for the infant include
    1. fruit juices.
    2. fruits.
    3. vegetables.
    4. dry infant cereals.

11. The risk of vitamin D deficiency to an infant is increased for those
    1. living in northern latitudes.
    2. living in southern latitudes.
    3. whose mothers do not drink milk.
    4. taken out into the sun regularly.

12. Vitamins/minerals that definitely need to be supplemented in the first four months of the exclusively breastfed infant include
    1. iron.
    2. fluoride.
    3. vitamin D.
    4. vitamin K.

For questions 13 to 16, choose the best answer from the following key:

   A. Zinc deficiency   C. Iron deficiency
   B. Vitamin B deficiency   D. Vitamin D deficiency

13. Nutritional rickets

14. Spoon nails

15. Cheilosis

16. Dermatitis, diarrhea, growth deficit

For questions 17 to 20, choose the best answer.

17. Identify the energy requirement for a two-month-old infant.
    A. 85 to 90 kcal/kg per day
    B. 90 to 120 kcal/kg per day
    C. 125 to 135 kcal/kg per day
    D. 140 to 145 kcal/kg per day

18. From birth to four months of age, there is a _____ in protein needs and a _____ in protein needs from 5 to 12 months of age.
    A. rapid increase; slow increase
    B. rapid increase; slow decrease
    C. rapid decrease; slow decrease
    D. rapid decrease; slow increase

19. From greatest to lowest, identify the bioavailability of zinc.
    A. breastmilk; cow milk-based formula; soy-based formula
    B. cow milk-based formula; soy-based formula; breastmilk
    C. soy-based formula; breastmilk; cow milk-based formula
    D. soy-based formula; cow milk-based formula; breastmilk

20. Vitamin K supplementation is recommended for the breastfed infant
    A. immediately after birth only.
    B. immediately after birth and every 5 to 7 days until two months old.
    C. immediately after birth, and during bouts of diarrhea a supplement should be given for 5 to 7 days for as long as the diarrhea persists.
    D. immediately after birth and at six months of age.

Introduction

The American Academy of Pediatrics recommends that infants be breastfed exclusively for the first four to six months of life (AAP, 1997), and the American Dietetic Association recommends exclusive breastfeeding for four to six months (ADA, 1997). Many are beginning to assert that exclusive breastfeeding can continue for longer in developed countries and most agree that in developing countries, extended, exclusive breastfeeding saves lives. Breastfeeding should be continued through the first two years of life as solid foods are introduced into the diet. In many parts of the world, breastfeeding continues until the birth of the next child, with tandem nursing not uncommon. Prolonged lactation is a concept foreign to many Western, industrialized countries but is recognized for its influence on reducing infant and child morbidity and mortality and child spacing by many researchers and policymakers (Hanson et al., 1994).

The purpose of this section is to briefly review the nutritional needs of the infant and the guidelines for feeding once solids are introduced into the breastfed infant's diet, differentiate between intake and growth in breastfed and formula-fed groups, and highlight nutrients of specific concern and/or controversy for the exclusively breastfed infant. Nutrition for the breastfed infant was included in this module rather than with the nutrition information on milk content and maternal diet in Module 3, *The Science of Breastfeeding*, because growth and development depend on nutrition and nutrition is essential to the successful management of breastfeeding.

This is not, however, intended to be a comprehensive discussion of infant nutrition. Several excellent resources for in-depth study are available already, including S. J. Fomon's (1993) *Nutrition for Normal Infants* and *Neonatal Nutrition and Metabolism*, edited by W. W. Hay, Jr. Module 2, *The Process of Breastfeeding*, Chapter 2, includes information on initiating lactation and assessing the adequacy of lactation in the early weeks, and Chapter 2 of this module discusses conditions of nutritional concern for the infant such as iron deficiency anemia and growth deficit—failure to thrive. Chapter 3 of this module discusses the nutritional needs of the preterm infant.

Nutritional Needs of the Infant

MACRONUTRIENT NEEDS

Rapid growth occurs during the first six months of life. During this time the infant is gaining weight and length and the brain continues to grow as exhibited by an increase in head circumference measurements. To support this growth, adequate calories must be consumed.

Energy

Energy guidelines for infants set in the 1970s and 1980s are now recognized to be substantially higher than what is needed for growth. The development, refinement, and application of a technique to measure infants' direct energy expenditure—doubly labeled water method (Prentice et al., 1988)—has yielded lower energy intake recommendations for infancy (Prentice et al., 1988; Whitehead, 1995). Early recommendations for energy intake by infants made by the World Health Organization/Food and Agriculture Organization (1973) were found to be as much as 25% higher than results of subsequent investigations (Lucas et al., 1987; Prentice et al., 1988; Whitehead et al., 1981). The 1985 WHO/FAO/UNU report on energy recognized the need to lower the energy recommendations, but the group was concerned about such a drastic reduction, and thus compromised by releasing a more moderate reduction guidelines (see Table 1C–1).

Whitehead (1995) explains the rationale for this conservative view as the need to err on the side of caution when making recommendations for young children because often such guidelines are used to prescribe a diet (this is particularly true for formula-fed infants). The use of higher energy recommendations, coupled with information on the energy content of human milk (approximately 70 kcal/ 100 mL) and an average peak breastmilk output of 750 mL to 850mL per day, led many to conclude that exclusive breastfeeding could not sustain growth beyond four to six months (see Table 1C–2). This concept has been challenged in a recent commentary (Borresen, 1995), and data published in the late 1980s (Lucas et al., 1987; Prentice et al., 1988) reported energy intake stabilized at substantially lower levels (85 kcal/kg body weight per day) than those recommended.

Krebs et al. (1994) also found that the mean energy intakes of healthy breastfed infants were lower through the first seven months of life than the current recommendations. The recommended energy needs of infants and the belief that breastmilk feeding alone could not meet these needs has been the basis for the recommendation to start solids between four to six months. In light of the new discussion regarding a lower energy requirement in infancy, many are reexamining the recommendation to begin solids this early. Ahn and Maclean (1980) reported on growth of exclusively breastfed infants in a La Leche League population (N = 96) and found the average duration of exclusive breastfeeding to be seven months and found no evidence to support the introduction of solid foods during the major part of the first year of life.

Salmenpera and associates (1985) studied 116 exclusively breastfed infants and found that at 7.5 months, 71 were exclusively breastfed; at nine months, 36 were

Table 1C–1   Energy Recommendations Based on Weight and Age of Infants During the First Year of Life

Report and Year Published	Months of Age	Energy in kcal (kJ)/kg body weight/day
WHO/FAO	0 to 3	120 (500)
1973[a]	4 to 6	115 (480)
DHSS (London)	0 to 3	100 (420)
1979[b]	4 to 6	100 (420)
Whitehead et al.	3	95 (400)
1981[c]	4	90 (360)
WHO/FAO/UNU	2 to 3	109 (450)
1985[d]	3 to 4	103 (430)
	4 to 5	99 (415)
IOM	0 to 6	108 (447)
1989[e]	6 to 12	98 (411)

[a]WHO/FAO (1973). Energy and protein requirements. World Health Organization Technical Report Series No. 522. Food and Agriculture Organization. Nutrition Meetings Report Series No. 52.

[b]Department of Health and Social Security (1979). Recommended daily amounts of food energy and nutrients for groups of people in the United Kingdom. *Reports on Health and Social Subjects, No. 15.* Her Majesty's Stationery Office: London.

[c]Whitehead, RG, Paul, AA, Cole, TJ (1981). A critical analysis of measured food energy intakes during infancy and early childhood in comparison with current international recommendations. *J Hum Nutr*, 35:339–48.

[d]World Health Organization (1985). Energy and protein requirements. Report of joint FAO/WHO/UNU meeting. World Health Organization (WHO) Technical Report Series, No. 724, Geneva.

[e]Institute of Medicine, National Academy of Sciences (1989). *Recommended Dietary Allowances*, 10th ed. Washington, DC: National Academy Press.

exclusively breastfed; and at 12 months, 7 were exclusively breastfed. No significant differences in height or weight were found between the exclusively breastfed infants and a control group weaned before six months, although the control group was one centimeter longer (not significant) and the breastfed group had a slightly higher weight for length ratio (also not significant).

Like adults, an infant's caloric need is based on many variables, including weight, sex, ambient temperature, and body size. How an infant is fed is also being recognized as a determinant of caloric need. Fat is absorbed less efficiently from artificial milk than from unheated human milk in early infancy (Widdowson, 1965), and total energy expenditure has been shown to be higher in artificially fed infants (Garza & Butte, 1990). So, it may be that what is needed are energy-intake recommendations based on how an infant is fed.

Table 1C–3 shows the breakdown of components to determine estimated caloric requirements. The recommendation of 90 to 120 kcal/kg per day given by Barness (1993) is more than sufficient to meet the needs of a full-term breastfed infant. Growth slows at six months of age; in response to this, the daily caloric requirement decreases as the infant ages (see Table 1C–4). But even these guidelines published by Fomon in 1993 may be higher than what the exclusively breastfed infant actually needs.

Table 1C–2   Estimated Energy Intake for Exclusively Breastfed Infants

Months	Weight[a] on Growth Charts[b]	Energy Intake in kcal/kg body weight/day Based on a Breastmilk Intake of 750–850 mL/day
2	4.9 kg	105–122
3	5.7 kg	90–105
4	6.4 kg	80–90
5	6.9 kg	74–87
6	7.5 kg	70–80
7	8.0 kg	64–75

[a]Weight at 50th percentile (average of males and females) assuming an intake of 750–850 mL of breastmilk per day and a breastmilk energy content of 70 kcal/100 mL

[b]Hamill, PVV, Drizd, TA, Johnson, CL, Reed, RB, Roche, AF, Moore, WM (1979). Physical growth: National Center for Health Statistics percentiles. *Am J Clin Nutr*, 32:607–29.

Table 1C–3   Estimated Calorie Requirements of Typical Growing Term Infant

Item	Number of kcal/kg/day
Resting caloric expenditure	40–60
Activity	15–25
Thermic effect of food	10
Fecal loss of calories	5
Growth	20
Total	90–120

Source: Barness, LA (1993). *Pediatric Nutrition Handbook*, p. 91. Copyright © 1993, AAP, Elk Grove Village, IL. Used with permission of the American Academy of Pediatrics.

Table 1C–4   Estimated Energy and Protein Requirements

Age Interval (months)	Energy* (kcal/kg^{-1}/d^{-1})	Mean Requirement Protein	Mean Requirement Protein g/100 kcal
0 to 1	115	1.98	1.7
1 to 2	112	1.71	1.5
2 to 3	100	1.46	1.5
3 to 4	94	1.27	1.4
4 to 5	94	1.18	1.3
5 to 6	92	1.18	1.3
6 to 9	92	1.17	1.3
9 to 12	92	1.14	1.2

Source: Fomon, SJ (1993). *Nutrition of Normal Infants*. St. Louis: Mosby, p. 137. Copyright © SJ Fomon. Reprinted with permission of author.

Infants consume enough calories to meet their needs to promote growth. This is the beauty of breastfeeding. When a healthy infant needs more calories, he or she signals to be fed and the mother responds. If an infant is ill or requires surgery, energy requirements may be altered.

Protein

Protein is required by the infant to meet the needs of growth and to provide essential amino acids. Growth accounts for an estimated 52% of the protein requirement during the first month of life. This decreases to 30% at 3 to 4 months and 18% at 9 to 12 months of age. The percentage continues to decrease as the child ages (Fomon, 1993). In relationship to this, there is a rapid decrease in protein requirements from birth to 4 months (1.7 to 1.4 g/100 kcal), which gradually decreases before leveling. See Table 1C–4 for protein requirements during the first year of life (Fomon, 1993).

Protein intake has been found to be 66% to 70% higher in formula-fed groups when compared to breastfed groups in the first six months of life (Heinig et al., 1993). Breastfed infants were also reported to gain more weight and lean body mass per gram of protein intake than their formula-fed counterparts (Heinig et al., 1993). Not all of the protein in human milk is used for nutritional purposes. Enzymes, hormones, immunologic components, and so on are composed of protein and perform nonnutritive functions. This further mystifies scientists as the total amount of protein in human milk is less than what is commonly believed to be needed to support growth. See Module 3, *The Science of Breastfeeding*, Chapter 2, for more information on protein constituents in human milk.

Fat

Fat is a concentrated source of energy. This is especially important because infants' intake may be low. Full-term infants have lower serum levels of essential fatty acids than toddlers. It is possible for full-term infants to develop a fatty-acid deficiency within one week of fat-free hyperalimentation (Friedman et al., 1977). Essential fatty acids (linoleic and linolenic acid) should comprise 3% or more of the total caloric intake (AAP, 1993a). Human milk contains 3% to 7% of its calories as linoleic acid while commercial formulas contain less than 10% of fat as linoleic acid (Barness, 1993). Human milk approaches 50% of total calories from fat. Breastmilk contains very long-chain polyunsaturated fatty acids (VLCPUFA) while formulas sold in the United States do not contain them. In Europe, Japan, and Israel, formulas with the VLCPUFA have been available for a few years. A Maryland-based company—Martek Biosciences—has culled the VLCPUFA from microscopic marine algae.

The AAP has not pushed for the addition of the fats, believing the evidence is not conclusive and because of concerns regarding the appropriate balance among the fatty acids. Growth can be influenced negatively if arachidonic acid metabolism is disturbed by the addition of an inappropriate mixture of fatty acids. Nevertheless, very-long-chain polyunsaturated fatty acids are essential for preterm infants and may also be essential for full-term infants. See Module 2, *The Science of Breastfeeding*, Chapter 2, for a further discussion of fatty acids requirements in infancy.

Carbohydrates

The primary form of carbohydrates for the infant is lactose, found in human- and cow's milk–based infant formulas. Infants who are lactose intolerant and receive soy-based formulas receive carbohydrates in the form of sucrose or corn syrup solids.

As solids are introduced into the infant's diet, carbohydrates are obtained from other sources, including cereal, fruits, and vegetables. There is not a recommended dietary allowance (RDA) for carbohydrates. Diets containing less than 10% of total calories from carbohydrate can result in *ketosis*—when ketones are used by the developing brain for energy, tissue damage can occur.

SELECTED MICRONUTRIENT NEEDS

Iron, vitamin K, vitamin D, and fluoride are discussed later in this chapter in the Nutrients of Specific Concern for the Breastfed Infant section. The micronutrient content of human milk is discussed in Module 3, *The Science of Breastfeeding*, Chapter 2.

Zinc

The recommended intake of zinc is 2.0 mg per day from birth to 12 months of age (Fomon, 1993). Zinc is added to infant formulas and is present in breastmilk. The bioavailability of zinc is greatest in breastmilk and it is higher in cow's milk–based formula than soy-based formula. Few other infant foods are fortified with zinc and the foods high in zinc (meats, organ meats, shellfish, wheat germ) are not usually fed to infants in sizeable portions. Requirements are higher during times of rapid growth; preterm infants have higher zinc requirements than full-term infants (Barness, 1993).

Zinc deficiency can depress growth (Hambidge et al., 1987). Because breastfed infants have shown differences in weight-for-age measurements during the first year of life when compared to formula-fed infants, some investigators have raised the possibility that marginal zinc intake at five to six months in exclusively breastfed infants may be involved (Krebs et al., 1994). For a group of breastfed infants given zinc supplements between four and nine months of age, greater linear growth and weight gain have been reported, although this report did not define the amount of breastfeeding or supplementary foods (Walravens et al., 1992). More study is needed before the role of zinc in the growth pattern of the exclusively breastfed infant can be fully understood.

Calcium

The RDA for calcium increases by 10% by the infant's first birthday. Milk products, tofu (calcium fortified), and cheese are the major sources of calcium in the diet. Cereals have low levels of calcium and are not a good source even though they are fortified. Orange juice fortified with calcium is now available and is a good source for the toddler but should not be given under one year of age, according to recommendations to avoid common allergens such as citrus foods until the first birthday. Module 3, *The Science of Breastfeeding*, Chapter 3, provides information on ways to increase the calcium intake and may be useful for the lactating mother or parent of a young child allergic to cow's milk, lactose intolerant, or who dislikes dairy products.

Sodium

Sodium is essential to maintain the extracellular fluid compartment and a normal blood pressure. Sodium is found naturally in most foods and is added to most processed foods. Recent data show older U.S. infants consume an average of 1020 mg per day of sodium. The six-month-old infant receives 1.2 mEq of sodium per 100 kcal (23 mg/mEq) and when unsalted foods are added, sodium intake increases to 1.3 to 1.9 mEq/100 kcal (Ernst & Rickard, 1990). The majority of the increase comes from adult table foods. Infants need some sodium but excessive sodium intake should be avoided.

INTAKE AND GROWTH OF THE BREASTFED INFANT

The mean quantities of breastmilk produced in the colostrum, transitional, and mature milk stages are reviewed in Module 2, *The Science of Breastfeeding*, Chapter 2. The reader should refer to that module for a discussion of the biochemical, immunologic, and nutritional composition of breastmilk and colostrum.

Infant demand is the main determinant of maternal milk supply. Adequate maternal supply of breastmilk, in turn, supports adequate growth. Growth should be monitored at regular intervals, including measurement of head circumference. The reader is directed to texts on anthropometrics for guidance on the correct methods for measuring weight, height, and head circumference in infancy and childhood (see Additional Readings). It is desirable for the breastfed infant to regain birth weight by two weeks of age (AAP, 1993a); failure to achieve this goal or continuous weight loss after ten days of life indicates further evaluation is needed. Breastfed infants should be weighed within three to five days of being discharged from the hospital or birthing center or at least one time after the delivery and within the first week of life in the case of a home delivery.

Many physicians are prone to recommend supplementing with formula when an infant has not regained his or her birth weight by two weeks of age. This is rarely necessary and it often is detrimental to the establishment of lactation. Unfortunately, until the knowledge of appropriate early lactation management is increased in the professional population, many mothers will continue to be advised to supplement. The lactation specialist can develop referral networks with family physicians, pediatricians, obstetricians, pediatric nursing specialists, WIC nutritionists, pediatric dietitians, and so on so that accurate information and literature can be distributed to the mother.

When a breastfeeding infant has not shown satisfactory weight gain during the early weeks, a lactation specialist should be consulted. Some questions to ask the mother in this case are shown in Table 1C–5 and are reviewed in detail in Module 2, *The Process of Breastfeeding*, Chapter 1. Also, see Chapter 2 of this module for a discussion of failure to thrive—growth deficit.

When compared to their formula-fed counterparts, breastfed infants exhibit different growth patterns. In an Australian study of 82 infants, formula-fed infants

Table 1C–5   Questions to Ask the Mother Whose Infant Has Not Gained Satisfactorily During the Neonatal Period

Maternal Considerations

- Did your breasts increase in size during pregnancy?
- Is your intake of calories at least 1800?
- Is there evidence of retained placental fragments?
- Are you on an antihistamine?
- How many times in a 24-hour period do you nurse?
- Do you experience leaking, uterine contractions, drowsiness, or thirst during or between breastfeedings?
- Is there evidence of Sheehan's syndrome or was there an excessive loss of blood during delivery?
- Did you deliver by cesarean section?
- Was there a long delay in the initiation of lactation?
- Is your zinc intake adequate to not influence milk zinc content?

Infant Considerations

- How many wet diapers is the infant having per 24 hours?
- What is the frequency, consistency, and color of the stools?
- Is the infant jaundiced?
- Is the infant spitting up or having projectile vomiting?
- Is the infant breastfeeding on one or both breasts at each feeding?
- What is the duration of a nursing?
- Is there evidence of milk transfer during a feeding (swallowing, milk leaking around the mouth during feeding)?
- Is the infant satisfied after a feeding?
- Does the infant have a medical problem?
- Is the infant being given supplemental or complementary feeds?

gained less weight between birth and 10 days of life when compared to totally breastfed infants. The formula-fed group had greater fat deposition in males and greater daily gains in lean body mass in females (Shepherd et al., 1988). Females tend to gain less weight than males whether they are breastfed or formula fed (Nelson et al., 1989). Others have found that breastfed and formula-fed infants have comparable weight gain throughout the first three months of life (Dewey et al., 1992). The mean weight of breastfed 6- to 8-month-old infants dropped below the National Center for Health Statistics median and was significantly lower than that of a matched 6- to 8-month-old formula-fed group (Dewey et al., 1992).

Breastfed infants have a lower energy intake between 3 and 12 months of age than those who are formula fed (Dewey et al., 1993; Heinig et al., 1993; Krebs et al., 1994). Energy intake averaged 113 kcal/kg per day at one month of age but decreased to 85 to 89 kcal/kg per day at five to six months of age for the breastfed group followed in the DARLING Study, whereas the energy intake of formula-fed infants was 93 to 98 kcal/kg per day (Dewey & Lonnerdal, 1983; Heinig et al., 1993).

The weight-gain difference between breastfed and formula-fed infants is reflected by a drop of one standard deviation point on the growth grids. It is important, however, for the health-care provider to keep in mind that growth grids are primarily based on formula-fed infants. Before recommending a mother initiate formula supplements or introducing solids, a health-care provider or LC should assess the lactation process.

The research is inconclusive on the length-for-age measurements between breastfed and formula-fed infants. The DARLING Study showed no significant difference between length and head circumference measurements of the two groups through one year (Dewey et al., 1992). However, Krebs and associates (1994) found a decrease for breastfed infants from the 43rd percentile at two weeks of age to the 28th percentile at seven months, and the 26th percentile at nine months of age for length.

The intake of the breastfed infant appears to peak at a mean of 750 mL around the third month of life and the infant is reported to sustain adequate continued growth without increasing the number of calories consumed (Garza & Butte, 1990). Breastfed infants' birth weight, weight at three months of age, and total breastfeeding time have been reported to be positively associated with intake (Dewey, 1991). The average daily weight gain in grams based on the 50th percentile of the growth charts is shown in Table 1C–6.

The general recommendation is for the exclusively breastfed infant to gain between 4 oz. to 7 oz. per week in the early months. This is equivalent to 448 g to 784 g per month or 16 oz. to 28 oz. per month. Another general recommendation for weight gain in the first few months is 15 g to 30 g per day. Length and head circumference gains in the early months should equal approximately 0.8 cm to 1.1 cm per week and 0.5 cm to 0.8 cm per week, respectively (Groh-Wargo et al., 1994).

If the growth of a breastfed infant slows or drops growth channels on growth grids more than what is expected at around three months, the health-care provider should do a complete assessment to ensure that there are no underlying medical problems. But until separate growth grids are available for exclusively breastfed infants, an awareness of the differences in weight gain between breastfed and formula-fed infants is needed. Infants grow rapidly throughout the first year of life; by 12 months of age, an infant's weight will triple and length will double.

Table 1C–6   Average Daily Weight Gain Based on 50th Percentile

Age (mo)	Male (g)	Female (g)
1 to 3	31	24
3 to 6	20	20
6 to 9	25	15
9 to 12	12	11

Suggested Guidelines for Feeding the Breastfed Infant

ASSESSING INTAKE

For a formula-fed infant, it is easy to assess intake—recommended intakes are listed in Table 1C–7. The assessment of intake for the breastfed infant is more dependent on infant indicators and is subjective unless a precise baby scale is used before and after feedings. Usually this is not necessary for the full-term infant because weight, length, and head circumference measurements can assist in determining the adequacy of feedings over a period of time. The use of baby scales for monitoring the intake of an individual feed is gaining acceptance for the newly discharged preterm infant because the scales are now more precise than earlier models and are available for home use.

Indicators of adequate feedings for the breastfed infant include the following:

- Six (disposable) to eight (cloth) wet diapers per day
- Frequent stools (two to three minimum) during the neonatal period, with a decrease in frequency after four to six weeks of age
- Eight to 12 nursing sessions per day
- Evidence of milk transfer
- Satisfaction after nursing
- Softening of the breast after a feeding
- Increases in infant growth parameters

Growth or appetite spurts occur at about 10 days to 2 weeks, 2 to 3 months, and 5 to 6 months. During these periods, the infant will breastfeed more frequently, possibly every one to one-and-one-half hours, often clustering several feedings within a short period of time followed by several longer sleep periods.

A mother should be counseled on appetite spurts to increase her knowledge of normal development and heighten her awareness of her infant's ability to regulate the feedings. It is important for a mother to understand that the introduction of

Table 1C–7   Suggested Number and Volume of Bottle Feedings for a Healthy, Full-Term Formula-Fed Infant

Age	Number	Volume
Birth to 1 week	6–10	30–90 mL
1 week to 3 months	7–8	60–120 mL
1 to 3 months	5–7	120–180 mL
3 to 6 months	4–5	180–210 mL
6 to 9 months	3–4	210–240 mL
10 to 12 months	3	210–240 mL

Source: Kelts, DG, Jones, EG (1984). *Manual of Pediatric Nutrition,* p. 38. Copyright © Little, Brown and Company, Boston. Reprinted with permission.

formula, juice, or solid foods during an early growth spurt is not indicated and will be detrimental to the maintenance of her milk supply.

PROGRESSING TO SOLIDS

Determining the best time for introducing solid foods into the baby's diet requires an understanding of several factors: the baby's ability to ingest food other than liquids; the baby's ability to digest and assimilate the foods ingested; the baby's growth and health status while still on mother's milk; and the presence of prematurity, disease, or injury affecting digestion, absorption, or metabolism.

Current practices involving the introduction of baby foods are greatly instigated by commercial industry. According to the Institute of Medicine (IOM, 1992) in their report *Nutrition During Lactation*:

Human milk serves as the nutritional standard for infants. . . . Providing the breastfed infant with supplemental foods has a complex effect on the total amount of nutrient absorbed. For example, infants consuming such foods as formula or infant cereal generally decrease their intake of human milk . . . and, thus, the nutrients and other specialized components it supplies. Thus, the intake of supplementary foods may add nutrients in a less available form, decrease the bioavailability of nutrients in human milk, and decrease the intake of other important factors in human milk.

Digestive Maturation

The presence, or lack of, specific digestive enzymes should also guide the timing of solid food introduction. As Lebenthal (1995) states:

In early infancy, pancreatic amylase is not available in the duodenal fluids during the first four months of life when the pancreatic lipase is also very low. In addition, during the immediate postnatal life, the pancreatic acinar cells are not responsive to pancreozymin, and bile salt levels in the duodenal fluids are low. These observations, and the fact that other gastrointestinal functions such as gastric acid secretion are still immature during early infancy, raise important questions about the relationship between the development of digestion and absorption and the feeding practices prior to and during the weaning period.

The infant's system can handle starches only when pancreatic maturity permits proper digestion. Adding starchy foods to an infant's diet under the age of six months may do harm to the internal structure of the small intestine, affecting development and increasing the likelihood of diarrhea in infancy. Permitting infants to have prolonged weaning periods protects the pancreatic functions from disruption, eliminating further possible damage to the gastrointestinal tract.

Early introduction of solid foods may cause excessive weight gain and may lead to obesity in later life. Baby food does not promote better sleeping habits, does not improve speech, does not accelerate growth, and generally exposes the infant to developing allergies. "Although a number of identifiable factors are involved in the pathogenesis of overnutrition, we feel that prolonged breastfeeding is a natural way to promote normal growth and possibly decrease the risk of later obesity" (Saarinen & Siimes, 1979).

Historically, weaning was a process of growth and change that occurred without much fanfare and effort. As children matured, they automatically imitated older members of the family and participated in mealtime. Baby food consisted of normal fare being mashed, chewed, or pounded into a consistency easily assimilated. Without the ability to sit up, chew, swallow, and reach for food, infants feed mostly on breastmilk.

An infant must be physiologically ready for solids before they are introduced into the diet. This includes the ability to transfer food from the front of the mouth to the back, and the ability to sit independently and to hold the head upright. These developmental events usually occur between four to six months of age. In infancy, the recommended caloric distribution for infants is 40% to 50% fat, 7% to 11% protein, and the remainder from carbohydrates (Fomon, 1993; IOM, 1989). Beyond infancy, the percentage of kcal from fat is reduced with much controversy over how low fat as a percentage of kcal should be in the diet of the toddler (one- to two-year-old) and young child.

Introducing Solids

Iron-fortified rice cereal should be the infant's first food. It should be prepared with breastmilk or formula preferably, although water can be used to make the cereal if an infant's growth is adequate. The iron availability of infant cereal is higher for the dried cereal than the ready-to-eat cereal available in the jar. Food should always be fed with a spoon and not put into the infant bottle or an infant feeder. The caregiver should look for symptoms of food allergy (fussiness, diarrhea, rash, spitting up, blood in stool, wheezing) after the introduction of a new food. If no symptoms occur after several days (two to four), introduction of new foods should continue. It is important to offer one new food at a time to assess for intolerance.

Vegetables should be added to the infant's diet after cereal. Because they are bland, vegetables are more acceptable to infants if offered before fruit. A recent study indicates that breastfed infants accept vegetables better than formula-fed infants (Sullivan et al., 1994). Flavors are passed into breastmilk and it is theorized that the breastfed infant has been experiencing a variety of flavors from his or her mother's milk and, thus, is more open to acceptance of vegetables. Fruit and juices can be added after a good variety of vegetables have been introduced. Juice should always be offered in the cup. The use of small amounts of juice in the cup initially is advised because the infant will experiment with turning the cup upside down and tossing it from the table while exploring the mealtime environment.

After the infant is accepting fruits, vegetables, and cereals, the introduction of other starches, such as pasta and grains, is advised. Broths and gravies can be added to liquify the texture as needed to improve acceptance and facilitate swallowing. Meat and egg yolk should be offered by nine months of age. To be able to identify any food intolerance, plain strained foods should be introduced before mixed foods. Plain foods are also recommended over commercial baby food dinners and desserts because they are nutritionally superior.

When strained foods are tolerated, the infant is ready to progress to foods with more texture. This can be well-mashed table foods or commercial junior infant foods. If table foods are used, they should not be flavored with fats or heavily seasoned. The caregiver should read labels on baby foods, selecting brands that do not add salt, sugar, and/or artificial flavorings and colorings whenever possible. As the infant becomes more coordinated, finger foods (toast, dry cereal, pieces of fruit or cooked vegetable, and so on) can be introduced.

By 12 months of age, an infant's meals can be similar to those of the rest of the family. By this time, the infant's caloric needs can be met through a variety of foods combined with breastfeeding. Texture advancements should be occurring to aid in chewing. Whole or 2% milk can be introduced, and its use is recommended through 24 months of age to ensure adequate fat intake.

Throughout the progression of introducing solids into the diet, the caregiver must be aware of the possibility of choking. An infant or toddler should not be allowed to eat without supervision nor should he or she be allowed to eat while crawling or walking around the home. Foods such as hot dogs, nuts, grapes, carrots, and round candies have been associated with choking and death (AAP, 1983).

As an infant grows, more calories are required to support continued growth. Introduction of solids will meet these needs. As solids are introduced the frequency and duration of breastfeedings will decline. Complete weaning should not occur before the mother and infant are ready. Breastfeeding provides comfort and security for the infant and weaning should not be rushed but instead be baby led.

The toddler is independent and strives for self-sufficiency. Usual feeding behaviors include self-feeding, refusal to be fed, and food jags. To promote this independence, foods should be easy to maneuver (e.g., finger foods and foods cut into bite-size pieces). The toddler also prefers single-item foods over casseroles and mixed dishes. Although toddlers need the same variety of foods as adults, the appropriate serving sizes are much smaller. One estimate is a tablespoon of food for each year of life. It is best to keep the portion sizes small so that the toddler does not become overwhelmed and refuse to eat any of the offered food. If the child is still hungry, he or she will indicate he or she wants more. Some toddlers refuse to eat foods if they are "touching" one another on the plate. This can be prevented if appropriate portion sizes are given. A small plate and appropriate-size utensils should be used during early childhood.

Snacks play an integral role in the diet of a toddler. To meet nutritional needs, two to three snacks should be planned during the day. These snacks should be comprised of nutrient-dense foods, not high-sugar or high-fat foods. Today, there are many excellent cookbooks and reference books for feeding small children available to the parent.

Snacks and beverages should be scheduled so as not to affect the mealtime appetite. If a toddler is hungry within 30 minutes of a planned meal or snack, water should be given to the child. If a child is consistently hungry more than an hour before the next scheduled feeding, the parent should look at the content of foods the child has been receiving to see if they have been limiting the portion sizes too much or not providing adequate fat for satiety. Today's parents are more aware of nutrition than ever before and many are very health conscious. In their zeal to improve their own habits, they may inappropriately restrict fat or kcal for their young child. Children with growth deficits often overconsume juice; when juice consumption is reduced, intake of solid foods, and thus calories, will increase.

Meals and snacks should be offered at the table. Children should have meals with other family members for the socialization. It is advisable to turn off the radio and television during mealtimes and encourage conversation. Conversation enhances family bonding and increases the length of the meal, which allows time for the body to recognize satiety cues. The development of eating habits begins early and mealtimes in the formative years of early childhood influence long-term eating

Table 1C–8 Guidelines for Progression to Solid Foods

Months of Age	Feeding Skills	Oral-Motor Skills	Suggested Types of Food	Suggested Activities
Birth to 4		Rooting reflex Sucking reflex Swallowing reflex Extrusion reflex	Breastmilk Infant formula	Breastfeed or bottle feed
5	Able to grasp objects voluntarily Learning to reach out with hands	Disappearance of extrusion reflex	Breastmilk Infant formula	Possible introduction of thinned cereal
6	Sits with balance while using hands	Transfers food from front of tongue	Infant cereal Strained fruits Strained vegetables	Prepare cereal with breastmilk or formula to make cereal to a semiliquid texture Use spoon Feed from a dish Advance to ⅓ to ½ cup cereal before adding fruits or vegetables
7	Improved grasp	Mashes food with lateral movements of jaw Learns side-to-side or "rotary" chewing	Infant cereal Strained to junior texture of fruits, vegetables, and meats	Thicken cereal to lumpier texture Sit in highchair with feet Introduce cup
8 to 10	Holds bottle without help Drinks from cup without spilling Decreases fluid intake and increases solids Coordinates hand–eye movements		Juices Soft, mashed, or minced table foods	Begin finger foods Do not add salt, sugar, or fats to foods Present soft foods in chunks ready for finger feeding
10 to 12	Feeds self Holds cup without help	Tooth eruption Improved ability to bite and chew	Soft, chopped table foods	Provide meals in pattern similar to rest of family Use cup at meals

Source: Barness, LA (1993). *Pediatric Nutrition Handbook*, p. 130. Copyright © 1993, AAP, Elk Grove Village, IL. Used with permission of the American Academy of Pediatrics.

habits. Table 1C–8 shows the AAP's 1993 (Barness, 1993) recommended schedule for progression to solids.

NUTRITIONAL NEEDS OF INFANTS AND CHILDREN

As a child grows, his or her nutritional needs increase to support that growth. The IOM's Recommended Dietary Allowances (1989) do not distinguish between the sexes until age 11. Tables 1C–9, 1C–10, and 1C–11 show the nutrient needs of infancy and childhood. Table 1C–12 shows estimated energy requirements for infants (0–11.9 months) and children (1–7.9 years).

Table 1C–9   Recommended Dietary Allowances

Category[a]	Age (years)	Weight[b] kg	lb	Height[b] cm	lb	Protein (g)	Vitamin A (µg RE)[c]	Vitamin D (µg)[d]	Vitamin E (mg a-TE)[e]	Vitamin K (µg)[e]
							Fat-Soluble Vitamins			
Infant	0.0–0.5	6	13	60	24	13	375	7.5	3	5
	0.5–1.0	9	20	71	28	14	375	10	4	10
Child	1–3	13	29	90	35	16	400	10	6	15
	4–6	20	44	112	44	24	500	10	7	20
	7–10	28	62	132	52	28	700	10	7	30

Water-Soluble Vitamins

Category	Age (years)	Vitamin C (mg)	Thiamin (B[1]) (mg)	Riboflavin (B[2]) (mg)	Niacin (B[3]) (mg NE)[f]	Vitamin B[6] (mg)	Folic Acid (µg)	Vitamin B[12] (µg)
Infant	0.0–0.5	30	0.3	0.4	5	0.3	25	0.3
	0.5–1.0	35	0.4	0.5	6	0.6	35	0.5
Child	1–3	40	0.7	0.8	9	1.0	50	0.7
	4–6	45	0.9	1.1	12	1.1	75	1.0
	7–10	45	1.0	1.2	13	1.4	100	1.4

Minerals

Category	Age (years)	Calcium (mg)	Phosphorus (mg)	Magnesium (mg)	Iron (mg)	Zinc (mg)	Iodine (µg)	Selenium (µg)
Infant	0.0–0.5	400	300	40	6	5	40	10
	0.5–1.0	600	500	60	10	5	50	15
Child	1–3	800	800	80	10	10	70	20
	4–6	800	800	120	10	10	90	20
	7–10	800	800	170	10	10	120	30

[a]The allowances, expressed as average daily intakes over time, are intended to provide for individual variations among most normal persons as they live in the United States under usual environmental stresses. Diets should be based on a variety of common foods in order to provide other nutrients for which human requirements have been less well defined.

[b]Weights and heights of Reference Adults are actual medians for the U.S. population of the designated age, as reported by NHANES II. The median weights and heights of those under 29 years of age were taken from Hamill et al. (1979). The use of these figures does not imply that the height-to-weight ratios are ideal.

[c]Retinol equivalents—1 retinol equivalent = 1 µg retinol or 6 µg B-carotene.

[d]As cholecalciferol—10 µg cholecalciferol = 400 IU of vitamin D.

[e]a-Tocopherol equivalents (TE)—1 mg d-a tocopherol = 1 a-TE.

[f]1 niacin equivalent (NE) is equal to 1 mg of niacin or 60 mg of dietary tryptophan.

Source: From Institute of Medicine (IOM)/National Academy of Sciences (1989). *Recommended Dietary Allowances*, 10th ed. Washington, DC: National Academy Press. Reprinted with permission.

EXTENDED LACTATION

Objections to prolonged breastfeeding fly in the face of national and international recommendations that all children exclusively breastfeed six months and continue to breastfeed while receiving complementary foods for up to two years and beyond. Breastfeeding can provide nutrients, strengthen immunity, and build relationships well past infancy. The average age of weaning worldwide is four years or older (Lawrence, 1989). Impediments to prolonged breastfeeding include viewing the breasts only as part of adult sexuality; concern over milk being dirty or unclean; viewing the practice as nasty; or worries over spoiling the infant, causing

Table 1C–10 Summary Table of Estimated Safe and Adequate Daily Dietary Intake of Selected Vitamins and Minerals

| | | Vitamins[a] | |
| | | Pantothenic Acid | |
Category	Age (yr)	Biotin (µg)	(mg)
Infants	0–0.5	10	2
	0.5–1	15	3
Children and	1–3	20	3
adolescents	4–6	25	3–4
	7–10	30	4–5
	11+	30–100	4–7

| | | Trace Elements[b] | | | | |
Category	Age (yr)	Copper (mg)	Manganese (mg)	Fluoride (mg)	Chromium (µg)	Molybdenum (µg)
Infants	0–0.5	0.4–0.6	0.3–0.6	0.1–0.5	10–40	15–30
	0.5–1	0.6–0.7	0.6–1.0	0.2–1.0	20–60	20–40
Children	1–3	0.7–1.0	1.0–1.5	0.5–1.5	20–80	25–50
and	4–6	1.0–1.5	1.5–2.0	1.0–2.5	20–120	30–75
adolescents	7–10	1.0–2.0	2.0–3.0	1.5–2.5	50–200	50–150
	11+	1.5–2.5	2.0–5.0	1.5–2.5	50–200	75–250

Source: Institute of Medicine (IOM)/National Academy of Sciences (1989). *Recommended Dietary Allowances,* 10th ed. Washington, DC: National Academy Press. Reprinted with permission.

[a]Because there is less information on which to base allowances, these figures are not given in the main table of RDA and are provided here in the form of ranges of recommended intakes.

[b]Since the toxic levels for many trace elements may be only several times usual intakes, the upper levels for the trace elements given in this table should not be habitually exceeded.

Table 1C–11 Estimated Sodium, Chloride, and Potassium Minimum Requirements for Healthy Persons

Age[a]	Weight (kg)	Sodium (mg)[b,c]	Chloride (mg)[b,c]	Potassium (mg)[d]
0–5 months	4.5	120	180	500
6–11 months	8.9	200	300	700
1 year	11.0	225	350	1,000
2–5 years	16.0	300	500	1,400
6–9 years	25.0	400	600	1,600
10–18 years	50.0	500	750	2,000

Source: Institute of Medicine (IOM)/National Academy of Sciences (1989). *Recommended Dietary Allowances,* 10th ed. Washington, DC: National Academy Press. Reprinted with permission.

[a]No allowance included for growth. Values for those below 18 years assume a growth rate at the 50th percentile reported by the National Center for Health Statistics (Hamill et al., 1979) and averaged for males and females.

[b]No allowance has been included for large prolonged losses from the skin through sweat.

[c]There is no evidence that higher intakes confer any health benefit.

[d]Desirable intakes of potassium may considerably exceed these values.

Table 1C–12   Energy Requirements

| Age[a] | Weight[b] (kg) | Mean Height (cm) | REE[c] (kcal/day) | Mean Activity Factor | Estimated Energy Allowances | | |
					By Time kcal/day (range) [MJ/day]	By Weight kcal/kg [kJ/kg]	By Height (kcal/cm)
Infants							
0–2.9 months	4.5	55	–	–	500 (400–700) [2.1][d]	110 [460]	9.1
3–5.9 months	6.6	64	–	–	650 (500–850) [2.7][d]	100 [420]	10.2
6–8.9 months	7.9	69	–	–	750 (600–1000) [3.1]	95 [400]	10.9
9–11.9 months	9.0	73	–	–	900 (700–1200) [3.8]	100 [420]	12.3
Children							
1–1.9 years	11	82	600	2.0	1200 (900–1600) [4.8]	105 [440]	14.0
2–3.9 years	14	96	700	2.0	1400 (1100–1900) [5.9]	100 [410]	14.6
4–5.9 years	18	109	830	2.0	1700 (1300–2300) [7.1]	92 [380]	15.6
6–7.9 years	22	121	930	2.0	1800 (1400–2400) [7.5]	83 [350]	14.9

[a]For persons ages <18 years, data originated from median heights and weights.
[b]Rounded to nearest kilogram for age >1 year.
[c]Based on equations for BMR with the age taken at the midpoint of age range for the group. The equation given for males was used for both sexes aged <10 years.
[d]For young children the estimated allowance is more suitably calculated from weight and allowance per kilogram body weight.

Source: Adapted from Pellett, PL (1990). Food energy requirements in humans. *Am J Clin Nutr*, 51:711–22. In: Barness, LA (1993). *Pediatric Nutrition Handbook*, p. 444. Copyright © 1993, AAP, Elk Grove Village, IL. Used with permission of the American Academy of Pediatrics.

neurotic attachments, homosexuality, or obesity. These views are based on cultural mores and concerns of the times, not on clinical evidence.

Several researchers have reviewed the available evidence on the possible advantages and disadvantages associated with breastfeeding the older infant after the introduction of solid foods (Hormann, 1993; Prentice, 1991). In poor areas of the developing world, the continuation of breastfeeding one to two years after solid-food introduction has several major benefits, including supply of nutrients (see Table 1C–13); delivery of protective, digestive, and trophic agents; extending the infertility of the mother; and reduction of infectious disease sensitivity in severely malnourished individuals (Prentice, 1991).

There is no evidence to support partial breastfeeding after solid-food introduction as a cause of poor growth performance. In fact, studies reviewed by Hormann (1993) show that in developing countries, the infants breastfed into the second year of life have higher intakes of energy than their nonbreastfed counterparts and substantial amounts of other nutrients are provided via breastmilk.

The immunological benefits from prolonged lactation include long-term protection against disease, day-to-day protection from pathogens, and reduced severity of infections. These benefits are discussed in Module 3, *The Science of Breastfeeding*, Chapter 2, and Module 1, *The Support of Breastfeeding*, Chapter 2.

WEANING

Responsive mothering is when the mother fulfills the child's needs. One child may wish to wean near the end of the first year while another may continue breast-

Table 1C–13   Breastmilk's Contributions to Toddlers' Diet

Benefits	Percentage
Higher energy than nonbreastfed toddlers at 12 to 18 months	25%
Higher energy than nonbreastfed toddlers >18 months	17%
Toddlers' calories provided by breastmilk	31%
Protein in a day	38%
Vitamin C in a day	95%
Vitamin A in a day	100%
Calcium in a day	44%
Niacin in a day	41%
Folic acid in a day	26%
Riboflavin in a day	21%
Iron in a day	50%

Source: Compiled from information in Cameron and Hofvander (1984) and McMillan et al. (1976).

feeding as he or she gets older. Mothers who are reluctant to practice baby-led weaning may find suggestions for gradual mother-led weaning helpful. *Mothering Your Nursing Toddler* (Bumgarner, 1990) provides guidance to couples breastfeeding a toddler, and *Still Nursing* (Diamond, 1982)—a La Leche League information sheet—also gives guidance in a supportive manner for parents contemplating weaning.

Weaning is the process of gradually introducing solid foods to a milk-fed infant or young child. Weaning is considered complete when the child no longer breastfeeds, drinks from a bottle, or uses milk as the main source of food. Among mammals, weaning times vary species to species depending on fat distribution of the body, brain complexity, and solute load of the mother's milk. The weaning time normally correlates with the ability of the young to obtain its own food (Lawrence, 1994), with the mother steadily reducing the frequency of sucking. Young elephants wean in their second year, seal pups at six weeks, porpoises at three years, primates at two to three years.

Weaning patterns in human cultures vary according to environmental and social influences. Cultures that retain some indigenous habits breastfeed their children at least two to four years. In industrialized countries, public and social pressures compel mothers to wean at earlier ages—six weeks to one year of age. Very few traditional societies wean under a year of age.

Sheila Kippley, in her book *Breast-feeding and Natural Child Spacing: How Ecological Breastfeeding Spaces Babies* (1989), presents comprehensive reports and compilations on the practice of breastfeeding as a contraceptive method. This information has been supported through historical investigation of population maintenance in indigenous societies and scientific research of lactation physiology. Unrestricted sucking suppresses estrogen levels in the mother and sustains elevated prolactin levels. The reproductive reflex involves sending nerve stimulation from the nipple to the hypothalamic and pituitary glands, which inhibits their activity. This activity increases prolactin secretion, which reduces progesterone secretion and has a direct effect on the ovaries. According to Kippley (1989):

There can be no doubt that hitherto breastfeeding has been the major factor holding human population growth in check; even today, it probably prevents more pregnancies the world over than all artificial forms of contraception put together.

Urbanization has been the force contributing most to the decrease in the use of breastfeeding as a contraceptive. Reducing the frequency of stimulation (scheduled feeds, using baby cribs, and infant seats) and using commercial baby foods and artificial means of feeds (baby bottles) have altered the effect of sucking in the induction of amenorrhea.

Technically, weaning begins when the infant begins to take any other form of nutrition other than mother's milk. This can take place in several forms:

1. To eliminate taking all human milk feeds directly from the breast; substituting an artificial nipple with a bottle filled with formula. This is known as abrupt weaning.
2. Dropping one breastfeeding session at a time and replacing it with a formula/bottle feeding. A method used for infants and young children still needing sucking activity.
3. To continue breastfeeding and gradually introduce solid foods into the infant's diet at a specific age. This is the most commonly preferred method among pediatricians.
4. To continue breastfeeding, gradually adding foods to the infant's diet when he or she shows readiness to eat; sitting up on his or her own; able to chew well; and developed hand-to-mouth coordination. This method is used by those who wish to breastfeed for an extended period of time.

Dietary guidelines as to first food choices typically have been based on environment selection and food availability. In industrialized countries, there are commercially manufactured baby foods to select from. Mothers of indigenous societies normally offer chewed foods from their mouths to their young. Generally, pediatricians suggest mothers begin with iron-fortified cereals and then vegetables and fruits, breads, with meats products last. Much speculation and investigation has been given to the sequence of offering foods to infants. Usually the mother decides which guidelines to follow—doctors, nutritionists, naturalists, or cultural.

Weaning is an emotional time for both mother and baby; much attention and concern should be included when counseling a breastfeeding couple. Abrupt weaning may leave subtle emotional scars on the infant and the mother may experience a grieving period that may last for years, even though the decision was for valid reasons. With gradual weaning, the baby may or may not resist and the emotional impact on the mother may not be as strong. With baby-led weaning, the impact is much lower because the breastfeeding couple is able to adapt slowly and fill the need for closeness with other activities.

As the child matures, his or her interest automatically turns to play, friends, other relatives, and so on, so feeding frequency diminishes as security levels expand. By the time a toddler is two years old, feeding frequency is usually only two or three times a day and the duration is brief. As older infants engage in activities with more people, the likelihood of infections and viruses increases. Breastfeeding at this stage still offers strong immunological protection, and in times of illness, may be the only source of nutrition for a child who is unable to eat.

There are a few instances when weaning abruptly is necessary. Maternal illness requiring medication incompatible with breastfeeding is the most common reason and with careful study, temporary weaning may be all that is needed. Beyond medically indicated situations, mothers mediate the timing of weaning based on their feelings, family support, and maturation of the baby. It is rare for children under a year to wean on their own. There are often other factors affecting early weaning such as mismanagement of breastfeeding during early infancy, prolonged mother–baby separation, misinterpreting older baby behavior, overuse of bottles and pacifiers, and/or any circumstance causing a break in the bonding cycle.

Nutrients of Specific Concern
for the Breastfed Infant

The question of the need for supplementation of the full-term, breastfed infant with vitamins or minerals before six months warrants discussion. The most widely available liquid, oral supplements include ones with vitamins A, C, D, E, with or without iron and fluoride. Table 1C–14 provides information about the content of a few common infant nutrient supplements available in the United States.

Table 1C–14   Content of Selected Liquid Nutrient Supplements

Mead-Johnson Tri-Vi-Sol (1 mL)
Vitamin A	1500 IU
Vitamin D	400 IU
Vitamin C	35 mg

Mead-Johnson Tri-Vi-Sol with Iron (1 mL)
Vitamin A	1500 IU
Vitamin D	400 IU
Vitamin C	35 mg
Iron	10 mg

Mead-Johnson Poly-Vi-Sol (1 mL)
Vitamin A	1500 IU
Vitamin D	400 IU
Vitamin E	5 IU
Vitamin C	35 mg
Thiamin	0.5 mg
Riboflavin	0.6 mg
Niacin	8 mg
Vitamin B_6	0.4 mg
Vitamin B_{12}	2 mcg

Mead-Johnson Poly-Vi-Sol with Iron (1 mL)
Vitamin A	1500 IU
Vitamin D	400 IU
Vitamin E	5 IU
Vitamin C	35 mg
Thiamin	0.5 mg
Riboflavin	0.6 mg
Niacin	8 mg
Vitamin B_6	0.4 mg
Iron	10 mg

Ross Vi-Daylin Multivitamin with Fluoride (1 mL)
Fluoride	0.25 mg
Vitamin A	1500 IU
Vitamin D	400 IU
Vitamin E	5 IU
Vitamin C	35 mg
Thiamin	0.5 mg
Riboflavin	0.6 mg
Niacin	8 mg
Vitamin B_6	0.4 mg

Ross Vi-Daylin Multivitamin with Fluoride and Iron (1 mL)
Fluoride	0.25 mg
Vitamin A	1500 IU
Vitamin D	400 IU
Vitamin E	5 IU
Vitamin C	35 mg
Thiamin	0.5 mg
Riboflavin	0.6 mg
Niacin	8 mg
Vitamin B_6	0.4 mg
Iron	10 mg

Ross Vi-Daylin Multivitamin (1 teaspoon—5.0 mL)
Vitamin A	2500 IU
Vitamin D	400 IU
Vitamin E	15 IU
Vitamin C	60 mg
Thiamin	1.05 mg
Riboflavin	1.2 mg
Niacin	13.5 mg
Vitamin B_6	1.05 mg
Vitamin B_{12}	4.5 mcg

Ross Vi-Daylin Multivitamin and Iron (1 teaspoon—5.0 mL)
Vitamin A	2500 IU
Vitamin D	400 IU
Vitamin E	15 IU
Vitamin C	60 mg
Thiamin	1.05 mg
Riboflavin	1.2 mg
Niacin	13.5 mg
Vitamin B_6	1.05 mg
Vitamin B_{12}	4.5 mcg
Iron	10 mg

Mead-Johnson Fer-in-Sol (0.6 mL)
Iron	15 mg

Ross Pediaflor (0.5 mL)
Fluoride	0.25 mg

The role of the maternal diet in influencing the composition of breastmilk's vitamins and minerals is discussed in detail in Module 3, *The Science of Breastfeeding*, Chapter 2. The following is a brief overview:

- Water-soluble vitamins are influenced by maternal diet.
- The vitamin D concentration of milk is low if the mother does not consume adequate dairy products or lives in northern latitudes where her sunlight exposure is limited.
- A minimum of 1800 kcal are needed for milk production to not be decreased.
- The type of fatty acids in the breastmilk is influenced by maternal diet.
- A Vitamin B_{12} deficiency has been reported in infants whose mothers are strict vegetarians.
- Malnourished mothers produce less milk.
- Breastmilk is a poor source of fluoride.
- Breastmilk iron is low but bioavailability is excellent and iron deficiency anemia is rare in exclusively breastfed infants in the first six months of life.
- At birth, the infant has a prolonged prothrombin time.

Given these conclusions, the following sections discuss general recommendations for some nutrients for healthy, full-term, exclusively breastfed infants. The last section gives suggestions for mothers who may have marginal diets.

VITAMIN D

Vitamin D is essential for bone mineralization and requirements are dependent on the length of exposure to the sun. Formula contains double the infant's requirement for vitamin D. Human milk vitamin D content depends on maternal diet and sunlight exposure.

The AAP recommends routine supplementation of vitamin D to selected groups of exclusively breastfed infants based on data that human milk vitamin D content is low. It is known that vitamin D in breastmilk is increased by an adequate maternal intake of the vitamin (AAP, 1997). Specker (1994) recommends that infants whose mothers do not consume dairy products, who are not taken out into the sunlight, or who live in northern latitudes be supplemented with vitamin D. Another consideration is ethnic background; the darker the skin pigmentation, the longer it takes for conversion of cholecalciferol to one of the vitamin D derivatives to occur (Specker, 1994). The AAP recommends supplementation with vitamin D for infants whose mothers are vitamin-D deficient or for those infants not exposed to adequate sunlight (AAP, 1997).

Careful history needs to be taken to determine whether supplementation is necessary. If the mother drinks dairy products supplemented with vitamin D, there is little reason for concern. The documentation of rickets in exclusively breastfed infants in recent literature has brought this issue to the attention of physicians who are now more likely to recommend vitamin D supplementation for the breastfed infant. For most infants, sunlight exposure approximately three times per week for ten minutes is an easy intervention. Sunscreens block ultraviolet rays in the range needed to convert cholecalciferol into a vitamin D precursor and should not be applied (if used) until after approximately ten minutes to allow adequate exposure time.

FLUORIDE

Fluoride plays a role in the prevention of dental caries. Over the past 10 to 15 years, there has been a marked reduction in the prevalence of caries in the United States and other countries. A major factor contributing to this significant public health success story appears to be the increased accessibility to fluorides, beginning in infancy, which is an inexpensive and highly effective preventive tool in the fight against caries.

Fluoride becomes incorporated in the mineral structure of the tooth, and its presence appears to prevent dental caries by increasing the tooth's resistance to acid dissolution, enhancing the process of remineralization (in effect, reversing early carious lesions), and reducing the potential of dental plaque to cause tooth decay. The benefits of fluorides can be acquired both systematically and topically. For infants and toddlers, the principal concern is that they receive an optimal level of systemic fluoride (Nowak & Crall, 1988).

The primary source of systemic fluoride is through naturally or artificially fluoridated drinking water. Fluoride consumed in this manner can safely reduce the incidence of caries by 40% to 50% in the primary dentition and by 50% to 65% in the permanent dentition (USDHEW, 1979). The recommended level for fluoride concentration of public drinking water is 0.7 to 1.0 parts per million (ppm).

Systemic fluoride supplementation, in the form of drops or chewable tablets, has been recommended in cases where adequate consumption of fluoridated water does not occur (AAP, 1979, 1986). Included in this category are the following:

1. Infants who derive all or most of their fluid intake from breastfeeding
2. Infants and children living in nonfluoridated communities or in communities with less than the optimum level of fluoride in the water supply (<0.7 ppm)
3. Cases in which the family utilizes bottled water or home filtration systems for their primary source of water for drinking and cooking

In 1995, the Committee on Nutrition *revised* this position. Fluoride supplementation is no longer recommended from birth. The level of water fluoride content when supplements are recommended was dropped from 0.7 to 0.6 ppm (AAP, 1995). The American Dental Association Council on Dental Therapeutics is reported to concur with the new recommendations (AAPD, 1995). See Table 1C–15 for the interim guidelines.

Topical fluoride, primarily that found in toothpastes, offers additional protection against tooth decay. However, infants and toddlers are not capable of expectorat-

Table 1C–15   Fluoride Supplementation

Age	Water <0.3 ppm	Fluoride Content (in ppm)	
		0.3–0.6	>0.6
Birth	0	0	0
6 months to 3 years	0.25 mg	0.25 mg	0
3 to 6 years	0.50 mg	0.25 mg	0
6 to 16 years	1.00 mg	0.50 mg	0

Source: AAP/Committee on Nutrition (1995). Fluoride supplementation for children: Interim policy recommendations. *Pediatrics*, 95(5):777. Used with permission of the American Academy of Pediatrics.

ing, so the topical fluoride soon becomes systemic as it is swallowed. The knowledge that this occurs, as well as the recent rise in the incidence of dental fluorosis (staining of the permanent teeth) has brought about a reexamination of recommendations regarding fluoride concentrations in toothpastes, frequency of toothpaste utilization, and levels of prescribed fluoride supplementation. In the future, the availability of children's-strength fluoridated toothpastes is likely. Pending the availability of new products and new guidelines, it is recommended that toothpaste be used sparingly (pea size or a smaller amount), and no more than once or twice a day when brushing the teeth of infants and toddlers. Preschool-age children should be supervised. New parents should seek advice from their pediatric dentist or pediatrician regarding the need for supplementation.

IRON

Breastmilk provides only slightly more than 0.3 mg/L of iron and approximately 50% is absorbed (Barness, 1993; IOM, 1992; Saarinen, 1977). This high absorption may be due to high levels of citrate and vitamin C as well as the protein/phosphorus ratios in human milk. Many believe that lactoferrin enhances iron absorption although studies do not support this contention. However, lactoferrin does bind iron and make it unavailable for bacteria. Increasing iron in the maternal diet does not influence breastmilk iron concentrations (IOM, 1992). Although the RDA of iron in infancy is not met by the amount in human milk, the exclusively breastfed infant is not considered at risk for iron deficiency anemia during the first six months of life thanks to fetal stores (Duncan et al., 1985; Schulz-Lell et al., 1987).

Most clinicians believe iron supplementation for full-term infants should begin at four to six months of age. This is based on data that show 10% to 30% of unsupplemented (with iron) breastfed infants need iron by nine months (Pizzarro et al., 1991; Siimes et al., 1984). For 40 infants fed only formula (N = 15) or human milk (N = 25) for the first six months, anemia was prevalent in 27.8% of the breastfed group and 7.1% of the formula-fed group (Calvo et al., 1992). Supplemental foods were given from the sixth to the ninth month; researchers emphasized to the mothers the importance of giving infants iron- and ascorbic-rich foods. Ferritin (storage iron) was absent in 27.8% of the breastfed group but in none of the formula-fed group (Calvo et al., 1992).

In a recent study of 30 infants who received no cow's milk, medicinal iron, or iron-enriched formula, plus cereal, and were breastfed until their first birthday, 30% were anemic at one year of age. However, for the nonanemic infants, the duration of exclusive breastfeeding was significantly longer—6.5 months versus 5.5 months. None of the infants who were exclusively breastfed for 7 or more months were anemic, although 43% of those who were breastfed for a shorter period of time were anemic. The infants exclusively breastfed for a prolonged period had good iron status at 12 and 24 months (Pisacane et al., 1995).

Clearly, the controversy of when to begin supplementing the breastfed infant with iron continues. Unfortunately, current screening mechanisms (hematocrit or hemoglobin) do not decline to abnormal levels until iron-deficiency anemia is evident, limiting the clinician's ability to recognize which breastfed infants are at risk for anemia. Newer measurement techniques, such as the transferrin receptor level, which detects early iron deficiency at the cellular level, are still being tested but show promise as screening tools.

The AAP (AAP, 1997) currently recommends that iron supplementation of exclusively breastfed infants begin when anemia is present or iron stores are low. The report by Pisacane and colleagues (1995), along with the realization of a lower energy requirement in infancy, has led many to question the practice of introducing solids at four to six months.

Whenever the clinician recommends beginning iron supplementation, the amount should be based on 1 mL/kg body weight per day (Barness, 1993). The most common form of supplementation is the use of iron-fortified formula and iron-fortified infant cereal. For the exclusively breastfed infant, iron-fortified cereal can be introduced at six months as the first solid food, or if the mother prefers to wait longer to introduce solid foods, oral vitamins with iron can be given although it appears that exclusive breastfeeding beyond seven months may be protective against iron deficiency.

If solid foods are added to an infant's diet prior to four to six months of age, iron supplementation may be necessary if high-iron foods are not given. The practice of early introduction of solid foods is not recommended, however. Use of iron-inhibitor foods (tea, sweetened powdered drinks, phytates, and so on) by the mother should be discouraged. See Module 3, *The Science of Breastfeeding*, Chapter 2, for foods that are high in iron; see Chapter 2 of this module for a discussion of iron deficiency anemia.

VITAMIN K

Vitamin K plays an important role in blood clotting. A vitamin K supplement, to restore the prolonged prothrombin time observed at birth, is recommended for the breastfed infant (AAP, 1993). Hemorrhagic disease of the newborn (HDN) is prevented by giving a prophylaxis of vitamin K because it prevents or minimizes the postnatal decline of the vitamin K–dependent coagulation factors (II, VII, IX, and X). It is given as a single, intramuscular dose of 0.5 mg to 1 mg or as an oral dose of 1.0 mg to 2.0 mg. Vitamin K prophylaxis is mandated by law in many states. If a breastfed infant has diarrhea for more than several days, the AAP recommends an intramuscular injection of 1.0 mg of vitamin K every five to seven days for as long as the diarrhea persists (AAP, 1993). After the initial newborn supplement, bottle-fed infants do not need supplements since vitamin K is present in cow's milk–based formula (AAP, 1993). Foods high in vitamin K include dark-green leafy vegetables, pork, and liver.

MOTHERS WITH MARGINAL DIETS

Infants of malnourished mothers; reformed alcoholic mothers who may not have adequate nutrient reserves; unsupplemented, strict vegetarian mothers; and teenage mothers with a poor food intake should be supplemented with a multivitamin because the vitamin content of human milk is influenced by these factors. Any mother who shows signs of having a marginal or unhealthy diet should be individually assessed to determine any supplementation needs for her and/or her baby.

POST-TEST

For questions 1 to 20, choose the best answer.

1. The diet of a full-term infant should be

   A. 40% to 50% carbohydrate, 7% to 10% fat, and the remainder in protein.
   B. 40% to 50% fat, 7% to 11% protein, and the remainder in carbohydrate.
   C. 20% to 30% fat, 7% to 10% protein, and the remainder in carbohydrate.
   D. 5% to 10% fat, 25% carbohydrate, and the remainder in protein.

2. The recommended first food to be introduced to an infant is

   A. fruit juice.
   B. vegetables.
   C. cereal.
   D. fruit.

3. Symptoms of Kwashiorkor include all of the following except

   A. fussiness.
   B. diarrhea.
   C. blood in the stool.
   D. vomiting.

4. The recommended feeding practice for infants includes all of the following except

   A. offering juice in bottle.
   B. offering single item foods prior to mixed foods.
   C. offering foods to the infant with a spoon.
   D. offering a new food for two to four days before offering another.

5. A four-month-old formula-fed infant will consume _____ amount of calories as a four-month-old breastfed infant.

   A. the same
   B. more
   C. less

6. When compared to formula-fed infants, breastfed infants will have _____ skin-fold at 9 to 15 months of age.

   A. the same
   B. a higher
   C. a lower

7. The growth of breastfed infants is adequately represented on standard growth grids.

   A. True
   B. False

8. Compare the four-month-old breastfed infant's growth to a formula-fed infant.

   A. The breastfed infant will have a lower weight/height.
   B. The breastfed infant will have a higher weight/height.
   C. The breastfed infant will have a similar weight/height.

9. All of the following are good indicators of adequate infant intake except

   A. increases in height, weight, and head circumference.
   B. evidence of milk transfer.

    C. six to eight wet diapers a day.

    D. feeding duration of one hour or more.

10. Good sources of protein for the infant include

    A. mixed vegetable–meat dinners.

    B. vegetables.

    C. single strained meat.

    D. fruits.

11. A breastfed infant of a mother who did not drink milk may be at higher risk for

    A. hyperlipidemia.

    B. scurvy.

    C. rickets.

    D. cheilosis.

12. Identify which vitamin(s) and mineral(s) must be supplemented in the exclusively breastfed infant between birth and four months of age.

    A. Iron

    B. Fluoride

    C. Vitamin K

    D. A and C

    E. All of the above

13. Spoon nails may be a symptom of

    A. iron deficiency.

    B. vitamin C deficiency.

    C. vitamin A deficiency.

    D. protein deficiency.

14. Vitamin B deficiency may result in

    A. osteoporosis.

    B. cheilosis.

    C. scurvy.

    D. growth deficit.

15. Which nutrient may be deficient in the diet of an infant who exhibits poor growth?

    A. Calcium

    B. Magnesium

    C. Zinc

    D. Fluoride

16. Fluoride appears to prevent dental caries by

    A. increasing the tooth's resistance to acid dissolution.

    B. enhancing the process of remineralization.

    C. reducing the potential of dental plaque to cause tooth decay.

    D. A and B

    E. All of the above

17. The energy requirement for an eight-month-old infant is

    A. 85 to 90 kcal/kg per day.

    B. 95 to 100 kcal/kg per day.

    C. 110 to 115 kcal/kg per day.

    D. 115 to 120 kcal/kg per day.

18. At birth, the protein requirement for an infant is
    A. 2.0 g/100 kcal.
    B. 1.7 g/100 kcal.
    C. 1.4 g/100 kcal.
    D. 1.0 g/100 kcal.

19. Linoleic acid is found in
    A. vegetable oil.
    B. strained fruits.
    C. strained meats.
    D. fruit juice.

20. The recommended daily intake for zinc remains constant at _____ throughout the first year of life.
    A. 1.0 mg per day
    B. 1.5 mg per day
    C. 2.0 mg per day
    D. 2.5 mg per day

References

Ahn, CH, Maclean, WC (1980). Growth of the exclusively breast-fed infant. *Am J Clin Nutr*, 33:183-92.

American Academy of Pediatrics (AAP), Committee on Nutrition (1979). Fluoride supplementation: revised dosage schedule. *Pediatrics*, 63:150-52.

AAP (1983). *Food and Choking in Children*. A report to the FDA resulting from a conference on foods and choking in children held in Elkridge, MD, August 4-5. Evanston, IL: AAP.

AAP/Committee on Nutrition (1986). Fluoride supplementation. *Pediatrics*, 77:758-61.

AAP (1997). Breastfeeding and the use of human milk. *Pediatrics*, 100(6):1035-39.

AAP/Vitamin K Ad Hoc Task Force (1993). Controversies concerning vitamin K and the newborn. *Pediatrics*, 91(5) 1001-3.

AAP/Committee on Nutrition (1995). Fluoride supplementation for children: interim policy recommendations. *Pediatrics*, 95(5):777.

American Academy of Pediatric Dentistry (AAPD) (1994-1995). *Pediatric Dentistry, Special Issue*. Reference Manual, 16:7-29.

American Dietetic Association (ADA) (1997). Promotion of breastfeeding. *J Am Dietetic Assoc*, 97:662-66.

Amiel-Tison, C (1968). Neurological evaluation of the maturity of newborn infants. *Arch Dis Child*, 43(227):89-93.

Anderson, GC (1988). Early infant–mother interaction (Lecture). Physicians Conference, LLLI, Miami.

Anderson, GC (1989). Skin-to-skin: kangaroo care in western Europe. *Am J Nurs*, May, 662-668.

Anderson, GC, Vidyasagar, D (1979). Development of sucking in premature infants from 1 to 7 days post birth. *Birth Defects. Original Article Series*, 15:7, 145-71.

Aono, J, Ueda, W, Manabe, M (1993). Alteration in glucose metabolism by crying in children. *N Engl J Med*, 329 (13):1129.

Babcock, CJ (1938). Feed flavors in milk and milk products. *J Dairy Sci*, 21:661-67.

Baranowski, T, Bee, DE, Rassin, DK, Richardson, CJ, Brown, JP, Guenther, N, Nadar, PR (1983). Social support, social influence, ethnicity and the breastfeeding decision. *Soc Sci Med*, 17:1599.

Barness, LA (Ed.) (1993). *Pediatric Nutrition Handbook*, 3rd ed. Elk Grove Village, IL: American Academy of Pediatrics.

Barr, RG (1990). The normal crying curve: what do we really know? *Dev Med Child Neurol*, 32:356-62.

Barr, RG, Woolridge, J, Hanley, J (1991). Effects of formula change on intestional hydrogen production and crying. *J Dev Behav Pediatr*, 12(4):248-53.

Beauchamp, GK, Cowart, B (1990). Preference for high salt concentrations among children. *Dev Psychol*, 261: 539-45.

Beauchamp, GK, Cowart, B, Moran, M (1986). Developmental changes in salt acceptability in human infants. *Dev Psychol*, 19:17-25.

Beauchamp, GK, Maone, TR, Mennella, JA (1991). The role of flavor in infant nutrition. In: Heird, WC (Ed.), *Nutritional Needs of the Six to Twelve Month Old Infant*. New York: Glendale/Raven Press, Ltd.

Bell, RQ (1966). Level of arousal in breast-fed and bottle-fed newborns. *Psychosomatic Med*, 28:177-80.

Berg, WK, Berg, KM (1987). Psychophysiological development in infancy: state, startle, and attention. In: Osofsky, J (Ed.), *Handbook of Infant Development*, 2nd ed. (pp. 238-317). New York: Wiley.

Bernal, J (1972). Crying during the first 10 days of life and maternal responses. *Dev Med Child Neurol*, 14:362-72.

Bernal, J, Richards, MP (1970). The effects of bottle and breast feeding on infant development. *J Psychosom Res*, 14:247-52.

Berlo, D (1960). *The Process of Communication*. New York: Holt, Rinehart and Winston.

Bernbaum, JC, Pereira, GR, Watkins, JB, Peckam, GJ (1983). Non-nutritive sucking during gavage feeding enhances growth and maturation in premature infants. *Pediatrics*, 71:41-45.

Beske, EJ, Garvis, MS (1982). Important factors in breast-feeding success. *MCN*, 7:174-79.

Bevan, ML, Mosley, D, Lobach, KS, Solimano, GR (1984). Factors influencing breastfeeding in an urban WIC program. *J Am Diet Assoc*, 84:564.

Black, RF, Blair, JP, Jones, VN, DuRant, RH (1990). Infant feeding decisions among pregnant women from a WIC population in Georgia. *J Am Diet Assoc*, 90:255-59.

Bocar, D, Moore, K (1987). Acquiring the parental role: a theoretical perspective. In: Auerbach, K (Ed.), *Lactation Consultant Series*. Franklin Park, IL: La Leche League.

Borresen, HC (1995). Rethinking current recommendations to introduce solid food between four and six months to exclusively breastfeeding infants. *J Hum Lact*, 11:201-14.

Bossey, J (1980). Development of olfactory and related structures in human embryos. *Anat Embryol*, 161:225-36.

Bradley, RM (1972). Development of the taste bud and gustatory papillae in human fetuses. In: Bosma, JF (Ed.), *The Third Symposium on Oral Sensation and Preception: The Mouth of the Infant* (pp. 137-62). Springfield, IL: Charles C. Thomas.

Bradley, RM, Stern, IN (1967). The development of the human taste bud during the foetal period. *Anat*, 101: 743-47.

Brazelton, TB (1962). Crying in infancy. *Pediatrics*, 29:579-88.

Brazelton, TB (1973). *A Neonatal Behavioral Assessment Scale*. Philadelphia: Lippincott.

Brazelton, TB (1984). *Neonatal Behavioral Assessment Scale*. Philadelphia: Lippincott.

Brazelton, TB (1992a). *On Becoming a Family: The Growth of Attachment Before and After Birth*. New York: Dell Publishing Co.

Brazelton, TB (1992b). *Touchpoints: Your Child's Emotional and Behavioral Development*. Reading, MA: Addison-Wesley Publishing Co.

Brown, M, Hurlock, J (1977). Mother the mother. *Am J Nurs*, 77:439-41.

Bu'Lock, F, Woolridge, MW, Baum, JD (1990). Development of coordination of sucking, swallowing and breathing: ultrasound study of term and preterm infants. *Dev Med Child Neurol*, 32(8):669-78.

Bumgarner, NJ (1990). *Mothering Your Nursing Toddler*. Franklin Park, IL: La Leche League.

Calvo, EB, Galindo, AC, Aspres, NB (1992). Iron status in exclusively breastfed infants. *Pediatrics*, 90(3):375-79.

Cameron, M, Hofvander, Y (1984). Problems associated with breast-milk substitutes. *Nurs J India*, 75(10):245-46.

Cannon, B, Bonnolly, E, Obregon, MJ, Nedergaard, J (1988). Perinatal activation of brown adipose tissue. In: Kanzel, W, Jensen, A (Eds.), *The Endocrine Control in the Fetus*. Berlin, Heidelberg: Springer-Verlag.

Cernoch, JM, Porter, RH (1985). Recognition of maternal axillary odors by infants. *Child Dev*, 56:1593-98.

Chapman, J, Macey, M, Keegan, M, Borum, P, Bennet, S (1985). Concerns of breast-feeding mothers from birth to 4 months. *Nurs Res*, 34:374-77.

Chisholm, J (1986). *Navajo Infancy: An Ethological Perspective*. New York: Aldine de Gruyer.

Chiva, M (1979). Comment la personne se construit en mangeant. *Communications*, 31:107-18.

Cho, F, Bhatia, J, Rassin, KD (1990). Amino-acid responses to dietary intake in the first 72 hours of life. *Nutrition*, 6(6):449-55.

Christensson, K, Siles, C, Moreno, L, Belaustequi, A, De la Fuente, P, Lagercranty, H, Puyol, P, Winberg, J (1992). Temperature, metabolic adaption and crying in healthy full-term newborns cared for skin-to-skin or in a cot. *Acta Paediatr*, 81:488-93.

Colman, AD, Colman, LL (1971). *Pregnancy: The Psychological Experience*. New York: Herder and Herder.

Coopersmith, S (1967). *The Antecedents of Self-Esteem*. San Francisco: Freeman.

Daly, SE, Owens, RA, Hartmann, PE (1993). The short-term synthesis and infant-regulated removal of milk in lactating women. *Exp Physiol*, 78:209-20.

deChateau, P, Holmberg, H, Jakobsoon, K, et al. (1977). A study of factors promoting and inhibiting lactation. *Dev Med Child Neurol*, 19:575-84.

Department of Health and Social Security (DHSS) (1979). Recommended daily amounts of food energy and nutrients for groups of people in the United Kingdom. *Reports on Health and Social Subjects, No. 15*. London: Her Majesty's Stationery Office.

Deson, JA, Maller, O, Turner, RE (1973). Taste in acceptance of sugars by human infants. *J Comp Physiol Psychol*, 84:496-501.

Dewey, KG, Heinig, M, Nommsen, L, Peerson, J, Lönnerdal, B (1992). Growth of breastfed and formula-fed infants from 0–18 months: The DARLING Study. *Pediatrics*, 89:1035-41.

Dewey, KG, Heinig, MJ, Nommsen, LA, Peerson, JM, Lonnerdal, B (1993). Breastfed infants are leaner than formula-fed infants at 1 year of age: The DARLING Study. *Am J Clin Nutr*, 57(2):140-45.

Dewey, KG, Lonnerdal, B (1983). Milk and nutrient intake of breast-fed infants from 1 to 6 months: relation to growth and fatness. *J Pediatr Gastroenterol Nutr*, 2(3): 497-506.

Diamond (1982). *Still Nursing?* La Leche League Report No. 97. Franklin Park, IL: LLLI.

DiPietro, JA, Larson, SK, Porges, SW (1987). Behavioral and heart rate pattern differences between breast-fed and bottle-fed neonates. *Dev Psychol*, 23:467-74.

Duncan, B, Schifman, RB, Corrigan, JJ, Jr., Schaefer, C (1985). Iron and the exclusively breast-fed infant from birth to six months. *J Pediatr Gastroenterolo Nutr*, 4(3):421-25.

Engen, T, Lipsitt, LP, Ray, H (1963). Olfactory responses and adaption in the human neonate. *J Comp Physiol*, 56:73-77.

Erikson, EH (1956). Problem of ego identity. *J Am Psychoanal Assoc*, 4:56-121.Erikson, EH (1963). *Childhood and Society*. New York: W. W. Norton & Co., Inc.

Erikson, EH (1963). *Childhood and Society*. New York: W. W. Norton & Co., Inc.

Ernst, JA, Rickard, KA (1990). Food and nutrient intake of 6- to 12-month-old infants fed formula or cow milk: a summary of four national surveys. *J Pediatr*, 117(2): S86-100.

Ernst, JA, Rickard, KA, Neal, PR, Yu, PL, Oei, TO, Lemons, JA (1989). Lack of improved growth outcome related to non-nutritive sucking in very low birth weight premature infants fed a controlled nutrient intake: a randomized prospective study. *Pediatrics*, 83:706-16.

Field, T, Rignatoff, E, Stringer, S, Brennan, J, Greenberg, R, Widmayer, S, Anderson, GC (1982). Nonnutritive sucking during tube feedings: effects on preterm neonates in an intensive care unit. *Pediatrics*, 70:381-84.

Fomon, S. (1993). *Nutrition of Normal Infants*. St. Louis: Mosby.

Frantz, RL (1965). Visual perception from birth, as shown by pattern sensitivity. *Ann NY Acad Sci*, 118:739-814.

Galef, BG, Clark, MM (1972). Mother's milk and adult presence: the factors determining initial dietary selection by weanling rats. *J Comp Physiol Psychol*, 78:220-25.

Galef, BG, Sherry, DF (1973). Mother's milk: a medium for transmission of cues reflecting the flavour of mother's diet. *J Comp Physiol Psychol*, 83:374-78.

Galinsky, E (1981). *Between Generations*. New York: Times Books.

Garza, C, Butte, NF (1990). Energy intakes of human milk-fed infants during the first year. *J Pediatr*, 117: S124-31.

Graef, P, McGhee, K, Rozycki, J, et al. (1988). Postpartum concerns of breastfeeding mothers. *Nurs Midwifery*, 33:62-66.

Groh-Wargo, S, Thompson, M, Cox, JH (1994). *Nutritional Care for High-Risk Newborns*. Chicago: Precept Press.

Hambidge, KM, Casey, CE, Krebs, NF (1987). Zinc. In: Mertz, W (Ed.), *Trace Elements in Human and Animal Nutrition*, 5th ed. (pp. 1-137). Orlando, FL: Academic Press.

Hamill, PVV, Drizd, TA, Johnson, CL, Reed, RB, Roche, AF, Moore, WM (1979). Physical growth: National Center for Health Statistics percentiles. *Am J Clin Nutr*, 32:607-29.

Hammarlund, K, Stromberg, B, Sedin, G (1986). Heat loss from the skin of preterm and fullterm newborn infants during the first weeks after birth. *Biol Neonate*, 50(1):1-10.

Hanson, LA, Ashraf, R, Zaman, S, Karlberg, J, Lindblad, BS, Jalil, F (1994). Breastfeeding is a natural contraceptive and prevents disease and death in infants, linking infant mortality and birth rates. *Acta Paediatr*, 83:3-6.

Hauser, GJ, Chitayat, JD, Berns, L, Braver, D, Mulbauer, B (1985). Peculiar odors in newborns and prenatal ingestion of spicey foods. *Eur J Pediatr*, 144:403.

Hay, WW (Ed.) (1991). *Neonatal Nutrition and Metabolism*. St. Louis: Mosby Year-Book.

Heffner, E (1978). *Mothering: The Emotional Experience of Motherhood after Freud and Feminism*. New York: Doubleday and Company.

Heinig, MJ, Nommsen, LA, Peerson, JM, Lonnerdal, B, Dewey, KG (1993). Energy and protein intakes of breastfed and formula-fed infants during the first year of life and their association with growth velocity: The DARLING Study. *Am J Clin Nutr*, 58:152-61.

Hepper, PG (1987). The amniotic fluid: an important priming role in kin recognition. *Animal Behav*, 35:1343-46.

Herbst, JJ (1981). Development of suck and swallowing. In: Lebenthal, E (Ed.), *Textbook of Gastroenterology and Nutrition in Infancy*. New York: Plenum Press.

Hormann, E (1993). Breastfeeding your older baby. *Mothering*, 84-88.

Humenick, S, Van Steenkiste, S (1983). Early indicators of breastfeeding progress. *Iss Comp Pediatr Nurs*, 6:205-15.

Hunziker, VA, Barr, RG (1986). Increased carrying reduces infant crying: a randomized controlled trial. *Pediatrics*, 77:641-48.

Institute of Medicine (IOM)/National Academy of Sciences (1992). *Nutrition During Lactation*. Washington, DC: National Academy Press.

IOM/National Academy of Sciences (1989). *Recommended Dietary Allowances*, 10th ed. Washington, DC: National Academy Press.

Jakobsson, I, Lindberg, T (1983). Cow's milk proteins cause infantile colic in breast-fed infants: a double-blind crossover study. *Pediatrics*, 71(2):268-71.

Jones, S (1992). *Crying Baby, Sleepless Nights: Why Your Baby Is Crying and What You Can Do About It*. Boston: Harvard Common Press.

Jordan, PL (1986). Laboring for relevance: expectant and new fatherhood. *Nurs Res*, 39:11-16.

Jordan, PL (1990). Breastfeeding as a risk factor for fathers. *JOGNN*, 15:94-97.

Jordan, PL (1991). *The Male Experience of Expectant and New Fatherhood*. Final Report of Grant No. NR01480 (pp. 60-63). Washington, DC: National Center for Nursing Research, National Institutes of Health.

Jordan, PL, Wall, VR (1990). Breastfeeding and fathers: illuminating the darker side. *Birth*, 17:210-13.

Jordan, PL, Wall, VR (1993). Commentaries: Supporting the father when an infant is breastfed. *J Hum Lact*, 9(1): 31-34.

Kearney, MH, Cronenwett, LR, Barrett, JA (1990). Breastfeeding problems in the first week postpartum. *Nurs Res*, 39(2):90-95.

Kelts, DG, Jones, EG (1984). *Manual of Pediatric Nutrition* (pp. 38, 132). Boston: Little, Brown and Co.

Kennell, J, Klaus, M (1987). *Parent-Infant Bonding* (pp. 30-31, 71). St. Louis: Mosby.

Kessen, W, Haith, MM, Salapatek, PH (1970). Human infancy: a bibliography guide. In: Mussen, PH (Ed.), *Carmichael's Manual to Child Psychology*. New York: John Wiley & Sons.

Kippley, SK (1989). *Breastfeeding and Natural Child Spacing: How Ecological Breastfeeding Spaces Babies* (pp. 53-64). New York: Penguin Books.

Kitzinger, S (1980). *Women as Mothers*. New York: Random House.

Klaus, MH, Kennell, JH (1970). Human maternal behavior at first contact with her young. *Pediatrics*, 46:187-92.

Klaus, MH, Kennell, JH (1976). *Maternal-Infant Bonding*. St. Louis: Mosby.

Klaus, MH, Kennell, JH (1982). *Parent-Infant Bonding*. St. Louis: Mosby.

Klaus, MH, Kennell, JH, Klaus, PH (1995). *Bonding: Building of Foundations of Secure Attachment and Independence*. Reading, MA: Addison-Wesley Publishing.

Korner, AF, Thomas, EB (1972). The relative efficacy of contact and vestibular proprioceptive stimulation in soothing neonates. *Child Dev*, 43:443-53.

Kostelc, JG, Preti, G, Zelson, PR, Tonzetich, J, Huggins, GR (1981). Volatiles of exogenous origin from the human oral cavity. *J Chromatogr*, 226:315-23.

Krebs, NE, Reidinger, CJ, Robertson, AD, Hambridge, KM (1994). Growth and intake of energy and zinc in infants fed human milk. *J Pediatr*, 124(1):32-39.

Lawrence, RA (1989). *Breastfeeding: A Guide for the Medical Profession*, 3rd ed. (pp. 148-160). St. Louis: Mosby.

Lawrence, RA (1994). *Breastfeeding: A Guide for the Medical Profession*, 4th ed. St. Louis: Mosby.

Lebenthal, E (1985). Impact of digestion and absorption in the weaning period on infant feeding practices. *Pediatrics*, 75(suppl):207-13.

Lester, BM (1984). A biosocial model of infant crying. In: Lipsitt, L (Ed.), *Advances in Infant Behavior and Development* (pp. 167-212). Norwood, NJ: Ablex.

Levanthal, AS, Lipsitt, LP (1964). Adaptation, pitch discrimination and sound localization in the neonate. *Child Dev*, 35:759-67.

Lewis, M (1969). Infant's responses to facial stimuli during the first year of life. *Dev Psychol*, 1:75-86.

Liedloff, J (1977). *The Continuum Concept*. New York: Addison-Wesley.

Liley, AW (1972). Disorders of amniotic fluid. In: Assali, NS (Ed.), *Pathophysiology of Gestation. Fetal Placental Disorders*, Vol. 2 (pp. 157-206). New York: Academic Press.

Locklin, MP, Naber, SJ (1993). Does breastfeeding empower women? Insights from a select group of educated, low-income, minority women. *Birth*, 20:30-35.

Lucas, A, Ewing, G, Roberts, SB, Coward, WA (1987). How much energy does the breast fed infant consume and expend? *Brit Med J*, 295:75-77.

MacFarlane, A (1975). Olfaction in the Development of Social Preferences in the Human Neonate: Parent–Infant Interaction, CIBA Foundation Symposium, No. 33.

Magid, K, McKelvey, CA (1987). *High Risk: Children Without a Conscience* (pp. 71-78, 245-56). New York: Bantam Books.

Mahler, MS (1967). *The Psychological Birth of the Human Infant*. New York: Basic Books.

Makin, JW (1987). Bottle feeding infants responsiveness to lactating maternal breast and axillary odors. Dissertation, Vanderbilt University.

Maone, TR, Mattes, RD, Bernbaum, JC, Beauchamp, GK (1990). A new method for delivering a taste without fluids to preterm and term infants. *Dev Psychobiol*, 23:179-91.

Martuis, J, Krohn, MA, Hillier, SL, Stamm, WE, Holmes, KK, Eschenbach, JDA (1988). Relationships of vaginal lactobacillus species Chlamydia trichomatis and bacterial vaginosis to pre-term birth. *Obstet Gynecol*, 71:89-95.

May, K, Solid, DT (1984). Unanticipated cesarean birth from the father's perspective. *Birth*, 11:87-95.

McKenna, J (1986). An anthropological perspective on the sudden infant death syndrome (SIDS): the role of parental breathing cues and speech breathing adaptations. *Med Anthropol*, 10(1):Special Issue.

McKenna, J (1993). Rethinking healthy infant sleep. *Breastfeeding Abstracts*, 12:3.

McKenna, J, Mosko, S, Dungy, C, McAnninch, J (1991). Sleep and arousal pattern among co-sleeping mother–infant pairs: implications for SIDS. *Am J Physical Anthropol*, 83:331-47.

McMillan, JA, Landaw, SA, Oski, FA (1976). Iron sufficiency in breast-fed infants and the availability of iron from human milk. *Pediatrics*, 58(5):686-91.

Mennella, JA, Beauchamp, GK (1991). The transfer of alcohol to human milk: effects on flavor and the infant's behavior. *N Engl J Med*, 325:8-13.

Mennella, JA, Beauchamp, GK (1993). Effects of beer on breast-fed infants. *JAMA*, 269(13):1635-36.

Mercer, RT (1981). The nurse and maternal tasks of early postpartum. *Am J Nurs*, 81:341-45.

Miller, AJ (1982). Deglutition. *Physiol Rev*, 62:129-84.

Montegue, A (1971). *Touching: the Significance of the Skin*. New York: Harper & Row.

Moore, JG, Krtoszynski, BK, O'Neill, HJ (1984). Fecal odorgrams: a method for partial reconstruction of ancient and modern diets. *Dig Dis Sci*, 29:907-11.

Neely, CA (1979). Effects of non-nutritive sucking upon the behavior arousal of the newborn. *Birth Defects* (Original Article Series, March of Dimes), 15:7, 173-200.

Nelson, SE, Roger, RR, Ziegler, EE, Fomon, SJ (1989). Gain in weight and length in early infancy. *Early Human Dev*, 19:223-39.

Oberlander, TF, Barr, RG, Young, SN, Brean, JA (1992). Short-term effects of feed composition on sleeping and crying in newborns. *Pediatrics*, 90(5):733-40.

O'Doherty, N (1986). *Neurological Examination of the Newborn* (pp. 1-2, 4, 5). Hingham, MA: MPT Press Limited.

Pellett, PL (1990). Food energy requirements in humans. *Am J Clin Nutr*, 51:711-22. In: Barness, LA (Ed.) (1993), *Pediatric Nutrition Handbook* (p. 444). Elk Grove Village, IL: AAP.

Peterson, GH, et al. (1979). The role of some birth-related variables in father attachment. *Am J Orthopsychiat*, 49:330-38.

Pinilla, T, Birch, L (1993). Help me make it through the night: behavioral entrainment of breast-fed infants' sleep patterns. *Pediatrics*, 91:436-44.

Pisacane, A, DeVizia, B, Valiante, A, Vaccaro, F, Russo, M, Grillo, G, Giustardi, A (1995). Iron status in breast-fed infants. *J Pediatr*, 127(3):429-31.

Pizzarro, F, Yip, R, Dallmann, PR, Olivares, M, Hertrampf, E, Walter, T (1991). Iron status with different infant feeding regimens: relevance to screening and prevention of iron deficiency. *J Pediatr*, 118:687-92.

Prentice, AM (1991). Breast feeding and the older infant. *Acta Paediatr Scand*, 374(Suppl.):78-88.

Prentice, AM, Lucas A, Vasquez-Velasquez, L, Davies, PSW, Whitehead, RG (1988). Are current dietary guidelines for young children a prescription for overfeeding? *Lancet*, 2(8619):1066-69.

Pritchard, JA (1965). Deglutition by normal and anencephalic fetuses. *Obstet Gynecol*, 25:289-97.

Pryor, K, Pryor, G (1991). *Nursing Your Baby*. New York: Pocket Books.

Raphael, D (1973). *The Tender Gift: Breastfeeding*. New York: Schocken Books.

Riesenfeld, T, Hammarlund, K, Sedin, G (1987). Respiratory water loss in relation to activity in full-term infants on their first day after birth. *Acta Paediatr Scand*, 76:889-93.

Righard, L, Alade, MO (1990). Effect of delivery room routines on success of first breastfeed. *Lancet*, 336(8723):1105-7.

Rosenstein, D, Oster, H (1990). Differential facial responses to four basic tastes in newborns. *Child Dev*, 59:1555-68.

Rubin, R (1961). Basic maternal behavior. *Nurs Outlook*, 19:683-86.

Rubin, R (1967a). Attainment of the maternal role, I. *Nurs Res*, 16:237-42.

Rubin, R (1967b). Attainment of the maternal role, II. *Nurs Res*, 16:342-46.

Saarinen, UM, Siimes, MA, Dallman, PR (1977). Iron absorption in infants: high bioavailability of breast milk iron as indicated by the extrinsic tag method of iron absorption and by the concentration of serum ferritin. *J Pediatr*, 91(1):36-39.

Saarinen, UM, Siimes, MA (1979). Role of prolonged breastfeeding in infant growth. *Acta Paediatr Scand*, 68:245-50.

Salmenpera, L, Perheentupa, J, Siimes, MA (1985). Exclusively breastfed healthy infants grow slower than reference infants. *Pediatr Res*, 19:307-12.

Sarbin, TR (1954). Role theory. In: Linzey, G (Ed.), *Handbook of Social Psychology*, Vol. 1. Cambridge, MA: Addison-Wesley.

Sastry, SD, Buck, KT, Janak, J, Dressler, M, Preti, G (1980). Volatiles emitted by humans. In: Wallert, GR, Dermer, OC (Eds.), *Biochemical Applications to Mass Spectrometry* (pp. 1085-129). New York: John Wiley.

Schaal, B (1988). Olfaction in infants and children: developmental and functional perspectives. *Chemical Senses*, 13:145-90.

Schaffer, JP (1910). The lateral wall of the cavum nasi in man with special reference to the various developmental stages. *J Morphol*, 21:613-17.

Schulz-Lell, G, Buss, R, Oldigs, HD, Dorner, K, Schaub, J (1987). Iron balances in infant nutrition. *Acta Paediatr Scand*, 76(4):585-91.

Self, PA, Horowitz, FD, Paden, LY (1972). Olfaction in newborn infants. *Dev Psychol*, 7:349-63.

Shepherd, RW, Oxborough, DB, Holt, TL, Thomas, BJ, Thong, YH (1988). Longitudinal study of the body composition of weight gain in exclusively breastfed and intake-measured whey-based formula-fed infants to age 3 months. *J Pediatr Gastroenterol Nutr*, 7(5):732-39.

Siimes, MA, Salmenpera, L, Perheentupa, J (1984). Exclusive breastfeeding for 9 months: risk of iron deficiency. *J Pediatr*, 104:196-99.

Specker, BL (1994). Do North American women need supplemental vitamin D during pregnancy or lactation? *Am J Clin Nutr*, 59(2 Suppl):S484-90.

Stafford, M, Horning, MC, Zlatkis, A (1976). Profiles of volatile metabolites in body fluids. *J Chromatogr*, 126:495-502.

Steinberg, LA, O'Connell, NC, Hatch, TF, Picciano, MF, Birch, LL (1992). Tryptophan intake influences infants' sleep latency. *J Nutr*, 122(9):1781-91.

Sugarman, M (1988). Contrasting mothering styles in infancy (Lecture). The Physicians Conference, LLLI, Miami.

Sullivan, SA, Birch, LL (1994). Infant dietary experience and acceptance of solid foods. *Pediatrics*, 93:271-77.

Thornton, R, Nardi, PM (1975). The dynamics of role acquisition. *Am J Social*, 80:870-85.

Tully, M, Overfield, ML (1996). Newborn reflexes and breastfeeding. Lactation Consultants of North Carolina, Raleigh.

Vasquez, M, Pearson, PB, Beauchamp, KG (1982). Flavor preferences in malnourished Mexican infants. *Physiol Behav*, 28:513-19.

Wallace, P (1977). Individual discrimination of humans by odor. *Physiol Behav*, 19:577-99.

Walravens, PA, Chakar, A, Mokni, R, Denise, J, Lemonnier, D (1992). Zinc supplements in breastfed infants. *Lancet*, 340:683-85.

Weir, NF (1976). Auditory frequency sensitivity in the neonate: a signal detection analysis. *J Exp Child Psychol*, 21:219-21.

Whitehead, RG (1995). For how long is exclusive breastfeeding adequate to satisfy the dietary energy needs of the average young baby? *Pediatr Res*, 37(2):239-43.

Whitehead, RG, Paul, AA, Cole, TJ (1981). A critical analysis of measured food energy intakes during infancy and early childhood in comparison with current international recommendations. *J Hum Nutr*, 35:339-48.

Widdowson, EM (1965). Absorption and excretion of fat, nitrogen, and mineral from "filled" milks by babies one week old. *Lancet*, ii(7422):1099-1105.

Woodson, R, Field, T, Greenberg, R (1983). Estimating neonatal oxygen consumption from heart rate. *Psychophysiology*, 20:558-61.

World Health Organization (WHO) (1985). Energy and protein requirements. Report of joint WHO/FAO/UNU meeting. WHO Technical Report Series, No. 724. Geneva: WHO.

WHO/Food and Agriculture Organization (FAO) (1973). Energy and protein requirements. WHO Technical Report Series, No. 522. Geneva: Food and Agriculture Organization, Nutrition Meetings Report Series No. 52.

Worobey, J, Lewis, M (1989). Individual differences in the reactivity of young infants. *Dev Psychol*, 25:663-67.

Yogman, MW, Zeisel, SA (1983). Diet and sleep patterns in newborn infants. *N Engl J Med*, 309:1147-49.

Zeskind, PS (1981). Behavioral dimensions and cry sounds of infants of differential fetal growth. *Infant Behavior Dev*, 4:321-30.

Zeskind, PS, Goff, DM, Marshall, TR (1991). Rhythmic organization of neonatal heart rate and its relation to atypical fetal growth. *Dev Psychobiol*, 24:413-29.

Zeskind, PS, Goff, DM, Marshall, TR (1992). Rhythmic organization of heart rate in breast-fed and bottle-fed newborn infants. *Early Dev Parenting*, 1(2):79-87.

Zeskind, PS, Lester, BM (1981). Analysis of cry features in newborns with differential fetal growth. *Child Dev*, 52:207-12.

ADDITIONAL READINGS

American Academy of Pediatrics (AAP)/Committee on Nutrition (1992). The use of whole cow's milk in infancy. *Pediatrics*, 89(6, Pt 1):1105-9.

Anderson, GC (1977). The mother and her newborn: mutual caregiver. *JOGNN*, Sept/Oct:50-57.

Barr, RG (1990). The "colic" enigma: prolonged episodes of normal predisposition to cry. *Infant Mental Health J*, 11:340-48.

Brazelton, TB (1986). *Infants and Mothers: differences in Development*. New York: Dell Publishing Co.

Brazelton, TB (1990). Crying and colic. *Infant Mental Health J*, 11:340-48.

Breastfeeding (1989). Kangaroo care and breastfeeding for preterm infants. *Breastfeeding Abstracts*, 9:9.

Caplan, F (1978). *The First Twelve Months of Life—Your Baby's Growth Month by Month*. New York: Bantam Books.

Capute, AJ (1976). Early neuromotor reflexes in infancy. *Pediatr Annals*, 15(3):217-26.

Carter, CS (1988). Patterns of infant feeding, the mother-infant interaction and stress management. In: Field, TM, McCabe, PM, Schneideman, N (Eds.), *Stress and Coping Across Development*. Hillsdale, NJ: Erlbaum.

Conine, TA, Carty, E, Safarik, PM (1988). *Aids and Adaptations for Parents with Physical or Sensory Disabilities*. Vancouver, BC: School of Rehabilitative Medicine, University of British Columbia.

DeCaper, AJ, Fifer, WP (1980). Of human bonding: newborns prefer their mothers' voices. *Science*, 208:1174-76.

Deutsch, JA, Moore, BO, Heinrichs, SC (1989). Unlearned specific appetite for protein. *Physiol Behav*, 46:619-24.

Dohl, LK (1958). Salt intake and salt need. *N Engl J Med*, 258:1205-8.

Emde, R, et al. (1975). Human wakefulness and biological rhythms after birth. *Arch Gen Psychiat*, 32:780-83.

Erikson, EH (1968). The ontogenesis of ritualization. *Psyche*, 22(7):4881-5002.

Freed, GL, Fraley, JK, Schanler, RJ (1992). Attitudes of expectant fathers regarding breast-feeding. *Pediatrics*, 90:224-27.

Kagan, J (1966). Infant's differential reactions to familiar and distorted faces. *Child Dev*, 36:519-32.

Kaitz, M, Lapidot, P, Bronner, R, Eidelman, AI (1992). Parturient women can recognize their infants by touch. *Dev Psychol*, 28:35-39.

Kuzela, AL, Stifter, CA, Worobey, J (1990). Breastfeeding and mother-infant interactions. *J Repro Infant Psychol*, 8: 185-94.

Lohman, TG, Foche, AF, Martorell, R (1988). *Anthropometric Standardization Reference Manual*. New York: Human Kinetics.

Makin, JW, Porter, RH (1989). Attractiveness of lactating females' breast odors to neonates. *Child Dev*, 60:803-10.

McKenna, JJ, Thoman, EB, Anders, TF, Sadeh, A, Schechtman, VL, Glotzbach, SF (1993). Infant parent co-sleeping in an evolutionary perspective: implications for infant development and the sudden infant death syndrome. *Sleep*, 16:263-82.

Morse, JM, Harrison, MJ (1987). Social coercion for weaning. *J Nurs Midwifery*, 32:205-10.

Mosko, S, Richard, C, McKenna, J, Drummond, S (1996). Infant sleep architecture during bedsharing and possible implications for SIDS. *Sleep*, 19:677-84.

Nowak, A, Crall, J (1988). Prevention of dental disease. In: Pinkham, JR (Ed.), *Pediatric Dentistry, Infancy through Adolescence* (p. 160). Philadelphia: W. B. Sanders.

Pridham, KF (1993). Anticipatory guidance of parents of new infants: potential contribution of the internal working model construct. *Image*, 25:49-56.

Queen, PM, Lang, CE (1993). *Handbook of Pediatric Nutrition*. Gaithersburg, MD: Aspen Publications.

Roopnarine, JL, Miller, BC (1985). Transitions to fatherhood. In: Hanson, SMH, Bozett, FW (Eds.), *Dimensions of Fatherhood* (pp. 57-58). Beverly Hills: Sage Publications.

Russell, MJ (1976). Human olfactory communication. *Nature*, 260:520-22.

Shipe, WF, Basette, R, Deane, DD, et al. (1978). Off flavors of milk: nomenclature, standards and bibliography. *J Dairy Sci*, 61:855-69.

Worobey, J (1989). Infant activity and irritability as influenced by breast- or bottle-feeding status. *FASEB J*, 3: A765.

CHAPTER 2

The Impact of Maternal and Infant Health Issues on Breastfeeding

SECTION A

Maternal Health Issues

Robin McRoberts, MS, RD/LD
Rebecca F. Black, MS, RD/LD, IBCLC

LEARNING OBJECTIVES

At the completion of this section, the learner will be able to do the following:

1. Discuss the influence of maternal cystic fibrosis, multiple sclerosis, phenylketonuria, diabetes, and hyperlipoproteinemia on milk production and milk composition.
2. Describe how viral and bacterial infections impact feeding.
3. List the advantages and disadvantages of various contraceptive methods for the lactating woman.
4. Identify the factors that influence the passage of drugs into human milk and the absorption of drugs by the infants.
5. Identify drugs that may impair or stimulate lactation.
6. Identify drugs that are contraindicated during lactation.
7. Cite the circumstances when breastfeeding is contraindicated.

OUTLINE

I. Maternal Diseases and Limitations

   A. Cystic fibrosis

   B. Diabetes mellitus

   C. Hyperlipoproteinemia

   D. Multiple sclerosis

   E. Hyperprolactinemia

   F. Sheehan's syndrome

PRE-TEST

For questions 1 to 9, choose the single best answer.

1. Changes in the milk fat composition may be found in the breastmilk of women
    A. with silicone implants.
    B. with hyperlipoproteinemia and cystic fibrosis.
    C. on estrogen-containing birth control pills.
    D. on metoclopramide.

2. When a woman with diabetes mellitus has serum glucose levels that are not within normal ranges the following may occur:

    A. Her colostrum will have higher than usual levels of lactose.
    B. Her infant will experience hyperglycemia.
    C. Her breastmilk will be low in protein.
    D. Lactogenesis may be delayed.

3. The bone mineral density of well-nourished, nonadolescent women in the United States is _____ during pregnancy and lactation and _____ after weaning.

    A. increased; decreased
    B. decreased; decreased
    C. increased; increased
    D. decreased; increased

4. Atypical connective tissue disease is a disease that has been attributed to

    A. silicone breast implants.
    B. hyperlipoproteinemia.
    C. diabetes mellitus.
    D. cystic fibrosis.

5. A premature infant with low antibody levels whose mother has cytomegalovirus (CMV)

    A. probably should not be breastfed.
    B. could be breastfed.

6. A woman with phenylketonuria _____ breastfeed.

    A. can totally
    B. can partially
    C. cannot

7. Lactation is contraindicated for the infant with which disorder?

    A. Phenylketonuria
    B. Diabetes mellitus
    C. Hyperlipoproteinemia
    D. Galactosemia

8. In mothers who have cystic fibrosis, breastmilk may be lacking in

    A. linoleic acid.
    B. arachidonic acid.
    C. docosahexaenoic acid.
    D. palmitic acid.

9. Which condition increases the risk of mastitis and Candida infection?

    A. Phenylketonuria
    B. Hyperlipoproteinemia
    C. Diabetes mellitus
    D. Cystic fibrosis

For questions 10 to 14, choose the single best answer from the following key:

    A. Galactorrhea
    B. Hepatitis B virus
    C. Human immunodeficiency virus type I
    D. Bromocriptine
    E. Metoclopramide

10. _____ is the virus that is contraindicated in developed countries but not in developing countries.

11. The secretion of lactose- and fat-containing fluid independent of pregnancy is _____.

12. The virus that is allowed once the infant receives the immunoglobulin and vaccine.

13. This medication inhibits lactation.

14. This medication stimulates lactation.

For questions 15 to 20, choose the answer from the following key:
   A. Can be used during breastfeeding
   B. Should not be used during breastfeeding

15. Metoclopramide

16. Norplant

17. Estrogen-containing birth control pills with levels greater than 50 mcg ethinyl estradiol

18. Progesterone-containing birth control pills

19. Depo Provera injection

20. Lactational Amenorrhea Method

INTRODUCTION

This section discusses maternal disease, silicone breast implants, maternal infections, contraception during lactation, maternal medication use, and contraindications to breastfeeding. The reader is encouraged to monitor the literature regularly because these areas are of high research interest and new developments may be reported each month.

Maternal Diseases and Limitations

CYSTIC FIBROSIS

Studies about the breastmilk of women with cystic fibrosis (CF) are limited. CF affects the fatty acid composition of tissues. Whether the breastmilk of the woman with CF has a fat content capable of supporting adequate growth of the infant has been questioned (Welch et al., 1981). A study done on the milk of six women with CF showed that the total milk fat content was slightly less when compared to milk of women without CF (Bitman et al., 1987). Even with this difference, it was determined adequate growth could be supported. Triglycerides comprised 98% of total fat, which is consistent with normal milk.

Significant differences also have been reported for the fatty acid composition of the breastmilk of women with CF. Linoleic acid was 75% less in the milk of CF mothers while other polyunsaturated fatty acids (PUFA) were higher (16:2 and 18:3 PUFAs were twice the concentration). Cholesterol levels in the milk of mothers with CF were similar to the milk of mothers without CF. In the phospholipid classes, differences were noted in sphingomyelin concentrations (CF mothers had lower levels) and phosphatidylethanolamine concentrations (CF mothers had higher levels), which may affect the milk fat globule membrane (Bitman et al., 1987).

If adequate calories are not consumed, linoleic acid may be used by the body to provide energy. Since linoleic acid plays a specific role in stabilizing membrane structure and prostaglandin synthesis, supplementation of it may be necessary for the lactating woman with CF (Hamosh & Bitman, 1992). The mother should be monitored closely to ensure adequate caloric intake to promote optimal maternal and infant health. Breastfeeding women with mild cases of cystic fibrosis have been reported to maintain their own weight and support growth of their healthy infants (Michel et al., 1994). Infants with cystic fibrosis can breastfeed. If they are having problems with malabsorption, enzyme replacement therapy can be initiated and breastfeeding continued (Gaskin et al., 1994).

DIABETES MELLITUS

Women with diabetes can breastfeed successfully. Immediately following delivery, usually within 24 hours, insulin needs drop before adjusting to a level lower than reported during pregnancy (Engelking & Page-Lieberman, 1986; National Diabetes Data Group, 1979). Because insulin is a large molecule, it does not pass into breastmilk.

Recommendations for establishing milk supply in the lactating woman with diabetes do not differ from those for nondiabetic mothers. Lactation should be initiated as soon after delivery as possible. To facilitate feeding on demand, rooming-in should be encouraged. If, due to hospital protocol or illness, the infant must remain in the nursery and breastfeeding is not possible, the mother should express her milk using an electric pump.

The lactating woman with diabetes may be at risk for mastitis (Ferris et al., 1988; Guthrie & Guthrie, 1982) and Candida infection (Riordan & Auerbach, 1993). However, there is no evidence proving a woman with good glycemic control is at an increased risk (Engelking & Page-Lieberman, 1986). Regardless, a mother should be educated on signs and treatment of plugged ducts, breast infection, and Candida infections.

To prevent hypoglycemic episodes, the lactating woman should continue monitoring blood glucose levels and follow her diet plan. Suggestions to manage these episodes include having available ready-to-eat meals and snacks and quick sugar sources (raisins, sugar cubes). Frequent hypoglycemic episodes may indicate the need to lower insulin or oral agent dosage(s) in the lactating woman who has an increased caloric expenditure.

Research on the quality of the breastmilk of a diabetic woman is limited. The milk of women with good glycemic control has few differences from nondiabetic breastmilk, when the two are compared. These differences primarily include an alteration of the lipid content (Bitman et al., 1989; Neubauer, 1990). Cholesterol levels have been reported to be lower in the breastmilk of diabetic women at both the onset of and during established lactation. Polyunsaturated fatty acids are present in higher concentrations, indicating increased chain elongation, while medium-chain fatty acids are decreased, indicating impairment of fatty acid synthesis in the mammary gland (Bitman et al., 1989). Other studies show no difference in cholesterol or fatty acid concentration in women with good glycemic control (van Beusekom et al., 1993).

Lactogenesis may be delayed in women with diabetes as indicated by a lower lactose content and a higher total nitrogen (Neubauer et al., 1993). This is especially true if the woman does not have good glycemic control. In the milk of women in tight control, there was no difference in the lactose concentration when compared to the milk of healthy women (van Beusekom et al., 1993). None of the alterations found in the breastmilk of women with diabetes should discourage breastfeeding. Mothers cannot pass their diabetes to their infants by breastfeeding (Engelking & Page-Lieberman, 1986). The health-care professional should provide support and education just as for any new mother. Emphasis should be placed on maintaining good glycemic control.

HYPERLIPOPROTEINEMIA

Type I hyperlipoproteinemia is characterized by an absence of lipoprotein lipase activity (Nikkila, 1983), so carriers of plasma triglyceride accumulate in the maternal circulation. The lactating mother experiences hypertriglyceridemia throughout lactation but triglycerides are not available to the mammary gland for milk fat synthesis because of the absence of lipoprotein lipase (Hamosh et al., 1970). The breastmilk of women with hyperlipoproteinemia has lower triglyceride levels and a lower proportion of long-chain fatty acids (C > 18:1) when compared to healthy control samples. As a result, the mammary gland produces higher concentrations of medium-chain fatty acids (C < 14) (Berger et al., 1983; Myher et al., 1984; Steiner et al., 1985).

MULTIPLE SCLEROSIS

Multiple sclerosis, a progressive degenerative neurologic disorder, is not considered a contraindication for breastfeeding, but it also has not been shown to protect against exacerbations. Women are affected twice as often as men, with the diagnosis often made between the ages of 20 to 40. In a recent study, patients with multiple sclerosis were less likely than controls to have been breastfed for a prolonged period of time (Pisacane et al., 1994). Lawrence (1994) reported an increased risk of exacerbations in multiple sclerosis during the postpartum period.

Nelson and colleagues (1988) studied 435 women with multiple sclerosis during pregnancy and lactation, including 191 who were pregnant while in a nonprogressive phase of the disease. The exacerbation risk during pregnancy was 10% and was three times higher at 34% in the first nine months postpartum. The rate of exacerbation was highest in the immediate postpartum period (three months). Of the 91 women who breastfed, the average duration was 6.3 months. The exacerbation rate was 37.5% for breastfeeding women and 31.5% for nonbreastfeeding women. The exacerbation pattern was similar in both groups with an average time of onset at 3.0 and 3.1 months, respectively. There was no correlation of exacerbation pattern with the duration of breastfeeding.

The mother with multiple sclerosis who chooses to breastfeed may need additional supportive help. The variability of sleep, frequent feedings, and need for adequate calories in the postpartum period may be especially difficult for her during the periods of deterioration, which are common during the first year after delivery.

HYPERPROLACTINEMIA

Hyperprolactinemia can result from physiologic, pharmacologic, pathologic, and functional causes. It may occur with or without galactorrhea. *Galactorrhea* is the secretion of a lactose- and fat-containing fluid that occurs independent of pregnancy. Increased prolactin concentrations or the removal of hypothalamic inhibition can cause galactorrhea (Vorherr, 1974). For women with hyperprolactinemia who achieve pregnancy, lactation is possible. Table 2A–1 lists causes of chronic female hyperprolactinemia.

Breastfeeding does not cause the rise in prolactin seen in women without hyperprolactemic disorders (Frantz & Wilson, 1985). Milk prolactin levels have been shown to be similar in women with and without galactorrhea (Adamopoulos & Kapolla, 1984). Plasma levels of prolactin vary while milk levels are relatively constant.

Table 2A-1 Causes of Chronic Hyperprolactinemia in the Female

Physiologic	Excessive breast manipulation
	Stress, surgery, venipuncture, etc.
Pharmacologic	Depletion of tuberoinfundibular dopamine stores (by extrusion from intracellular granule to cytosol)
	• Reserpine
	Blockade of dopamine receptor binding
	• Phenothiazines (Thorazine, Mellaril, Compazine, Trilafon, Stelazine)
	• Thioxanthenes (Taractan)
	• Butyrophenones (Haldol)
	• Benzamines (metoclopramide, sulpiride)
	• Dibenzoxapine antidepressants (amoxapine)
	Inhibition of dopamine release
	• Chronic opiate use (methadone, morphine)
	Blockade of histamine (H_2) receptor binding
	• Cimetidine
	Estrogen-containing oral contraceptives
	Interference with the synthesis of dopamine
	• a-Methyldopa
	Calcium channel blockers
	• Verapamil
	Mechanism unknown
	• Tricyclic antidepressants (imipramine, amitriptiline, etc.)
	• Papaverine derivatives
Pathologic	Primary hypothyroidism
	Hypothalamic disorders
	• Neoplastic, infectious, vascular, degenerative, or granulomatous hypothalamic lesions
	Pituitary stalk section
	Pituitary disorders
	• Prolactin-secreting adenoma
	• Acromegaly, Cushing's disease, Nelson syndrome
	Ectopic production of prolactin
	• Bronchogenic carcinoma, hypernephroma
	Chronic renal failure
	Chest wall lesions
	• Surgical scars, herpes zoster
Functional	Idiopathic (no demonstrable tumor)

Sources: Lawrence, RA (1994). *Breastfeeding: A Guide for the Medical Profession*, 3rd ed., p. 497; St. Louis: Mosby. Katz, E, Adashi, EY (1990). Hyperprolactinemic disorders, *Clin Obstet Gynecol*, 33:623. Reprinted with permission of Mosby-Year Book, Inc., and Lippincott-Raven Publishers.

SHEEHAN'S SYNDROME

Sheehan's syndrome is an endocrine disorder associated with lactation failure (Adamopoulos & Kapolla, 1984). It is caused by severe postpartum hemorrhage with hypotension that leads to pituitary thrombotic infarction and necrosis or other vascular injury such as hypoperfusion. The syndrome's occurrence is 0.01% to 0.02% in postpartum women. A key clinical indicator of the syndrome is the failure to lactate postpartumly. Other signs include diabetes insipidus, amenorrhea, hypothyroidism, loss of auxiliary hair, and/or sparse regrowth of pubic hair postpartum (Lawrence, 1994). According to Lawrence (1994), some women with Sheehan's syndrome do succeed at lactation through the use of prolactin-stimulating drugs such as sulpiride and the use of nasal syntocin spray.

OSTEOPOROSIS

Prolactin has a beneficial effect on bone mineralization. Estrogen normally inhibits bone resorption and thus its decrease during lactation allows bone resorption so that calcium can be released for lactation. During lactation, the body may also maximize absorption of calcium and minimize its excretion. Alterations in absorption, metabolism, and excretion may conserve calcium when requirements increase.

Some studies report bone demineralization and increased bone turnover during pregnancy and lactation, but the relationship to diet is unknown because most studies have not looked at calcium intake. Bone demineralization during pregnancy and lactation can be influenced by changed activity patterns, altered bone loading due to changes in body weight and regional body composition, and modified bone turnover rates. Another study reports decreased urinary excretion and increased bone resorption, but not increased intestinal absorption of calcium, of 8 women (Specker et al., 1994).

Several studies that have followed women into the weaning period have found no long-term effects of pregnancy and lactation on bone density. Recovery of bone loss has been observed in a recent study of women who breastfed for an extended length of time and consumed high-calcium diets—1,966 mg per day (SD 179 mg) during pregnancy and 1,840 mg per day (SD 90 mg) during lactation (Sowers et al., 1993). Kent and colleagues (1993) found that the bone mineral content of the lumbar spine decreases approximately 3.5% during lactation and increases 4.8% after weaning.

Koetting and Wardlaw (1988) studied the relationship between long-term lactation (> 10 months) and the bone density of 28 women, aged 26 to 37. Ten of the women lactated long-term for 1 to 2 children, 8 lactated long-term for 3 to 4 children, and 10 were nulliparous. There was no significant difference among the women in height, weight, percentage of ideal weight, usual caffeine or calcium intake, or duration of oral contraceptive use. Bone density was measured at five sites, including the wrist, spine, and hip. They did not find lactation history to be associated with significant differences in bone density in any bone site. In another study, which looked at the relationships of parity, breastfeeding, the use of birth control pills, and bone densities, breastfeeding was found to increase lumbar spine density by 1.5% per breastfed child (Hreshchyshyn et al., 1988).

Sowers and colleagues (1995) report that well-nourished women who practice extended lactation followed closely by pregnancy are not at risk for failure of bone recovery to prelactation levels. Blaauw and associates (1994) report that the odds that a woman with osteoporosis did not breastfeed her baby is four times higher than for a woman in a control group. These studies suggest that bone mineral density losses associated with lactation are temporary and reversible.

PHYSICAL LIMITATIONS

Baby care guidelines for physically challenged mothers compiled from the work of Conine et al. (1988), Kirshbaum (1990), Minami (1990), Nursing Mothers' Association of Australia (1982), Riordan and Auerbach (1993), include the following:

- Arrange a particular living area for breastfeeding that is easily accessible and comfortable for the mother.
- If the mother is confined to a wheelchair, have her use a harness or a wide belt with a long strip of adhesive to lift and retrieve a crawling baby from the floor.
- A small baby can be laid diagonally across the mother's knees on a pillow to breastfeed; support the mother's feet with a nursing stool or large books.
- Adapt changing tables and cribs so that they are accessible from a wheelchair, and arrange the room so that moving about is minimized. For the mother who cannot lift, a low-sided pram or baby stroller makes it easier for her to slide the baby out onto her lap.
- When the mother has unilateral weakness or paralysis (e.g., from a stroke), have her use a baby sling during breastfeeding, which allows the mother's arms to be free.
- Keep track of a mobile child by tying a bell to the baby's shoes.
- Teach a toddler how to climb on his or her mother's knee for a ride and to sit still while the wheelchair is moving.
- Touching in bed at night gives the baby the extra cuddling needed if there are barriers to physical contact during the day.
- Infant overalls with crossed straps make it easier to lean over and pick her or him up.
- Use a nursing bra with an easy-to-fasten clip or adhesive strap that can be fastened with one hand and that opens in the front, instead of the back.
- Have maternity clothes altered or buy ones that have openings or large ring zippers.
- Schedule rest periods during the day and sit up to do work (cooking, cleaning, etc.) whenever possible.
- Put the infant in bed with the mother at night and/or have the father or someone bring the baby to the mother to breastfeed during the night.
- Use an intercom system that picks up the sound of the baby crying and can be transformed into flashing light signals for the deaf mother.
- The mother can spend the day on a carpeted or padded floor to enable feeding, changing, and playing with the baby if she can not lift him or her. A bean bag chair or large pillows can provide support for breastfeeding.

Silicone Breast Implants and Breastfeeding

Silicone is a naturally occurring element; it is the second most common element in the earth's crust. In its natural state, silicone is not hazardous to humans. Silicone compounds are used in cosmetics, antacids, and for the coating of fruits and vegetables (Mohrbacher, 1994). It is used to lubricate syringes and for bottle nipples and pacifiers. Mylicon drops have the same polymer as silicone breast implants and are given to infants with colic. Due to its presence in the environment, it is difficult to distinguish between normal and abnormal maternal levels. Even so, several articles reporting on immunologic responses to silicone and clinical syndromes associated with silicone have been published in peer-reviewed journals.

Silicone-associated atypical connective-tissue disease is recognized by rheumatologists as an actual disease (Goldman, 1995; Seibold, 1993; Sergent et al., 1993). Solomon and associates (1994) have reported on over 3,000 patients with silicone breast implants who are symptomatic. Between 850,000 and 1 million women had breast implants by 1989 (Bright et al., 1993). Human adjuvant disease was the name given by Japanese investigators in the 1970s and early 1980s to describe symptomatic patients with silicone breast implants (Kumagai et al., 1984).

Little research has been done on the effects of silicone implants on lactation. Areas of concern are as follows:

- The possibility of implants leaking materials into the breastmilk
- The possibility of a maternal immunologic response
- If silicone gets into the milk, will the baby absorb it?
- Does breastfeeding add an additional risk of infant exposure to silicone?

In a study of six breastmilk samples, there was not a significant difference in levels of polydimethylsiloxane (the silicone polymer in implants) when compared to water blanks and a control milk sample (Bejarano & Zimmer, 1991). Polydimethylsiloxane has a molecular weight of 14,000 to 21,000 kdaltons (McEvoy, 1992), and it is believed to be unlikely that the molecule passes into the milk. One chemist at a California laboratory tested the breastmilk of women whose implants ruptured and found no silicone in the milk (Mohrbacher, 1994).

Sclerodermalike esophageal disease has been reported in a study of children, some of whom were breastfed. During the study of 11 children (8 breastfed and 3 formula-fed), 5 breastfed children showed alterations in esophageal motility (Levine & Ilowite, 1994). A reduction in the movement of food from the esophagus to the stomach was noted as the child matured. The researchers postulated that this could be due to the silicone itself or a maternal immunologic response that the infant reacted to. The U.S. Food and Drug Administration cautioned against extrapolating conclusions from this one study, pointing out the limitations of the study size and selection bias (FDA, 1994). It will be many years before scientists know conclusively if silicone-gel breast implants are associated with an increase in immune disorders among the women who received them, and potential adverse effects associated with breastfeeding are yet to be confirmed (Flick, 1994).

The Human Milk Banking Association of North America (HMBANA) has taken the position that, because of their obligation to provide the safest product possible to its recipient infants, mothers with silicone breast implants will not be accepted as donors (HMBANA, 1994). Since research about breastfeeding and silicone breast implants is limited, it is difficult to reach conclusions. Whether health problems occur more often in the children of mothers with implants than in the children of mothers without implants must first be shown. If this does occur, the question then becomes, Does breastfeeding add a risk of silicone exposure that pregnancy does not? The potential health risks of artificial feeding have been shown (Cunningham et al., 1991), and until there is better evidence, women with breast implants should still be encouraged to breastfeed.

For those desiring to test breastmilk for silicon and its breakdown products, the National Medical Service laboratory can be of assistance (2300 Stratford Ave., Willowgrove, PA 19090; 800/522-6671 or 215/657-4900).

Maternal Infections

Much has been learned in the past decade regarding the transmission of viruses in breastmilk. Viruses that have been studied include cytomegalovirus (CMV); rubella; the herpes simplex and zoster viruses; hepatitis A, B, and C; human T-lymphotrophic viruses (types I and II); and human immunodeficiency virus, types 1 and 2 (HIV-1 and HIV-2). For some of these viruses, it has been established that breastfeeding is a route of transmission while for others the passage of maternal antibody is believed to protect the infant from symptomatic disease. Table 2A–2 lists management suggestions for infectious disease in the breastfeeding mother and Table 2A–3 shows preventive measure guidelines when chickenpox exposure in the nursery or maternity ward is an issue.

CYTOMEGALOVIRUS

Cytomegalovirus has been isolated from breastmilk (Diosi et al., 1967; Dworsky et al., 1983; Hayes et al., 1972), with more frequent shedding of the virus noted in later milk than in colostrum (Dworsky et al., 1983; Hayes et al., 1972). The reactivation of CMV in the breastmilk has been reported to increase between 2 and 12 weeks (Yeager et al., 1983). However, infants breastfed by seropositive mothers do not usually have symptomatic disease, which is attributed to the maternal CMV antibody (Alford, 1991). Maternal CMV seropositivity is not a contraindication to breastfeeding (Ruff, 1994). There are, however, a few groups of infants who may have a higher risk of contracting symptomatic disease through breastfeeding. According to Ruff (1994), these include the following:

- Premature infants with low levels of antibodies acquired transplacentally
- Infants of seronegative mothers who subsequently seroconvert during lactation
- Immunocompromised infants

RUBELLA

The wild and vaccine strains of rubella have been isolated from human milk (Buimovici-Klein et al., 1977; Klein et al., 1980; Landes et al., 1980; Losonsky et al., 1982a, 1982b). Transmission is believed to be primarily by the respiratory route and no significant disease has been associated with the presence of rubella in milk (Ruff, 1994). Acquired rubella and receipt of the rubella vaccine are not considered contraindications to breastfeeding (Ruff, 1994).

Table 2A–2 Management of Infectious Disease

Organism	Condition	Isolate from Mother	Mother Can Visit Nursery	Mother Can Breastfeed	Infant: Immediate Treatment	Contact with Pregnant Women Allowed
Bacteria	Premature rupture of membranes; longer than 24 hr without fever					
	Full-term infant	No	Yes	Yes	Observe	Yes
	Premature infant	No	Yes	Yes	Treat with antibiotics	Yes
	Maternal fever > 38°C twice, 4 hr apart, 24 hr before to 24 hr after delivery, or endometriosis; full-term or premature infant	Yes, until mother afebrile 24 hr if not breastfeeding	No, until mother afebrile 24 hr	Yes	Treat with antibiotics	Yes
Salmonella, Shigella		No	Yes, if culture negative	Yes, if culture negative	In most cases	Yes
Staphylococcus		No	Yes	Yes	Yes	Yes
Group B ß-streptococcus	Mother with possible cervical culture but otherwise negative obstetric history	No	Yes	Yes		Yes
	Mother with possible cervical culture and obstetric history of fever, premature rupture of membranes > 24 hr, fetal distress, meconium, low Apgar score, any symptoms of prematurity	No	Yes	Yes, after treatment	Treat with antibiotics	Yes
	Infant with surface colonizing	No	Yes	Yes, after treatment	Treat with antibiotics	Yes
	Negative history and physical examination	No	Yes	Yes	Observe	Yes
	With premature rupture of membrane or maternal infection	No	Yes	Yes	Treat with penicillin	Yes
Group A streptococcus	Mother with infection	Yes	Not in acute stage	Not in acute stage; after 24-hr treatment	Prophylactic penicillin for 10 days	Yes
Gonorrhea	Mother with positive smear or culture	No	Yes, after treatment	Yes, after treatment		
	Infant well				Antibiotic to the eyes, once in delivery room and once in nursery	Yes

Organism	Condition	Isolate from Mother	Mother Can Visit Nursery	Mother Can Breastfeed	Infant: Immediate Treatment	Contact with Pregnant Women Allowed
Gonorrhea (continued)	Infant with conjunctivitis	No	Yes, after treatment	Yes, after treatment	Penicillin IM or IV, plus chloramphenicol drops topically to eyes	Yes
Syphilis	Mother with positive VDRL test or clinical disease not treated	Only if mother with second-stage disease or with skin lesions	No, if skin lesions; yes, otherwise	Yes	Penicillin IM or IV after workup done; follow-up after discharge	Yes
Tuberculosis	Mother treated	No	Yes	Yes		Yes
	Mother with inactive disease	No	Yes	Yes	Consider BCG if follow-up in doubt	Yes
	Mother with active disease	Yes	No	No, until RX established	Prophylactic	No
Hepatitis	Mother had in first trimester, well at delivery	No	Yes	Yes		Yes
	Mother with active hepatitis at delivery or in third trimester	No, may room-in after good hand-wash technique followed	No	Yes, after HBIG and Heptavax	HBIG and immunization with Heptavax	Yes
	Mother is chronic carrier	No	Yes, not kiss other infants	Ask for infectious disease opinion	Immunization	Yes
Protozoa Toxoplasma	Toxoplasmosis	No	Yes	Yes		No

Source: Lawrence, R (1994). *Breastfeeding: A Guide for the Medical Profession*, 3rd ed., pp. 478-79. St. Louis: Mosby. Reprinted with permission of Mosby-Year Book, Inc..

Table 2A–3 Guidelines for Preventive Measures after Exposure to Chickenpox in the Nursery or Maternity Ward

Type of Exposure or Disease	Chickenpox Lesions Present		Disposition
	Mother	Neonate	
A. Siblings at home have active chickenpox when neonate and mother are ready for discharge from hospital	No	No	1. Mother: if she has a previous history of chickenpox, she may return home. Without a history, she should be tested for V-Z antibody titer. If test is positive, she may return home. If test is negative, VZIG is administered, and she is discharged home. 2. Neonate: may be discharged home with mother if mother has history of varicella or is V-Z antibody–positive. If mother is susceptible, administer VZIG to infant and discharge home or place in protective isolation.
B. Mother with no history of chickenpox; exposed during period 6–20 days antepartum*	No	No	1. Exposed mother and infant: send home at earliest date unless siblings at home have communicable chickenpox. If so, may administer VZIG and discharge home, as above. 2. Other mothers and infants: no special management indicated. 3. Hospital personnel: no precautions indicated if there is history of chickenpox or zoster. In absence of history, immediate serologic testing** is indicated to determine immune status. Nonimmune personnel should be excluded from patient contact until 21 days after an exposure. 4. If mother develops varicella one to two days postpartum, infant should be given VZIG†
C. Onset of maternal chickenpox antepartum§ or postpartum	Yes	No	1. Infected mother: isolate until no longer clinically infectious. 2. Infected mother's infant: administer VZIG to neonates born to mothers with onset of chickenpox < 5 days before delivery and isolate separately from mother. Send home with mother if no lesions develop by the time mother is noninfectious. 3. Other mothers and infants: send home at earliest date. VZIG† may be given to exposed neonates. 4. Hospital personnel: same as B-3.
D. Onset of maternal chickenpox antepartum§	No	No	1. Mother: isolation unnecessary 2. Infant: isolate from other infants but not from mother. 3. Other mothers and infants: same as C-3 (if exposed). 4. Hospital personnel: same as B-3 (if exposed).

Table 2A–3   *Continued*

Type of Exposure or Disease	Chickenpox Lesions Present		Disposition
	Mother	Neonate	
E. Congenital chickenpox	No	Yes	1. Infected infant and his or her mother: same as D-1 and 2.
			2. Other mothers and infants: same as C-3.
			3. Hospital personnel: same as B-3.

* If exposure occurred less than 6 days antepartum, mother would not be potentially infectious until at least 72 hours postpartum.

** Send serum to virus diagnostic laboratory for determination of antibodies to V-Z virus by a sensitive technique such as FAMA or ELISA. Personnel may continue to work for 8 days after exposure pending serologic results because they are not potentially infectious during this period. Antibodies to V-Z virus > 1:4 probably are indicative of immunity.

†VZIG is available through the American Red Cross. The dose for a newborn is 1.25 mL.

§Considered noninfectious when no new vesicles have appeared for 72 hr and all lesions have progressed to the stage of crusts.

Source: Gershon, AA (1995). Chickenpox, measles, mumps. In: Remington, JS, Klein, JO (Eds.). *Infectious Diseases of the Fetus and Newborn Infant*, p. 590. Philadelphia: Saunders. Reprinted with permission of W.B. Saunders and authors.

HERPES SIMPLEX AND ZOSTER VIRUSES

Neonatal herpes simplex virus (HSV-1) is most often transmitted during delivery through an infected maternal genital tract or through an ascending infection. One case report of postnatal HSV-1 transmission via breastmilk, which has been documented (Dunkle et al., 1979), has been questioned because transmission during delivery could not be ruled out (Ruff, 1994). One case of the fatal infection of an infant breastfed from birth has been reported in which the mother developed a skin sore on the areola of the left breast (she had no other lesions) on the third day (Quinn & Lofberg, 1978). The father had a history of recurrent oral–labial herpes and a report of oral breast contact 3 weeks prior to delivery was obtained.

HSV-1 transmission in the presence of maternal breast lesions after breastfeeding has also been reported (Sullivan-Boyai et al., 1983). It is believed that transmission through breastfeeding in the absence of breast lesions is unlikely (Ruff, 1994). Women with active herpetic lesions on their breasts are advised not to breastfeed (Ruff, 1994). Mothers with genital or oral lesions but no herpetic lesions on the breast may breastfeed (AAP, 1991). They should be cautioned to practice handwashing, clean covering of the lesions, and no fondling or kissing of the infant until the lesions are dried.

HEPATITIS

Hepatitis A virus (HAV), hepatitis B virus (HBV), and hepatitis C virus (HCV) are the three major types of hepatitis. Hepatitis D is a less common type of hepatitis that is associated with infection by HBV and HIV, type 1. Hepatitis E is less common, is transmitted by the fecal–oral route, and causes an acute illness. Table 2A–4 summarizes the common hepatitis types.

HAV is often called infectious hepatitis; it causes an acute febrile illness with jaundice, anorexia, nausea, and malaise. HBV can cause an asymptomatic seroconversion

Table 2A–4 Summary of Common Hepatitis Types

Virus Type	Route of Transmission	Detected in Milk	Recommendations for Feeding
HAV	Oral–fecal route	Yes	Mother can breastfeed. Immune globulin given to the infant if mother is ill and icteric—0.02 mL/kg at delivery.
HBV	Blood, sexual activity, perinatal transmission	Yes	If mother is HBsAG positive—give infants hepatitis B immune globulin (HBIG)—0.5 mL. Also give infant 3 doses of hepatitis vaccine (Heptavax)—one after delivery; the second and third doses are given 1 and 6 months later.
HCV	Parenteral drug use, blood, sexual activity, perinatal transmissions	Yes	Committee on Infectious Disease of the Academy of Pediatrics states breastfeeding is contra-indicated (1991) but in 1994 the AAP *1994 Red Book* states that perinatal transmission probably occurs, with undefined risks and consequences. However, prominent pediatric infectious disease specialists report breastfeeding is not contra-indicated (Berlin, 1995; Gardner & Ruff, 1995; Polywka et al., 1997).

in which the mother is a carrier to fatal hepatitis. HBV contains several antigens: hepatitis B surface antigen (HBsAG), hepatitis B core antigen (HBcAG), and hepatitis Be antigen (HBeAG). Current infection is indicated by the presence of HBsAG.

It is recommended that all infants receive the hepatitis vaccine (Heptavax) at birth regardless of the mother's status (AAP/Committee on Infectious Disease, 1991). Hepatitis B immune globulin (HBIG) is also given at birth to all infants whose mothers have active hepatitis B; this is believed to effectively decrease any risk of transmission of HBV through breastfeeding. In countries where HBIG and Heptavax are not available and the morbidity and mortality are high from diarrhea, breastfeeding is still recommended for infants born to mothers who are HBV seropositive.

Hepatitis C infection causes a slowly developing disease, and the risk of chronic liver disease is high. Treatment measures to reduce or eliminate the hepatic inflammation have not been successful. HCV perinatal transmission is more frequent for infants born to HIV-coinfected mothers than to mothers not infected with HIV (Paccagnini et al., 1995), and the risk of vertical transmission from mother to infant is correlated with the titer of HCV RNA in the mother (Ohto et al., 1994). In the absence of effective therapy and HCV's probable transmission in breastmilk, breastfeeding is not recommended (AAP, 1991). However, in lectures given at international meetings, pediatric researchers have begun to propose that hepatitis C may be compatible with breastfeeding (Berlin, 1995; Gardner & Ruff, 1995).

HUMAN T-LYMPHOTROPHIC VIRUSES, TYPES I AND II

Human T-Lymphotrophic Virus Type I (HTLV-I) has been associated with tropical spastic paraparesis, T-cell leukemia, urethritis, arthritis in adults (Manns & Blattner, 1991), and infective dermatitis in children (LaGrenade et al., 1990). HTLV-I antigen-positive lymphocytes have been found in the breastmilk of women seropositive for the virus (Kinoshita et al., 1984). Longer duration of breastfeeding, advanced maternal age, and higher maternal anti-HTLV-I antibody titers have been associated with maternal–infant transmission of HTLV-I (Takahashi et al., 1991; Wiktor et al., 1993). The CDC (1993) recommends that women with HTLV-I not breastfeed.

Human T-Lymphotrophic Virus Type II (HTLV-II) has been detected in breastmilk by polymerase chain reaction (PCR) (Heneine et al., 1992). There are few studies of HTLV-II seropositive women and the vertical transmission rate to their infants of the virus. The additional risk as a result of breastfeeding is not known. Van Dyke and colleagues (1994) report 14% of breastfed and 3.6% of nonbreastfed children were infected. Little is known about this disease spectrum or the risk to the infant of contracting the virus if breastfed. The current recommendation is that women seropositive for HTLV-II not breastfeed.

HUMAN IMMUNODEFICIENCY VIRUS, TYPE 1

Maternal–infant transmission of HIV-1 occurs in utero, intrapartum, and postpartum (Mofenson & Wolinsky, 1994; Oxtoby, 1994). HIV-1 is the virus that causes acquired immunodeficiency disease syndrome (AIDS). Case studies, laboratory detection of HIV-1 in milk, and epidemiological studies suggest breastfeeding as a means of transmission of HIV-1 (Goldfarb, 1993; Oxtoby, 1988; Ruff et al., 1992; Van de Perre et al., 1992). High viral load associated with seroconversion and advanced illness may increase the risk of HIV-1 transmission during breastfeeding (Ruff, 1994). The picture is not as clear for HIV-1 seropositive but well women who enter pregnancy. The determination of the additional risk (over pregnancy and delivery) of contracting HIV-1 via breastfeeding remains unclear. Because infants retain the maternal antibody to HIV-1 for 15 to 18 months and viral cultures and/or PCR and ICD p24 antigen tests cannot be detected immediately at birth, the question of whether the infant was infected during pregnancy or during the intrapartum period remains unanswered.

The large prospective cohort studies, which might be able to answer the question, unfortunately have been conducted in one of two scenarios: either in industrialized countries where HIV-1 seropositive women are advised not to breastfeed or in developing countries where breastfeeding is the norm. This results in HIV-1 transmission rates for very different populations that probably are not comparable (Ruff, 1994). Nevertheless, such a comparison has been done and the attributable risk of breastfeeding on HIV-transmission by women infected prenatally is estimated at 14% (Dunn et al., 1992).

HIV-1 DNA has been found in the cell-free fraction (Armstrong, 1991; Thiry et al., 1985), histiocytes (Armstrong, 1991), and colostrum and later milk samples (Ruff, 1994; Van de Perre, 1993) by PCR. There appears to be intermittent viral shedding (Ruff, 1994). Polymerase chain reaction may not mean the virus is actively replicating—it detects the presence of viral fragments. HIV-1 p24 antigen (believed to indicate the presence of actively replicating virus) has been found in 24% of colostrum samples and none of the later milk samples (Ruff, 1994). Confounding this are reports that higher rates of transmission have been associated with prolonged breastfeeding (de Martino et al., 1992; Embree et al., 1993). There are HIV-1–specific antibodies in the milk of seropositive women (de Martino et al., 1992) and a persistence of HIV-1–specific IgM has been associated with a significantly lower rate of HIV-1 transmission.

Other factors, which may influence virus infection or virus expression, have been identified in human milk, including glycosaminoglycans that inhibit binding of the HIV-1 envelope glycoproteins to CD_4 molecules (Newburg et al., 1992) and other lipid-associated factors (Orloff et al., 1993). Lipids have activity against viral envelopes as documented by Isaacs and associates (1986). Breastmilk also contains generous amounts of antioxidants, which have been shown to negatively influence the expression of the virus at the nuclear membrane level (Baker, 1992; Beg et al., 1993; Menon et al., 1993). Oral or intestinal mucosal breakdown from trauma, or infection in the mother or infant, increases the risk of HIV-1 transmission through breastmilk, thus also needing consideration (Bartlett et al., 1992; Blau et al., 1983; Moyer et al., 1990; Ruff, 1994).

Many questions remain unanswered. In developing countries, the risk of dying from infectious disease or malnutrition if not breastfed are higher than the risk of contracting HIV-1 from a seropositive mother, so breastfeeding is still recommended by the World Health Organization (WHO, 1992). In industrialized countries, HIV-1–infected women are advised not to breastfeed (CDC, 1985).

HUMAN IMMUNODEFICIENCY VIRUS, TYPE 2

HIV-2 is also associated with the development of AIDS and is transmitted through sexual contact, blood transfusions, and needle sharing. Maternal–infant HIV-2 transmission has been reported (Gayle et al., 1992; Matherson et al., 1990; Morgan et al., 1990) although prospective studies of seropositive pregnant women have failed to detect any infected infants (Andreasson et al., 1993; French Collaborative Study Group, 1994; Poulsen et al., 1992). The role of breastfeeding in maternal–infant HIV-2 transmission is unknown.

Contraception During Lactation

Breastfeeding is known to be the optimal food for newborns. The breastfed infant is less likely to suffer from diarrhea and other neonatal complications. These have a direct relationship on the health of the child as he or she ages. Child spacing also has a direct relationship to the health of the child.

Throughout the world, the leading cause of weaning is pregnancy (Thappa et al., 1988). During pregnancy, the composition as well as the taste of breastmilk may change. In many cultures, it is unacceptable to breastfeed while pregnant. The child is quickly weaned onto a nutritionally inadequate diet, resulting in the development of Kwashiorkor, a protein deficiency (Labbok, 1989a).

LACTATIONAL AMENORRHEA

After delivery, placental hormones decrease rapidly. If there is no nipple stimulation, plasma levels of follicle stimulating hormone (FSH) and luteinizing hormone (LH) return to normal within four weeks after delivery (Glasier et al., 1983). Sleep increases the LH level via a pulse release system, which is necessary for ovulation (Liu & Pack, 1988).

During lactation, levels of FSH return to normal four weeks postpartum (Glasier et al., 1983). Follicle growth occurs but the follicle does not rupture and may become cystic or atretic. This is due to the insufficient pulsatile LH release (McNeilly, 1993; McNeilly et al., 1994). Nipple stimulation by the infant's sucking decreases the normal pattern of release of gonadotrophin-releasing hormone (GnRH) by the hypothalamus (Glasier et al., 1986; McNeilly, 1993; McNeilly et al., 1994).

Prolactin is released by the anterior pituitary in response to nipple stimulation. Prolactin levels are high during the first three- to four-postpartum months and drop with decreased sucking, and levels peak at night (Diaz et al., 1989). This may be why night feeds are related to lactational amenorrhea.

LACTATIONAL AMENORRHEA METHOD

A study of totally breastfeeding women showed ovulation rates of 37% at 6 months and 97% at 12 months postpartum. During amenorrhea, 67% of the ovulations occurred. The risk of ovulation and pregnancy in amenorrhea was 27% and 0.97%, respectively, at 6 months postpartum (Diaz et al., 1992). A woman who is exclusively breastfeeding may be protected from pregnancy without using any other contraceptive methods; this method of protection is called the *Lactational Amenorrhea Method* (LAM).

In 1988, the Bellagio Consensus Conference developed the LAM guidelines as a contraceptive method for the first 6 postpartum months. Researchers have determined that a totally breastfeeding mother who is amenorrhoeic has a < 2% chance of another pregnancy up to 6 months postpartum (Kennedy et al., 1989; Kennedy & Visness, 1992). See Figure 2A–1 for the recommended use of the LAM. In Chile, a

Figure 2A–1

How to determine if a woman can use breast-feeding as a child spacing method.

Source: Labbok, M (1989b). *Breastfeeding and Fertility, Mothers and Children Supplement* (8:1), American Public Health Association, Washington, DC. Reprinted with permission.

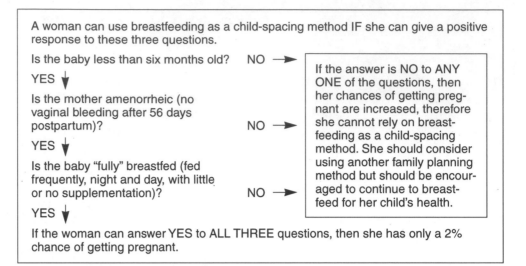

A woman can use breastfeeding as a child-spacing method IF she can give a positive response to these three questions.

Is the baby less than six months old?   NO →

YES ↓

Is the mother amenorrheic (no vaginal bleeding after 56 days postpartum)?   NO →

YES ↓

Is the baby "fully" breastfed (fed frequently, night and day, with little or no supplementation)?   NO →

YES ↓

If the woman can answer YES to ALL THREE questions, then she has only a 2% chance of getting pregnant.

If the answer is NO to ANY ONE of the questions, then her chances of getting pregnant are increased, therefore she cannot rely on breastfeeding as a child-spacing method. She should consider using another family planning method but should be encouraged to continue to breastfeed for her child's health.

study of the effectiveness of LAM showed one pregnancy at six months in a group of 422 lactating women. This corresponded to a pregnancy rate of 0.45% for women who relied on LAM as their only method of contraception (Perez et al., 1992).

It is important to note that researchers recommend at least five breastfeeding sessions a day for a total of more than 65 minutes to rely on LAM for contraception (McNeilly et al., 1983). The amount of supplementation, if any, and night feeds also need to be assessed by the health-care provider.

ORAL CONTRACEPTIVES

If a woman chooses to use oral contraceptives during lactation, a progestogen-only mini-pill such as MicroNor®, Nor-Q-D®, or Ovrette® should be used. There is no effect on milk production or infant growth and development. A combined estrogen–progestogen pill may decrease milk volume, resulting in earlier weaning, and may alter milk composition (Fraser, 1991). Breast enlargement in a breastfed male whose mother was taking a combined oral contraceptive was reported by Curtis (1964). The infant's breasts returned to normal after weaning. Folate deficiency in a infant of a healthy breastfeeding woman taking a combined birth control pill has been reported in Israel (Mandell & Berant, 1985). Progestogen-only pill use should be initiated at six weeks postpartum (Diaz & Croxatto, 1993). It is unlikely that ovulation will occur prior to then and lactation should be well established.

BARRIER METHODS

Use of barrier methods (condoms, diaphragms, IUDs) do not affect lactation because no chemicals are absorbed by the body. When used correctly these methods can be effective. Diaphragms should be fitted after the uterus returns to pre-pregnancy size. Because of hormonal changes, extra lubrication may be needed when latex condoms are used.

Intrauterine devices inserted during amenorrhea are safe. If correctly inserted into a woman at low risk for sexually transmitted diseases, there is little risk of pelvic inflammatory disease (Burkman, 1981). Copper-based IUDs prevent conception because of their effect on the sperm (Croxatto, 1992).

Levonorgestrel (Norplant System®) and medoxyprogesterone acetate (Depo Provera®) are safe to use during lactation. There is little effect on milk production, volume, and composition. Use should begin by six weeks after delivery to ensure protection from pregnancy. Table 2A–5 summarizes family planning options (contraceptive use) during lactation and Table 2A–6 shows the effects of contraceptive agents on milk yield and infant development.

Table 2A–5   Family Planning Options as They Relate to the Specific Concerns of Breastfeeding Women

FIRST CHOICE: NON-HORMONAL COMPLEMENTARY METHODS

Method	Breastfeeding Considerations	Advantages	Disadvantages
Lactational Amenorrhea Method—LAM	• Supports optimal breastfeeding	• Does not require a physical examination. • Improved infant health through breastfeeding. • No action required at time of sexual intercourse. • No commodities needed. • 99% or more effective for up to 6 months.	• Introductory method, is only effective in the postpartum period. • If the mother and child are separated for extended periods, family planning efficacy may be decreased.
Condoms	• No effect on breastfeeding. • No risk to mother or child.	• Does not require a physical examination. • Generally available. • Provides some protection against sexually transmitted diseases (STD) • 95-97% effective when used correctly.	• Requires action at time of sexual intercourse.
Diaphragm (with spermicide)	• No effect on breastfeeding • No risk to mother or child. *See Spermicides.*	• May have some STD protective effect. • 94% effective when used correctly.	• Size requirements may change during the first months postpartum. • Requires action at time of sexual intercourse.
Spermicides	• No effect on breastfeeding. • Minuscule amounts may be absorbed into maternal blood and there may be some passage into milk; there is no known effect on the infant.	• Does not require a physical examination. • Provides some STD protection. • Provides additional lubrication—vagina may be dry during breastfeeding. • 94% effective when used correctly.	• May cause local irritation to both men and women. • Requires action at time of sexual intercourse.
Intrauterine devices (non-hormonal IUD)	• No effect of IUD itself, nor the copper in some IUDs, on breastfeeding. • No effect on infant.	• Less discomfort when inserted during breastfeeding. • No action required at time of sexual intercourse. • 99.4-99.9% effective.	• Requires experienced health-care worker to insert and counsel. • Expulsion and complications may be higher if inserted after 2-4 days and before 4-8 weeks postpartum. *continued*

Table 2A–5   Family Planning Options as They Relate to the Specific Concerns of Breastfeeding Women
continued

FIRST CHOICE: NON-HORMONAL COMPLEMENTARY METHODS

Method	Breastfeeding Considerations	Advantages	Disadvantages
Natural family planning (periodic abstinence)	• No effect on breastfeeding. • May require additional training to ensure accurate interpretation of fertility signs and symptoms.	• Only method acceptable to some groups. • No commercial commodities needed. • 91-99% effective when done correctly.	• Fertility signs and symptoms may be difficult to interpret during breastfeeding. • May require extended periods of abstinence. • Calendar/rhythm method does not apply during amenorrhea. • Training is necessary.
Vasectomy (male voluntary surgical sterilization)	• No effect on breastfeeding. • No risk to mother or child.	• Permanent. • Mother and child are not disturbed. • No action required at time of sexual intercourse. • Recommended if no more children are desired. • 99.9% effective.	• Irreversible, surgical procedure with risk of side effects. • Counseling recommended.
Tubal ligation (female voluntary surgical sterilization)	• No effect on breastfeeding. • May involve short-term mother–infant separation. • If a period of separation is foreseen, necessary to express and store breastmilk before the procedure.	• Permanent. • No action required at time of sexual intercourse. • Recommended if no more children are desired. • 99.6% effective.	• Irreversible, surgical procedure with risk of side effects. • Counseling recommended. • Breastmilk supply must be maintained during mother–infant separation.

SECOND CHOICE: HORMONAL COMPLEMENTARY METHODS

Method	Breastfeeding Considerations	Advantages	Disadvantages
Mini-Pill, Injectables, Implants (Norplant®)	• Study results vary: Some hormone may pass into breastmilk. There is currently no evidence of adverse effects on the infant from the very small amount of hormone that passes into the milk. • These methods should be considered on an individual basis, taking the planned breastfeeding pattern into consideration since milk production may be reduced if given prior to 8 weeks.	• No action required at time of sexual intercourse. • Norplant provides up to 5 years of protection. • Mini-pill: 99.5% effective. • Injectables: 99.7% effective. • Implants: 99.9% effective.	• Studies of use prior to 8 weeks with full breastfeeding reflect possible negative effect on milk volume. • Some hormone may pass into the breastmilk. It is unclear how well the hormone is metabolized by the infant in the first weeks of life. • Injectables require injections monthly or every 3 months. Users may have irregular menstrual cycles. Hormone passes easily into the breastmilk; passive absorption by the infant is not well studied.

Table 2A–5 *Continued*

SECOND CHOICE: HORMONAL COMPLEMENTARY METHODS

Mini-pill, Injectables, Implants (Norplant®) *cont.*	• WHO/A.I.D. recommend method use be delayed until at least 6 weeks postpartum.

THIRD CHOICE: METHODS CONTAINING ESTROGEN

Method	Breastfeeding Considerations	Advantages	Disadvantages
Combined oral contra-ceptives, combined injectables (estrogen and progestin)	• Estrogen may reduce milk supply. • Some hormones may pass into breastmilk—there is no immediate nor long-term negative effect shown on infants. • In some women, decreased milk supply can lead to earlier cessation of breast-feeding. • Breastfeeding can and should continue as it supplies important health and nutritional benefits for the infant and toddler.	• No action required at time of sexual intercourse. • Decreased ovarian cancer and decreased anemia when used during men-strual cycle. • 99.9% effective.	• Estrogens may reduce milk supply, resulting in early supplementation and early cessation of full breastfeeding with con-comitant risks. • WHO/A.I.D. recommend this method's use be delayed until at least 6 months postpartum.

Source: Labbok, M, Cooney, K, Coly, S (1994). *Guidelines: Breastfeeding, Family Planning, and the Lactational Amenorrhea Method–LAM*, pp. 11–13. Washington, DC: Institute for Reproductive Health. Reprinted with permission.

Table 2A–6 Effects of Contraceptive Agents on Milk Yield and Infant Development

Agent	Milk Yield	Effect on Infant
Combined estrogen/progestin	Moderate inhibitory effect Shorter breastfeeding Milk concentration unchanged Small amount of steroid in milk	Slower weight gain No long-term effects
Progestin only	No effect on volume	No effect on weight gain
Mini-pill (Micronor, Nory-D)	No effect on duration Small amount of steroid in milk	No reported long-term effects
Injectable depot midroxy	Breastfeeding lasts longer	No long-term effects
Progesterone acetate, DMPA, Depo-Provera, and norethindrone enanthate (NET-EN, NORIS-TERAT)	? Change in milk—protein increased, fat decreased Steroid present in milk	
Norplant implants	No effect Small amount of steroids in milk	Normal growth No long-term effects
Vaginal rings containing natural hormone progesterone	No significant differences	No effect on growth Long-term effects under study

Source: Lawrence, R (1994). *Breastfeeding: A Guide for the Medical Profession*, 3rd ed., p. 589. St. Louis: Mosby. Modified from Winikoff, B, Semeraro, P, Zimmerman, M (1987). *Contraception During Lactation.* New York: Population Council Publishers. Reprinted with permission of Mosby-Year Book, Inc., and Population Council Publishers.

Maternal Medication Use During Lactation

Maternal use of medications during lactation and the assessment of the risk of such use to the infant is one of the most common problems physicians face when working with breastfeeding patients. The decision about prescription medication use during lactation falls to physicians, but LCs must be informed regarding the issues involved and the resources available to direct clinical decision makers who may call on their expertise for information. Specific information on hundreds of drugs has been reported and numerous reviews have been written. The American Academy of Pediatrics Committee on Drugs (1994) publishes a listing of drugs, which is updated on a regular basis, considered compatible, contraindicated, or requiring temporary cessation of breastfeeding (see Appendix).

The University of Rochester maintains a free drug information service as does the CDC in Atlanta, Georgia. The Rocky Mountain Drug Consultation Center has established a 1-900 line for drug inquiries (a fee-for-service line). Several texts have excellent chapters on using drugs during lactation, including *Breastfeeding: A Guide for the Medical Profession* (1994) by Ruth Lawrence, M.D., and *Breastfeeding and Human Lactation* (1993) by Jan Riordan, Ed.D., and Kathleen Auerbach, Ph.D. *Medications and Mothers' Milk* (1996) is a handy and easy-to-use reference book, which is written and updated regularly by Thomas Hale, R.Ph., Ph.D., that can easily fit into a lab coat.

Factors to consider when prescribing drugs to lactating women include the necessity of the drug therapy. This often requires communication between the physicians taking care of the mother and the baby to identify the medication that can meet the mother's needs while ensuring the lowest risk to the baby. When a drug is used that raises concerns for the infant's safety, a plan for monitoring the baby should be documented and communicated to the caregiver. Often the LC is in a unique position to bring together the obstetrician, gynecologist, family practice specialist, and neonatologist–pediatrician to make decisions about drug choice. The LC also may be the first professional to identify a problem in an infant of a mother taking illicit drugs or over-the-counter (OTC) medications.

Decisions or advice given to lactating women should be done carefully and with specific knowledge of the medication and the mother's and infant's medical conditions. To discontinue breastfeeding because the mother is taking a medication when it is unnecessary is inappropriate, but so is dismissing concerns over a medication taken during lactation when it is contraindicated or warrants close monitoring of the infant.

FACTORS THAT INFLUENCE THE PASSAGE OF DRUGS INTO BREASTMILK

Drugs can be administered orally, intramuscularly, or intravenously. The availability of the drug for secretion into breastmilk is influenced by the following:

- Dosage and timing
- Absorption from the gastrointestinal tract or from the muscular tissue
- Half-life or peak serum time for the drug depending on the route of administration
- Dissociation constant

- Volume distribution of the drug in maternal plasma
- Presence of renal dysfunction in the mother

Almost all drugs and chemicals are capable of getting into breastmilk. Exceptions are extremely large molecules such as heparin and insulin.

To most easily grasp an understanding of maternal drug transfer to breastmilk, consider the mother's blood to be one compartment and the milk in the alveolar lumen to be another compartment. Between the two compartments are the barriers of the interstitial tissue, basement membrane, and the layer of alveolar cells. Under ideal conditions, a chemical diffuses from the mother's blood into the milk until the concentration in the milk equals that in the blood. Then the milk–plasma ratio is 1:0, which indicates equal concentrations on both sides of the barrier. Thus, the milk–plasma ratio is the ratio of the concentration of the substance in milk to the concentration of the substance in plasma, which is < 1 unless there are properties of the drug that trap it in the milk compartment. The typical milk-to-plasma ratio is .005:.05 (0.5%:5%).

The concentration of any drug in breastmilk is influenced by the following:

- Molecular weight (size of the molecule) < 500 daltons—most can cross biological membranes
- Solubility of drugs in lipids and water
- Ability to bind protein—if there is an increased binding in serum to proteins, the drug may not cross the membrane into the milk
- Degree of ionization—highly charged drugs will not cross biological membranes
- pH of plasma (7.4) and breastmilk (6.35–7.65; average is 7.08)
- Diffusion rates
- Rate of milk secretion
- Volume of milk secreted

Protein binding is one of the most important factors influencing the amount of drug that gets into breastmilk. Only free (unbound) chemicals can be transferred across the barrier. A common protein that binds drugs is albumin, which is too large to participate in diffusion. The binding of drugs to milk proteins is very small relative to plasma protein binding. Two examples of drugs that are highly protein-bound are phenytoin (Nau, et al., 1982) and oxprenolol (Sioufi et al., 1984).

Dosing and Timing

The dosage and timing of drug administration can be coordinated with feeding time, and in some instances drug half-lifes or peak serum times, to minimize exposure of the breastmilk to the drug. Many clinicians recommend that women on medications breastfeed just before their usual dose is to be taken to achieve the maximum interval between the previous dose and the feeding.

Ionizability of Drugs

When most drugs enter the mammary alveolar cells, they are in a nonionized, nonprotein-bound form. The ionizability of a drug influences how subject it is to trapping. Milk is generally more acidic than maternal blood is. Thus for basic chemicals, the degree of ionization in breastmilk is close to twice that in blood and ionized chemicals are concentrated in the milk. For acidic drugs, about half as much drug is ionized in breastmilk as in blood. Therefore, unless they are bound to plasma proteins, weak bases can be trapped in the milk. Decreases in the plasma pH, such as what occurs in respiratory acidosis, result in less ionization of an acidic drug and an increased milk-to-plasma ratio. Examples of weak bases that are concentrated in breastmilk are the B-blockers—atenolol and metoprolol (Liedholm et al., 1981), metoclopramide (Lewis et al., 1980), and terbutaline (Boreus et al., 1982).

Lipid Solubility

Drugs that are highly soluble in fat may be physically dissolved into all fatty tissues of the mother. The fat in breastmilk is the only fat reservoir that is periodically emptied. Thus the lipid droplets of newly forming breastmilk are excretion routes of some chemical agents. One example of this is industrial chemicals known as polychlorinated biphenyls (PCBs). Milk is believed to be an important PCB excretion route because new lipid droplets from the alveolar cells dissolve their share of PCBs, which are available in the maternal circulation due to maternal fatty-tissue breakdown (Rogan et al., 1986). Children's PCB levels have been documented to increase with duration of breastfeeding (Kuwabara et al., 1979).

When women have extensive exposure to PCBs, changes in children's nails, gums, and teeth have been documented and presumed to be related to PCB intoxication through breastmilk (Kuwabara et al., 1979). But, for the majority of infants whose exposure to PCBs in human milk is lower, the risk is not believed to outweigh the benefits of breastfeeding (Rogan et al., 1987). In summary, drugs that are transferred most readily into human milk include the following:

- Compounds that have low molecular weights
- Compounds that are nonionized at pH of 7.4 (maternal plasma pH)
- Compounds that have a high lipid solubility

FACTORS THAT INFLUENCE NEONATE DRUG ABSORPTION

The amount of drug appearing in the maternal milk is very low and depends on many factors, as outlined in the previous section. An additional set of parameters must be taken into consideration when determining whether the infant is exposed to a small amount of a drug that may have made its way into the milk, including the following: frequency of feeding, time interval between maternal dosing and feeding, rate and manner of infant's drug absorption, and volume of a feeding.

Drug Absorption from the Infant's Gastrointestinal Tract

Infancy is a rapid period of growth and the manner in which drugs are absorbed, distributed, and metabolized can vary within a very short period of time. The functional readiness of the gastrointestinal (GI) tract—the presence of a higher gastric pH and increased permeability of the gastrointestinal mucosa in the newborn when compared to the older infant—may allow drugs that are normally too large to be absorbed, or that are usually destroyed in the gut, to reach the systemic circulation of the newborn. Generally, gastric emptying time is prolonged and a slower transit time in the upper small intestine, which may enhance the absorption of certain drugs, has been observed in the newborn. Drugs like tetracycline form complexes with components in breastmilk that limit their absorption; aminoglycosides are not absorbed to any extent in the GI tract. Although neither of these reach the systemic system, they may exert an effect on the GI tract by altering gastrointestinal bacterial flora. The smaller pool of bile salts available in the infant's GI tract may decrease drug absorption because bile salts facilitate solubility of some agents.

Drug Distribution in the Infant

The distribution of drugs in the infant is different from adults because infants have a larger extracellular fluid volume and a smaller deposition of fat. Therefore, drugs such as gentamicin, tobramycin, ampicillin, and ticarcillin, which are confined to extracellular fluid, will have larger distribution volumes in the newborn (Green et al., 1984). Infants have a lower total serum protein concentration than adults, thus they have limited available protein-binding sites. When limited protein binding is present, more free or unbound drug is available; it is in the unbound state that drugs can diffuse across cell membranes to exert pharmacologic activity. A more profound response, secondary to an elevated free fraction of drug despite overall low drug concentrations, can result; Wilson (1983) has documented this for phenytoin (Dilantin), theophylline (aminophylline), and diazepam (Valium). Jaundice occurring as a result of sulfonamide therapy is caused by displacing of bilirubin from the plasma protein-binding sites (Gardner, 1987).

In early infancy, kidney function and drug metabolizing pathways are not fully developed. For about the first two months of life, the glomerular filtration rate is significantly less in the newborn than it is in the adult. The hepatic microsomal P-450 enzyme system in infants is immature, prolonging the half-lives of certain drugs and increasing infants' susceptibility to toxicity from drug accumulation.

Caffeine elimination is an example of the deleterious effects of hepatic immaturity. For the adult, the half-life of this drug is about five hours. For term infants, the half-life of caffeine is 80 hours, and it is 100 hours for premature infants (Berlin, 1981). With high maternal doses of caffeine, accumulation of significant amounts in the neonate from the small fraction excreted in breastmilk can result. Some infants' irritability and insomnia have been attributed to heavy consumption of caffeine by breastfeeding mothers (Hill et al., 1977). Slower elimination of chloramphenicol (Green et al., 1984) and hyperbilirubinemia resulting from estrogen ingestion by the breastfeeding infant (Wong & Wood, 1971) are both believed to be due to neonates' poorly developed liver metabolism. Concerns have also been expressed over the sensitizing of susceptible infants through very low doses to potential allergens such as the penicillins.

Calculating Drug Levels Neonates May Receive

To minimize the dose of a drug received by an infant in breastmilk, the lowest effective dose should be prescribed for the shortest period of time possible. Drugs that diffuse from blood to milk can also diffuse from milk back to blood when the concentration of the drug in the mother's blood declines (Scialli, 1991). So the amount of chemical ingested by the infant very much depends on when feeding occurs in relation to the mother's exposure to that chemical. For patients on chronic drug therapy, doses should be scheduled in a way that the infant is not fed at times of peak milk drug levels, which are generally one to two hours after the dose. Therefore, feeding the infant just prior to taking a medication or just prior to the infant's longest sleep period helps minimize the dose of a drug received via the milk.

If there is a concern that an infant may be receiving infant pharmacological amounts of a drug via the breastmilk, estimates of the amount of the dose received can be made (Gardner, 1987). Knowledge about the maternal serum level of a drug and the milk-to-plasma concentration ratio (M:P) allows calculation of the concentration of a drug in breastmilk:

$$\text{Maternal drug concentration} \times \text{Milk} \div \text{Plasma ratio} = \text{Milk drug concentration}$$

Then an estimate of the volume of milk an infant consumes in a 24-hour period is necessary to determine the infant's daily dose:

$$\text{Milk volume (mg/kg per day)} \times \text{Milk concentration} = \text{Infant dose (mg/kg per day)}$$

Once the infant dose in mg/kg per day has been calculated, a comparison with recommended pediatric dosages can be made. Monitoring infant plasma levels may be necessary, particularly if adverse effects are exhibited or if the therapeutic range is very narrow.

This calculation method has its limitations—most notably the fact that milk plasma concentrations are often static measurements in time because as milk composition and pH change (even over the course of the same feeding), the milk plasma concentration changes. Also, the manner in which the M:P ratio is derived may affect the results. Often the peak milk concentration is compared to the peak plasma concentration, yet these two concentrations are not taken at the same time. Simultaneous collection over time will give data to calculate the time–concentration curves for milk and plasma. A ratio based on the area under the time–concentration curve is more accurate than an M:P ratio from a static measurement.

Other things to consider when determining infants' dose exposure include the production of biotransformation products of the parent drug (which may include the active ingredient), differences seen in concentrations in milk and plasma with chronic dosing versus acute exposures (important for drugs that accumulate in milk, such as cimetidine), and whether the M:P ratio has been derived from a single subject or small groups of subjects. In light of these drawbacks, the best help the M:P ratio can give the clinician is that the drug appears in milk in concentrations much less than in plasma (M:P < 1), that the levels in milk are similar to those in plasma (M:P = 1), or that the drug is concentrated in the milk (M:P > 1) (Scialli, 1991).

COUNSELING BREASTFEEDING MOTHERS ABOUT DRUG THERAPY

The possibility that a drug can be withheld until breastfeeding is completed or that an alternative therapy can be used should always be given careful study when mothers consider drug therapy during lactation. The risk to the mother of not receiving the drug must be weighed against the risk to the infant of receiving the drug via the mother's milk. Much is now known regarding the pharmacological factors influencing the passage of drugs into human milk and very few drugs have been classified as contraindicated during lactation. The clinician usually can feel comfortable about continuing any medication a mother safely took during pregnancy because the newborn will have been exposed to higher levels of the drug during pregnancy than he or she will be exposed to during the subsequent lactational period. Sometimes drug therapy consists of only a few doses, and pumping and discarding the milk to maintain breastmilk flow until the mother can resume nursing can be employed if necessary.

The safety of OTC medications is often a question that LCs find themselves fielding. According to Backas (1994) and Nice (1992), the following are some general guidelines to use in answering the question:

- Avoid recommending combination medications; single-acting OTC drugs are more advisable for nursing mothers.
- Avoid recommending "extra-strength" and long-acting forms of OTC medications (see Table 2A–7).
- Recommend a nondrug or nonsystemic approach (i.e., topical preparations or nonabsorbing drugs that do not actually enter the bloodstream) for symptom management, if possible.
- Inform the mother about possible side effects of drugs used during childbirth and that she must monitor her infant as well as herself.

One aspect of intense interest to lactation consultants is the effect on the infant of medications provided to the mother during labor. Table 2A–8 summarizes commonly used medications and their advantages and disadvantages for the mother; much less is known about drugs' effect on infants. Most hospital LCs agree that the degree of infant alertness is altered by many labor medications. A diminished suck may also be a side effect. Research is underway to determine the effect of medications on infants so that mothers can be informed of possible side effects prior to use of a particular drug during labor.

DRUGS THAT IMPAIR OR STIMULATE MILK PRODUCTION

The most recent pharmacologic strategies to inhibit lactation are directed toward preventing prolactin secretion. The ergot alkaloid derivative, bromocriptine (Parlodel), activates dopamine receptors, taking advantage of the physiologic function of dopamine as a prolactin-inhibitory factor and decreases blood flow to the breast through vasoconstriction. Case reports of hypertension, seizure, myocardial infarction, severe headache, mania, and stroke in women using this agent in the puerperium have been reported (Eickman, 1992; Fisher et al., 1991; Gittleman, 1991; Kulig et al., 1991).

The U.S. Food and Drug Administration has issued warnings that the side effects of bromocriptine mesylate for lactation suppression have been deemed dangerous (de Jong-van den Berg & Mintzes, 1995; Rayburn, 1996). Current research focuses on dopamine agonists for the treatment of hyperprolactinemia and lactation suppression (European Multicentre Study Group for Cabergoline in Lactation Inhibition, 1991; Ferrari et al., 1995; Rains et al., 1995; van der Heijden et al., 1991, Webster, 1996).

Drugs that produce vasoconstriction may impair the amount of milk available because the blood supply to the alveoli is the primary source of water, which is the most abundant component of milk. Drugs that interfere with the blood supply to the breast include sympathomemetic amines like those in cold remedies, nicotine from cigarette smoke (Vorherr, 1974), and thiazide diuretics (however, several of these are considered safe when breastfeeding) (AAP, Committee on Drugs, 1994).

Metoclopramide (Reglan) is a gastrointestinal drug used primarily to stimulate gastric emptying and intestinal motility or used following cancer chemotherapy as an anti-emetic. Studies have reported it to be a potent stimulator of prolactin release and useful for assisting mothers with inadequate milk output (deGazelle et al., 1983; Ehrenkranz & Ackerman, 1986; Gupta & Gupta, 1985; Guzman, 1979; Kauppila et al., 1981; Sousa, 1975). The dose of metoclopramide to significantly increase milk supply is reported to be 10 mg orally two to three times per day (deGazelle et al., 1983). Because it is a potent CNS drug, the AAP Committee on Drugs has recommended caution when lactating women use the agent. New research exploring the use of human growth hormone (hGH) injections for increasing the milk of mothers with premature infants has been reported and is discussed in Section A, Breastfeeding the Premature Infant, in Chapter 3 of this module.

Table 2A–7   Common Over-the-Counter Drugs Used During Breastfeeding

Medication (Brand Name and Generic)*	Effects on Lactation and/or Infant
Analgesics (avoid extra-strength formulas)	
Actron, Orudis KT (Ketoprofen), Aleve (Naproxen)	Not harmful for short-term use
Anacin-3 Regular Strength, Datril, Excedrin, Tempra	Not harmful for short-term use
Tylenol (acetaminophen)	Not harmful
Motrin, Nuprin (ibuprofen)	Not harmful when dose is 400 mg or less
Anacin, Bayer, Bufferin, Ecotrin (aspirin)	Chronic use may lower infant blood clotting level, or may cause Reye's syndrome in ill infant.
Antacids and Digestive Aids	
Lact-Aid (lactobacillus acidophilus), Maalox, Mylanta, Mylicon, Tums	Not harmful
Alka-Seltzer, baking soda (sodium or potassium bicarbonate)	Systemic antacids should be avoided.
Tagamet HB (Cimetidine), Zantac (Ranitidine), Peptid AC (Famotidine)	Drugs are concentrated in milk, but no adverse effects have been reported.
Antidiarrheal Preparations	
Donnagel, Kaopectate, K-Pek (Kaolin-pectin, attapulgite), Pepto-Bismol (bismuth subsalicylate)	Not harmful
Imodium A-D, Maalox Anti-diarrheal, Pepto Diarrhea Control (loperamide HCL)	Not harmful—do not take medication for more than 2 days.
Artificial Sweeteners	
Equal, Nutrasweet (aspartame)	Use with caution in PKU infants and carriers.
Sweet 'N' Low (saccharin)	Avoid; data on safety unavailable
Cold and Allergy Preparations (use single ingredients, short-acting agents)	
Actifed, Benadryl Decongestant, Benylin, Chlor-Trimeton (short-acting), Dimetapp, Novahistine, Sudafed, Sudafed Plus, Triaminic	Not harmful; monitor for infant drowsiness or decrease in milk supply. Mother should drink plenty of fluids and discontinue medicine if milk supply drops.
Actifed Plus, Allerest, Alka-Seltzer Plus, Benadryl Allergy Sinus, CoADVIL, Comtrex Allergy, Contac, Dimetapp Extentabs, Dristan, Efidac/24, Excedrin Sinus, Sinarest, Sine-Aid, Sine-Off, Sinutab, Sudafed Sinus, Triaminic 12, Tylenol Cold Medication, Tylenol Maximum Strength Sinus	Avoid if at all possible when breastfeeding. Contain multiple or long-acting ingredients that can cause infant drowsiness and a decrease in milk supply.

Table 2A–7 *Continued*

Medication (Brand Name and Generic)	Effects on Lactation and/or Infant
Cough Syrups (avoid products with alcohol content over 20%)	
Benylin Cough Syrup, Robitussin, Robitussin DM, PE, Triaminic expectorant	Not harmful. Monitor milk levels and infant drowsiness.
Contac Cough Formula, Robitussin-CF/Night Relief, Robitussin Cold & Cough Liqui-Gels, Sudafed Cough, Triaminic DM, Vicks Formula 44 and 44D cough medicine, Vicks Nyquil	Avoid if at all possible when breastfeeding. May have same side effects as cold remedies.
Hemorrhoid Preparations	
Anusol, Preparation H, Tucks	Not harmful
Laxatives	
Colace, Surfak (docusate)	Not harmful, increase oral fluids
Fleets (Sodium biphosphate enema)	Not harmful
Glycerin suppositories	Not harmful
Metamucil (first choice), Maalox Daily Fiber, Citrucel	Not harmful
Correctol, Ex-lax, Doxidan, Dulcolax, Modane, Peri-colace (bisacodyl, cascara sagrada, phenolphthalein)	Avoid; may cause colic and/or diarrhea in infant
Castor oil, magnesium citrate	
Nasal Decongestant Sprays (short-acting best)	
NaSal (salt water nose drops)	Not harmful
Neo-Sinephrine, Sinex (phenylephrine)	Monitor milk supply; increase oral fluids.
Afrin, Dristan, Otrivin	Avoid
Nausea and Vomiting and/or Motion Sickness (do not use if pregnant)	
Emetrol (phosphorated CHO), Benadryl, Dramamine, Trip Tone (diphenhydramine, dimenhydrinate)	Not harmful. Monitor infant for drowsiness; breastfeed before taking dose.
Dramamine II, Marezine, Bonine (cyclizine, meclizine)	Avoid; safety not determined
Sleep Preparations	
Benadryl, Nytol QuickCaps, Sominex Formula 2, Unisom Maximum Strength Sleepgels (diphenhydramine)	Not harmful. Monitor for possible drowsiness in infant.
Nytol Maximum Strength, Unisom (doxylamine)	Avoid
Stimulants	
Caffeine (coffee, tea, cola) 1-2 cups, NODOZ, Vivarin	Not harmful in doses less than 150 mg per day. May cause infant to be irritable in higher doses.
Weight-Control Products	
Acutrim, Dexatrim, Dynatrim	Avoid. No data on effects of chronic use. Contain large amounts of caffeine.
Herbal preparations (e.g., Chromium Picolinate)	Avoid. May contain harmful ingredients.

*Manufacturers frequently change active ingredients. Read the label or ask your pharmacist/provider.

The following references were used to compile this information: Briggs, GR, Freeman, RK, Yaffe, SJ (1994). *Drugs in Pregnancy and Lactation,* 4th ed. Baltimore: Williams & Wilkins; Lawrence, RA (1994). *Breastfeeding: A Guide for the Medical Profession,* 4th ed. St. Louis: Mosby; Nice, FJ (Nov. 1995). OTC medications and breastfeeding: an update. *Pharmacy Times,* 17-22; Nice, FJ (Dec. 1995). OTC medications and breastfeeding: an update. *Pharmacy Times,* 29-31; American Academy of Pediatrics (1994). The transfer of drugs and other chemicals into human milk. *Pediatrics* 93(1), 137-145.

Source: Copyright © 1996. Christine Hoey, RN, IRCLC, and Sally Morton, PharmD. Adapted from Cardwell, P, Pharm, C, Hoey, C (1994). Common over-the-counter drugs used during breastfeeding. Paper presented at the International Lactation Consultants Association Annual Meeting, Atlanta, GA. Reprinted with permission of authors.

Table 2A–8 Pain Relief During Childbirth

Classification of Drug and Method of Administration	When Used	Positive Benefits	Negative Side Effects
SEDATIVES			
Barbiturate family Administered by oral pill, intramuscular, or intravenous injection	Latent phase of labor	Allow rest while uterine contractions not yet regular, coordinated, or effective	Drowsiness, no pain relief; neurobehavioral depression (decreased alertness, sucking, and motor activity) in newborn if administered within a few hours before birth
	Active labor	Decrease anxiety in extremely anxious woman	As above
TRANQUILIZERS			
Valium, Vistaril, Phenergan Administered by intramuscular or intravenous injection	Latent and active labor	Decrease anxiety Enhance effect of narcotics Alleviate nausea and vomiting (Vistaril and Phenergan)	No pain relief if used alone Valium concentrates in fetus, commonly causes neurobehavioral depression (decreased alertness, sucking, motor activity) in newborn
AMNESICS			
Scopolamine Administered by intramuscular or intravenous injection	Active labor (virtually never used in current practice)	Marked amnesia, if such is desirable	May cause wild, irrational maternal behavior, preventing active participation in birth Amnesia for birth experience
ANALGESICS			
Narcotics Demerol, Sublimaze, Nubain, Stadol, Morphine Adminstered by intramuscular or intravenous injection	Active labor Cesarean birth Postpartum or postoperative	Good pain relief with higher dosages	Sedation, drowsiness Sometimes causes decrease in strength and/or frequency of contractions Depending on when the medication is administered, respiratory or neurobehavioral depression may occur in newborn
Inhalants (In lower concentration than for general anesthesia) Administered by face mask	Late first stage of labor; second stage of labor	Moderately good pain relief	Maternal unconsciousness may occur See General Anesthetics for other maternal and fetal effects
REGIONAL ANESTHETICS			
"-caine" family			Drugs in the -caine family can cause rare maternal allergic or dose-related toxic effects (including anxiety, hypotension, seizures, cardiac or respiratory depression) and fetal cardiac depression or hypotension
Local infiltration of perineum	At birth	Quick and easy to administer No known effect on newborn	Effective only in area where anesthetic is injected

Classification of Drug and Method of Administration	When Used	Positive Benefits	Negative Side Effects
Pudendal block (injected through vaginal wall and sacrospinous ligament on each side)	Second stage of labor (very frequently used in otherwise unmedicated childbirth)	Relief of perineal pain; no interference with urge or ability to push Adequate for performance and repair of episiotomy, if indicated	Completely effective 80% of time
Paracervical block (injected into cervical–vaginal junction on each side)	Late first stage of labor	No interference with urge or ability to push	Completely effective 60–70% of the time Must be repeated every 45–60 minutes to retain effect. 10–70% incidence of decrease in fetal heart rate—usually transient but rarely can be fatal to fetus
Caudal or epidural block (injected outside spinal canal through a catheter which remains in place until after delivery)	Active labor Forceps delivery Cesarean birth	Usually gives good relief of labor pain; can be adjusted to provide perineal pain relief for delivery Readministration of anesthetic agent through catheter is easy, painless, and effective Provides pain relief without sedation for surgery, allowing for maternal alertness during cesarean birth	Administration is uncomfortable (needle-puncture, awkward position for about 5-10 minutes, another 10-20 minutes before it takes full effect) Occasional "patchy" block and incomplete pain relief Strength and frequency of contractions may decrease, especially in early labor; use of oxytocin may be necessary Loss of pelvic muscle tone can lead to persistence of unfavorable head position in posterior or transverse position May lower mother's blood pressure, resulting in decreased blood flow to the fetus Loss of urge to push and forceps delivery more frequent than without block
Spinal or saddle block (injected through dura membrane into spinal canal)	Forceps delivery Cesarean birth	Complete lower abdominal and perineal pain relief (depending on technique, may also extend to legs and feet) Can be used to relieve discomfort of forceps delivery	Administration is uncomfortable (needle-puncture, awkward position) Loss of urge and ability to push (necessitating forceps delivery) May lower mother's blood pressure, resulting in decreased blood flow to the fetus; occasional (2–5%) spinal headache Very rare injury or meningitis

GENERAL ANESTHETICS

Nitrous oxide, halogenated ethers (sedatives and/or narcotics usually administered concurrently) Administered by endotracheal intubation	Difficult vaginal birth Cesarean birth	Complete pain relief	Maternal unconsciousness; rare maternal aspiration of vomitus—can be fatal; possible cardiac or respiratory depression in mother or newborn; may cause decreased alertness in newborn

Contraindications to Breastfeeding

Several of the contraindications to breastfeeding have already been discussed earlier in this section, including HIV-1, HIV-2, HTLV-I, HTLV-II, and HCV seropositivity in the mother (see the section on viruses because the thinking is changing on hepatitis C). In certain situations, mothers with CMV may be discouraged from breastfeeding (see discussion in Maternal Infections). Medications that are contraindicated during lactation are listed in Table 2APP–1 and 2APP–2. Drug abuse is another contraindication, especially for women who use intravenous drugs (IOM, 1991). If the mother has a life-threatening illness, breastfeeding may not be possible or desired (Berger, 1981).

Classical galactosemia is an inherited metabolic disorder. If an infant has galactosemia, breastfeeding is contraindicated. The predominant carbohydrate of human milk is lactose (a disaccharide made up of glucose and galactose). Galactosemia is a disorder with low or absent activity of galactose-1-phosphate uridyl transferase (which is an enzyme necessary to break down galactose) and elevated galactose-1-phosphate concentration in red blood cells (Koch et al., 1982). Therefore, in infants with galactosemia, the clinical symptoms of persistent vomiting, jaundice, weight loss, and hepatomegaly occur within the first few days of life after an infant has ingested breastmilk or lactose-containing formulas (Donnell et al., 1980). Screening for this disorder reduces the severity of the clinical picture by identifying infants early so that feeding can be modified.

Appendix: Drugs and Breastfeeding

The information in this appendix was first published by the AAP in 1983[1] and a revised version was published in 1989.[2] The latest revision (AAP, 1994[†]) was "intended to revise the lists of agents transferred into human milk and describe their possible effects on the infant or on lactation, if known." The article also states the following:

Information about the transfer of drugs and chemicals into human milk continues to become available. . . . The fact that a pharmacologic or chemical agent does not appear on the lists is not meant to imply that it is not transferred into human milk or that it does not have an effect on the infant; it only indicates that there were no reports found in the literature.

The tables here should be helpful to the LC when counseling a breastfeeding mother when she "has a condition for which a drug is medically indicated." For more specific information on the drugs, consult the numbered reference that appears in the right-hand column. The complete list of references starts on page 130 after the tables, all of which have been excerpted from the publication noted in the footnote below.

Table 2APP-1   Drugs That Are Contraindicated During Breastfeeding

Drug	Reason for Concern, Reported Sign or Symptom in Infant, or Effect on Lactation	Ref. No.
Bromocriptine	Suppresses lactation; may be hazardous to the mother	3, 4
Cocaine	Cocaine intoxication	5
Cyclophosphamide	Possible immune suppression; unknown effect on growth or association with carcinogenesis; neutropenia	6, 7
Cyclosporine	Possible immune suppression; unknown effect on growth or association with carcinogenesis	8
Doxorubicin*	Possible immune suppression; unknown effect on growth or association with carcinogenesis	9
Ergotamine	Vomiting, diarrhea, convulsions (doses used in migraine medications)	10
Lithium	One-third to one-half therapeutic blood concentration in infants	11–13
Methotrexate	Possible immune suppression; unknown effect on growth or association with carcinogenesis; neutropenia	14
Phencyclidine (PCP)	Potent hallucinogen	15
Phenindione	Anticoagulant; increased prothrombin and partial thromboplastin time in one infant; not used in United States	16

[†]Drug is concentrated in human milk.

[†]AAP, Committee on Drugs (1994). The transfer of drugs and other chemicals into human milk. *Pediatrics*, 93(1):137-50. Copyright © 1994 by the American Academy of Pediatrics. Used with permission. *Note:* Superscript numbers in first paragraph above refer to references on p. 130.

Table 2APP–2   Drugs of Abuse: Contraindicated During Breastfeeding

Drug* Reference	Reported Effect or Reasons for Concern	Ref. No.
Amphetamine[†]	Irritability, poor sleeping pattern	17
Cocaine	Cocaine intoxication	5
Heroin	Tremors, restlessness, vomiting, poor feeding	18
Marijuana	Only one report in literature; no effect mentioned	19
Nicotine (smoking)	Shock, vomiting, diarrhea, rapid heart rate, restlessness; decreased milk production	20–26
Phencyclidine	Potent hallucinogen	15

*Drug is concentrated in human milk.

[†]The Committee on Drugs strongly believes that nursing mothers should not ingest any compounds listed in this table. Not only are they hazardous to the nursing infant, but they are also detrimental to the physical and emotional health of the mother. This list is obviously not complete; no drug of abuse should be ingested by nursing mothers even though adverse reports are not in the literature.

Table 2APP–3   Radioactive Compounds That Require Temporary Cessation of Breastfeeding

Drug*	Recommended Time for Cessation of Breastfeeding	Ref. No.
Copper 64 (^{64}Cu)	Radioactivity in milk present at 50 hr	27
Gallium 67 (^{67}Ga)	Radioactivity in milk present for 2 wk	28
Indium 111 (^{111}In)	Very small amount present at 20 hr	29
Iodine 123 (^{123}I)	Radioactivity in milk present up to 36 hr	30
Iodine 125 (^{125}I)	Radioactivity in milk present for 12 days	31
Iodine 131 (^{131}I)	Radioactivity in milk present for 2–14 days, depending on study	32–35
Radioactive sodium	Radioactivity in milk present 96 hr	36
Technetium-99m (^{99m}Tc), ^{99m}Rc macro-aggregates, ^{99m}Tc O4	Radioactivity in milk present 15 hr to 3 day	37–42

*Consult nuclear medicine physician before performing diagnostic study so that radionuclide that has shortest excretion time in breast-milk can be used. Before study, the mother should pump her breast and store enough milk in freezer for feeding the infant; after study, the mother should pump her breast to maintain milk production but discard all milk pumped for the required time that radioactivity is present in milk. Milk samples can be screened by radiology department for radioactivity before resumption of nursing.

Psychotropic drugs, the compounds listed under antianxiety, antidepressant, and antipsychotic categories, are a special concern when given to nursing mothers for long periods. Although there are no case reports of adverse effects in breastfeeding infants, these drugs do appear in human milk and thus could conceivably alter short-term and long-term central nervous system function.[43]

Table 2APP–4   Drugs Whose Effect on Nursing Infants Is Unknown but May Be of Concern

Drug	Reported or Possible Effect	Ref. No.
Antianxiety		
Diazepam	None	44–46
Lorazepam	None	47
Midazolam	...	48
Perphenazine	None	49
Prazepam*	None	50
Quazepam	None	51
Temazepam	...	52
Antidepressants		
Amitriptyline	None	53, 54
Amoxapine	None	55
Desipramine	None	56, 57
Dothiepin	None	58, 59
Doxepin	None	60
Fluoxetine	...	61
Fluvoxamine	...	62
Imipramine	None	56
Trazodone	None	63
Antipsychotic		
Chlorpromazine	Galactorrhea in adult; drowsiness and lethargy in infant	64, 65
Chlorprothixene	None	66
Haloperidol	None	67, 68
Mesoridazine	None	69
Chloramphenicol	Possible idiosyncratic bone marrow suppression	70, 71
Metoclopramide*	None described; dopaminergic blocking agent	72, 73
Metronidazole	In vitro mutagen; may discontinue breastfeeding 12–24 hr to allow excretion of dose when single-dose therapy given to mother	74, 75
Tinidazole	See metronidazole	76

* Drug is concentrated in human milk.

Table 2APP–5   Drugs That Have Been Associated with Significant Effects on Some Nursing Infants and Should Be Given to Nursing Mothers with Caution

Drug*	Reported Effect	Ref. No.
5-Aminosalicylic acid	Diarrhea (1 case)	77, 78
Aspirin (salicylates)	Metabolic acidosis (1 case)	79–81
Clemastine	Drowsiness, irritability, refusal to feed, high-pitched cry, neck stiffness (1 case)	82
Phenobarbital	Sedation; infantile spasms after weaning from milk containing phenobarbital, methemoglobinemia (1 case)	83–87
Primidone	Sedation, feeding problems	83, 84
Sulfasalazine (salicyl-azosulfapyridine)	Bloody diarrhea (1 case)	88

*Measure blood concentration in the infant when possible.

Table 2APP–6 Maternal Medication Usually Compatible with Breastfeeding

Drug*	Reported Sign or Symptom in Infant or Effect on Lactation	Ref. No.
Acebutolol	None	89
Acetaminophen	None	90–92
Acetazolamide	None	93
Acitretin	...	94
Acyclovir[†]	None	95, 96
Alcohol (ethanol)	With large amounts drowsiness, diaphoresis, deep sleep, weakness, decrease in linear growth, abnormal weight gain; maternal ingestion of 1 g/kg daily decreases milk-ejection reflex	20, 97–100
Allopurinol	...	101
Amoxicillin	None	102
Antimony	...	103
Atenolol	None	104–106
Atropine	None	107
Azapropazone (apazone)	...	108
Aztreonam	None	109
B₁ (thiamin)	None	110
B₆ (pyridoxine)	None	111-113
B₁₂	None	114
Baclofen	None	115
Barbiturate	See Table 2APP–5	
Bendroflumethiazide	Suppresses lactation	116
Bishydroxycoumarin (dicumarol)	None	117
Bromide	Rash, weakness, absence of cry with maternal intake of 5.4 g/day	118
Butorphanol	None	119
Caffeine	Irritability, poor sleeping pattern, excreted slowly; no effect with usual amount of caffeine beverages	120–125
Captopril	None	126
Carbamazepine	None	127, 128
Carbimazole	Goiter	129, 130
Cascara	None	131
Cefadroxil	None	102
Cefazolin	None	132
Cefotaxime	None	133
Cefoxitin	None	133
Cefprozil	...	134
Ceftazidime	None	135
Ceftriaxone	None	136
Chloral hydrate	Sleepiness	137
Chloroform	None	138
Chloroquine	None	139–141
Chlorothiazide	None	142–143
Chlorthalidone	Excreted slowly	144
Cimetidine[†]	None	145
Cisapride	None	146
Cisplatin	Not found in milk	9
Clindamycin	None	147
Clogestone	None	148
Clomipramine	...	149
Codeine	None	92, 107
Colchicine	...	15
Contraceptive pill with estrogen/progesterone	Rare breast enlargement; decrease in milk production and protein content (not confirmed in several studies)	151–158

B_1 (thiamin), B_6 (pyridoxine), B_{12}

Table 2APP–6   *Continued*

Drug*	Reported Sign or Symptom in Infant or Effect on Lactation	Ref. No.
Cycloserine	None	159
D (Vitamin)	None; follow up infant's serum calcium level if mother receives pharmacological doses	160–162
Danthron	Increased bowel activity	163
Dapsone	None; sulfonamide detected in infant's urine	141, 164
Dexbrompheniramine maleate with *d*-isoephedrine	Crying, poor sleeping patterns, irritability	165
Digoxin	None	166, 167
Diltiazem	None	168
Dipyrone	None	169
Disopyramide	None	170–171
Domperidone	None	172
Dyphylline[1]	None	173
Enalapril	...	174
Erythromycin†	None	175
Estradiol	Withdrawal, vaginal bleeding	176
Ethambutol	None	159
Ethanol (cf. alcohol)	...	
Ethosuximide	None, drug appears in infant serum	127, 177
Fentanyl	...	178
Flecainide	...	179, 180
Flufenamic acid	None	181
Fluorescein	...	182
Folic acid	None	183
Gold salts	None	184–188
Halothane	None	189
Hydralazine	None	190
Hydrochlorothiazide	...	142, 143
Hydroxychloroquine†	None	191, 192
Ibuprofen	None	193, 194
Indomethacin	Seizure (1 case)	195–197
Iodides	May affect thyroid activity; see miscellaneous iodine	198
Iodine (providone-iodine/vaginal douche)	Elevated iodine levels in breastmilk, odor of iodine on infant's skin	198
Iodine	Goiter; see miscellaneous, iodine	198
Iopanoic acid	None	199
Isoniazid	None; acetyl metabolite also secreted; ? hepatotoxic	159, 200
K₁ (Vitamin)	None	201, 202
Kanamycin	None	159
Ketorolac	...	203
Labetalol	None	204, 205
Levonorgestrel	...	206–209
Lidocaine	None	210
Loperamide	...	211
Magnesium sulfate	None	212
Medroxyprogesterone	None	148
Mefenamic acid	None	213
Methadone	None if mother receiving ≤ 20 mg/24 h	214, 215
Methimazole (active metabolite of carbimazole)	None	216
Methocarbamol	None	217

continued

Table 2APP–6 Maternal Medication Usually Compatible with Breastfeeding *Continued*

Drug*	Reported Sign or Symptom in Infant or Effect on Lactation	Ref. No.
Methyldopa	None	218
Methyprylon	Drowsiness	219
Metoprolol†	None	104
Metrizamide	None	220
Mexiletine	None	221
Minoxidil	None	222
Morphine	None; infant may have significant blood concentration	223, 224
Moxalactam	None	225
Nadolol†	None	226
Nalidixic acid	Hemolysis in infant with glucose-6-phosphate dehydrogenase (G-6-PD) deficiency	227
Naproxen	...	228
Nefopam	None	229
Nifedipine	...	230
Nitrofurantoin	Hemolysis in infant with G-6-PD deficiency	231
Norethynodrel	None	232
Norsteroids	None	233
Noscapine	None	234
Oxprenolol	None	235, 236
Phenylbutazone	None	237
Phenytoin	Methemoglobinemia (1 case)	85, 127, 238
Piroxicam	None	239
Prednisone	None	241
Procainamide	None	242
Progesterone	None	243
Propoxyphene	None	244
Propranolol	None	245–247
Propylthiouracil	None	248
Pseudoephedrine†	None	249
Pyridostigmine	None	250
Pyrimethamine	None	141, 251
Quinidine	None	252
Quinine	None	223
Riboflavin	None	110
Rifampin	None	159
Scopolamine	...	107
Secobarbital	None	253
Senna	None	254
Sotalol	...	180, 255
Spironolactone	None	256
Streptomycin	None	159
Sulbactam	None	257
Sulfapyridine	Caution in infant with jaundice or G-6-PD deficiency, and ill, stressed, or premature infant; appears in infant's milk	258, 259
Sulfisoxazole	Caution in infant with jaundice or G-6-PD deficiency, and ill, stressed, or premature infant; appears in infant's milk	260
Suprofen	None	261
Terbutaline	None	262
Tetracycline	None; negligible absorption by infant	263, 264
Theophylline	Irritability	120, 265
Thiopental	None	86, 266
Thiouracil	None mentioned; drug not used in United States	267
Ticarcillin	None	268
Timolol	None	236

Table 2APP–6   *Continued*

Drug*	Reported Sign or Symptom in Infant or Effect on Lactation	Ref. No.
Tolbutamide	Possible jaundice	269
Tolmetin	None	270
Trimethoprim/ sulfamethoxazole	None	271, 272
Triprolidine	None	249
Valproic acid	None	127, 273, 274
Verapamil	None	275
Warfarin	None	276
Zolpidem	None	277

*Drugs listed have been reported in the literature as having the effects listed or no effect. The word *none* means that no observable change was seen in the nursing infant while the mother was ingesting the compound. It is emphasized that most of the literature citations concern single case reports or small series of infants.

†Drug is concentrated in human milk.

Table 2APP–7   Food and Environmental Agents: Effect on Breastfeeding

Agent	Reported Sign or Symptom in Infant or Effect on Lactation	Ref. No.
Aflatoxin	None	278–280
Aspartame	Caution if mother or infant has phenylketonuria	281
Bromide (photo-graphic laboratory)	Potential absorption and bromide transfer into milk; see Table 2APP–6	282
Cadmium	None reported	283
Chlordane	None reported	284
Chocolate (theobromine)	Irritability or increased bowel activity if excess amounts (16 oz./day) consumed by mother	120, 285
DDT, benzenehexa-chlorides, dieldrin, aldrin, hepata-chlorepoxide	None	286–293
Fava beans	Hemolysis in patient with glucose-6-phosphate dehydrogenase (G-6-PD) deficiency	294
Fluorides	None	295, 296
Hexachlorobenzene	Skin rash, diarrhea, vomiting, dark urine, neurotoxicity, death	297, 298
Hexachlorophene	None, possible contamination of milk from nipple washing	299
Lead	Possible neurotoxicity	300–301
Methyl mercury, mercury	May affect neurodevelopment	302–304
Monosodium glutamate	None	305
Polychlorinated biphenyls and polybrominated biphenyls	Lack of endurance, hypotonia, sullen expressionless faces	306–310
Tetrachlorethylene-cleaning fluid (perchloroethylene)	Obstructive jaundice, dark urine	311
Vegetarian diet	Signs of B_{12} deficiency	312

APPENDIX REFERENCES

1. American Academy of Pediatrics, Committee on Drugs. *Pediatrics*, 1983;72:375-383.
2. American Academy of Pediatrics, Committee on Drugs. *Pediatrics*, 1989;84:924-936.
3. Kulski JK, Hartmann PE, Martin JD, et al. *Obstet Gynecol*, 1978;52:38.
4. Katz M, Kroti D, Pak I, et al. *Obstet Gynecol*, 1985;66:822-824.
5. Chasnoff IJ, Lewis DE, Squires L. *Pediatrics*, 1987;80:836-838.
6. Wiernik PH, Duncan JH. *Lancet*, 1971;1:912.
7. Amato D, Niblett JS. *Med J Aust*, 1977;1:383.
8. Fletcher SM, Katz AR, Rogers AJ, et al. *Am J Kidney Dis*, 1985;5:60.
9. Egan PC, Costanza ME, Dodion P, et al. *Cancer Treat Rep*, 1985;69:1387.
10. Fomina PI. *Arch Gynecol*, 1934;157:279.
11. Schou M, Amdisen A. *Br Med J*, 1973;2:138.
12. Tunnessen WW Jr, Hertz C. *J Pediatr*, 1972;81:804.
13. Sykes PA, Quarrie J, Alexander FW. *Br Med J*, 1976;2:1299.
14. Johns DG, Rutherford LD, Leighton PC, et al. *Am J Obstet Gynecol*, 1972;112:978.
15. Kaufman KR, Petrucha RA, Pitts FN Jr, et al. *J Clin Psychiatry*, 1983;44:269.
16. Eckstein HB, Jack B. *Lancet*, 1970;1:672.
17. Steiner E, Villen T, Hallberg M, et al. *Eur J Clin Pharmacol*, 1984;27:123.
18. Cobrinik RW, Hood RT Jr, Chusid E. *Pediatrics*, 1959;24:288.
19. Perez-Reyes M, Wall ME. *N Engl J Med*, 1982;307:819.
20. Bisdom W. *JAMA*, 1937;109:178.
21. Ferguson BB, Wilson DJ, Schaffner W. *AJDC*, 1976;130:837.
22. Luck W, Nau H. *Eur J Pediatr*, 1987:146:21-26.
23. Luck W, Nau H. *Br J Clin Pharmacol*, 1984;18:9-15.
24. Luck W, Nau H. *J Pediatr*, 1985;107:816-820.
25. Labrecque M, Marcoux S, Weber J-P, et al. *Pediatrics*, 1989;83:93-97.
26. Schwartz-Bickenbach D, Schulte-Hobein B, Abt S, et al. *Toxicol Lett*, 1987;35:73-81.
27. McArdle HJ, Danks DM. *J Trace Elem Exp Med*, 1991;4:81-84.
28. Tobin RE, Schneider PB. *J Nucl Med*, 1976;17:1055.
29. Butt O, Szaz KF. *Br J Radiol*, 1986;59:80.
30. Hedrick WR, DiSimone RN, Keen RL. *J Nucl Med*,1986;27:1569-1571.
31. Palmer KE. *Br J Radiol*, 1979;52:672.
32. Honour AJ, Myant NB, Rowlands EN. *Clin Sci*, 1952;11:447.
33. Karjalainen P, Penttila LM, Pystynen P. *Acta Obstet Gynecol Scand*, 1971;50:357.
34. Bland EP, Crawford JS, Docker MF, et al. *Lancet*, 1969;2:1039.
35. Nurnberger CE, Lipscomb A. *JAMA*, 1952;150:1398.
36. Pommerenke WT, Hahn PF. *Proc Soc Exp Biol Med*, 1943;52:223.
37. O'Connell MEA, Sutton H. *Br J Radiol*, 1976;49:377.
38. Berke RA, Hoops EC, Kereiakes JC, et al. *J Nucl Med*,1973;14:51.
39. Vagenakis AG, Abreau CM, Braverman LE. *J Nucl Med*, 1971;12:188.
40. Wyburn JR. *J Nucl Med*, 1973;14:115.
41. Pittard WB III, Merkatz R, Fletcher BD. *Pediatrics*, 1982;70:231.
42. Maisels MJ, Gilcher RO. *Pediatrics*, 1983;71:841.
43. American Academy of Pediatrics, Committee on Drugs. *Pediatrics*, 1982;69:241-244.
44. Patrick MJ, Tilstone WJH, Reavey P. *Lancet*, 1972;1:542.
45. Cole AP, Hailey DM. *Arch Dis Child*, 1975;50:741.
46. Dusci LJ, Goods M, Hall RW, et al. *Br J Clin Pharmacol*, 1990;29:123-126.
47. Summerfield RJ, Nielson MS. *Br J Anaesth*, 1985;57:1042.
48. Matheson L, Lunde PK, Bredesan JE. *Br J Clin Pharmacol*, 1990;30:787-793.
49. Olesen OV, Bartels U, Poulsen JH. *Am J Psychiatry*, 1990;147:1378-1379.
50. Brodie RR, Chasseaud LF, Taylor T. *Biopharm Drug Dispos*, 1981;2:59.
51. Hilbert JM, Gural RP, Symchowicz S, et al. *J Clin Pharmacol*, 1984;24:457.
52. Lebedevs TH, Wojnar-Horton RE, Yapp P, et al. *Br J Clin Pharmacol*, 1992;33:204-206.
53. Bader TF, Newman K. *Am J Psychiatry*, 1980;137:855.
54. Erickson SH, Smith GH, Heidrich T. *Am J Psychiatry*, 1979;136:1483.
55. Gelenberg AJ. *J Nerv Ment Dis*, 1979;167:635.

56. Sovner R, Orsulak PJ. *Am J Psychiatry*,1979;136:451.
57. Stancer HC, Reed KL. *Am J Psychiatry*, 1986;143:1597.
58. Rees JA, Glass RC, Sporne GA. *Practitioner*, 1976;217:686.
59. Ilett KF, Lebedevs TH, Wojnar-Horton RE, et al. *Br J Clin Pharmacol*,1992;33:635-639.
60. Kemp J, Ilett KF, Booth J, et al. *Br J Clin Pharmacol*, 1988;20:497.
61. Burch KJ, Wells BG. *Pediatrics*, 1992;88:676-677.
62. Wright S, Dawling S, Ashford JJ. *Br J Clin Pharmacol*, 1991;31:209.
63. Verbeeck RK, Ross SG, McKenna EA. *Br J Clin Pharmacol*, 1986;22:367.
64. Polishuk WZ, Kulcsar SA. *J Clin Endocrinol Metab*, 1956;16:292.
65. Wiles DH, Orr MW, Kolakowska T. *Br J Clin Pharmacol*, 1978;5:272.
66. Matheson I, Evang A, Fredricson Overo K, et al. *Eur J Clin Pharmacol*, 1984;27:611.
67. Stewart RB, Karas B, Springer PK. *Am J Psychiatry*, 1980;137:849.
68. Whalley LJ, Blain PG, Prime JK. *Br Med J*, 1981;282:1746.
69. Ananth J. *Am J Psychiatry*, 1978;135:801.
70. Havelka J, Hejzlar M, Popov V. *Chemotherapy*, 1968;13:204.
71. Smadel JE, Woodward TE, Ley HL Jr, et al. *J Clin Invest*, 1949;28:1196.
72. Gupta AP, Gupta PK. *Clin Pediatr*, 1985; 24:269.
73. Kauppela A, Arvela P, Kolvisto M, et al. *Eur J Clin Pharmacol*, 1983;25:819.
74. Erickson SH, Oppenheim GL, Smith GL. *Obstet Gynecol*, 1981;57:48.
75. Heisterberg L, Branebjerg PE. *J Perinat Med*, 1983;11:114.
76. Evaldson GR, Lindgren S, Nord CE, et al. *Br J Clin Pharmacol*, 1985;19:503.
77. Nelis GF. *Lancet*,1989;383.
78. Jenss M, Weber P, Hartmann F. *Am J Gastroenterol*, 1990;85:331.
79. Clark JH, Wilson WG. *Clin Pediatr*, 1981;20:53.
80. Levy G. *Basic and Therapeutic Aspects of Perinatal Pharmacol*, 1975:311.
81. Fakhredding J, Keshavarz E. *Int J Pharm*, 1981;8:285.
82. Kok THHG, Taitz LS, Bennett MJ. *Lancet*, 1982;1:914.
83. Nua H, Ratlig D, Hauser I, et al. *Eur J Clin Pharmacol*, 1980;18:31.
84. Kuhnz W, Koch S, Helge H, et al., *Dev Pharmacol Ther*, 1988;11:147.
85. Finch E, Lorber J. *J Obstet Gynaecol Br Emp*, 1954;61:833.
86. Tyson RM, Shrader EA, Perlman HH. *J Pediatr*, 1938;13:86.
87. Knott C, Reynolds F, Clayden G. *Lancet*, 1987;2:272.
88. Branski D, Kerem E, Gross-Kieselstein E, et al. *J Pediatr Gastroenterol Nutr*, 1986;5:316.
89. Boutroy MJ, Bianchetti G, Dubruc C, et al. *Eur J Clin Pharmacol*, 1986;30:737.
90. Berlin CM Jr, Yaffe SJ, Ragni M. *Pediatr Pharmacol*, 1980;1:135.
91. Bitzen PO, Gustafsson B, Jostell KG, et al. *Eur J Clin Pharmacol*, 1981;20:123.
92. Findlay JWA, DeAngelis RL, Kearney MF, et al. *Clin Pharmacol Ther*, 1981;29:625.
93. Soderman P, Hartvig P, Fagerlund C. *Br J Clin Pharmacol*, 1984;17:599.
94. Rollman O, Pihl-Lundin I. *Acta Derm Venereol (Stockh)*, 1990;70:487-490.
95. Lau RJ, Emery MG, Galinsky RE. *Obstet Gynecol*, 1987;69:468-471.
96. Meyer LJ, de Miranda P, Sheth N, et al. *Am J Obstet Gynecol*, 1988;158:586-588.
97. Binkiewicz A, Robinson MJ, Senior B. *J Pediatr*, 1978;93:965.
98. Cobo E. *Am J Obstet Gynecol*, 1973;115:817.
99. Kesaniemi YA. *J Obstet Gynaecol Br Comm*, 1974;81:84.
100. Little RE, Anderson KW, Ervin CH, et al. *N Engl J Med*, 1989;321:425-430.
101. Kamilli I, Gresser U, Schaefer C., et al. *Adv Exp Med Biol*, 1991;309A:143-145.
102. Kafetzis DA, Siafas CA, Georgakopoulos PA, et al. *Acta Paediatr Scand*, 1981;70:285.
103. Berman JD, Melby PC, Neva FA. *Trans R Soc Trop Med Hyg*, 1989;83:784-785.
104. Liedholm H, Melander A, Bitzen P-O, et al. *Eur J Clin Pharmacol*, 1981;20:229.
105. Schimmel MS, Edelman AI, Wilschanski MA, et al. *J Pediatr*, 1989;114:476-478.
106. Thorley KJ, McAinsh J. *Biopharm Drug Dispos*, 1983;4:299-301.
107. Sapeika N. *J Obstet Gynaecol Br Comm*, 1947;54:426.
108. Bald R, Bernbeck-Betthauser E-M, Spahn H, et al. *Eur J Clin Pharmacol*, 1990;39:271-273.
109. Fleiss PM, Richwald GA, Gordon J, et al. *Br J Clin Pharmacol*, 1985;19:509.
110. Nail PA, Thomas MR, Eakin R. *Am J Clin Nutr*, 1980;33:198.
111. Roepke JLB, Kirksey A. *Am J Clin Nutr*, 1979;32:2249.
112. West KD, Kirksey A. *Am J Clin Nutr*, 1976;29:961.
113. Greentree LB. *N Engl J Med*, 1979; 300:141.

Appendix References   *Continued*

114. Samson RR, McClelland DBL. *Acta Paediatr Scand,* 1980;69:93.
115. Eriksson G, Swahn CG. *Scand J Clin Lab Invest,* 1981;41:185.
116. Healy M. *Lancet,* 1961;1:1353.
117. Brambel CE, Hunter RE. *Am J Obstet Gynecol,* 1950;39:1153.
118. Tyson RM, Shrader EA, Perlman HH. *J Pediatr,* 1938;13:91.
119. Pittman KA, Smyth RD, Losada M, et al. *Am J Obstet Gynecol,* 1980;138:797.
120. Berlin CM Jr. *Semin Perinatol,* 1981;5:389.
121. Tyrala EE, Dodson WE. *Arch Dis Child,* 1979;54:787.
122. Hildebrandt R, Gundert-Remy V. *Pediatr Pharmacol,* 1983;3:237.
123. Berlin CM Jr, Denson HM, Daniel CH, Ward RM. *Pediatrics,* 1984;73:59-63.
124. Ryu JE. *Dev Pharmacol Ther,* 1985;8:329.
125. Ryu JE. *Dev Pharmacol Ther,* 1985;8:355.
126. Devlin, RG, Fleiss PM. *J Clin Pharmacol,* 1981;21:110.
127. Nau H, Kuhnz W, Egger JH, et al. *Clin Pharmacokinet,* 1982;7:508.
128. Pynnonen S, Kanto J, Sillanpaa M, et al. *Acta Pharmacol Toxocol,* 1977;41:244.
129. Cooper DS. *Am J Obstet Gynecol,* 1987;157:234.
130. Lamberg B-A, Ikonen E, Österlund K, et al. *Clin Endocrinol,* 1984;21:81-87.
131. Tyson RM, Shrader EA, Perlman HH. *J Pediatr,* 1937;11:824.
132. Yoshioka H, Cho K, Takimoto M, et al. *J Pediatr,* 1979;94:151.
133. Dresse A, Lambotte R, Dubois M, et al. *J Clin Pharmacol,* 1983;23:438.
134. Shyu WC, Shah VR, Campbell DA, et al. *Antimicrob Agents Chemother,* 1992;36:938-941.
135. Blanco JD, Jorgensen JH, Casteneda YS, et al. *Antimicrob Agents Chemother,* 1983;23:479.
136. Kafetzis DA, Brater DC, Fanourgakis JE, et al. *Antimicrob Agents Chemother,* 1983;23:870.
137. Lacey JH. *Br Med J,* 1971;4:684.
138. Reed CB. *Surg Gynecol Obstet,* 1908;6:514.
139. Soares R, Paulini E, Pereira JP. *Rev Bras Malariol Doencas Trop,* 1957;9:19.
140. Ogunbona FA, Onyizi CO, Bolaji OO, et al. *Br J Clin Pharmacol,* 1987;23:476.
141. Edstein MD, Veenendaal JR, Newman K, et al. *Br J Clin Pharmacol,* 1986;22:733.
142. Werthmann MW Jr, Krees SV. *J Pediatr,* 1972;81:781.
143. Miller EM, Cohn RD, Burghart PH. *J Pediatr,* 1982;101:789.
144. Mulley BA, Parr GD, Pau WK, et al. *Eur J Clin Pharmacol,* 1978;13:129.
145. Somogyi A, Gugler R. *Br J Clin Pharmacol,* 1979;7:627.
146. Hofmeyr GJ, Sonnendecker EWW. *Eur J Clin Pharmacol,* 1986;30:735.
147. Smith JA, Morgan JR, Rachlis AR, et al. *Can Med Assoc J,* 1975;112:806.
148. Zacharias S, Aguillern E, Assenzo JR, et al. *Contraception,* 1986;33:203.
149. Schimmell MS, Katz EZ, Shaag Y, et al. *J Toxicol Clin Toxicol,* 1991;29:479-484.
150. Milunsky JM. *J Pediatr,* 1991;119:164.
151. Nilsson S, Mellbin T, Hofvander Y, et al. *Contraception,* 1986;34:443.
152. Nilsson S, Nygren KG. *Res Reprod,* 1979;11:1.
153. American Academy of Pediatrics, Committee on Drugs. *Pediatrics,* 1981;68:138-140.
154. Barsivala VM, Virkar KD. *Contraception,* 1973;7:307.
155. Borglin NE, Sandholm LE. *Fertil Steril,* 1971;22:39.
156. Curtis EM. *Obstet Gynecol,* 1964;23:295.
157. Kora SJ. *Fertil Steril,* 1969;20:419.
158. Toaff R, Ashkenazi H, Schwartz A, et al. *J Reprod Fertil,* 1969;19:475.
159. Snyder DR Jr, Powell KE. *Arch Intern Med,* 1984;144:589.
160. Cancela L, LeBoulch N, Miravet L. *J Endocrinol,* 1986;110:43.
161. Rothberg AD, Pettifor JM, Cohen DF, et al. *J Pediatr,* 1982;101:500.
162. Greer FR, Hollis BW, Napoli JL. *J Pediatr,* 1984;105:61.
163. Greenhalf JO, Leonard HSD. *Practitioner,* 1973;210:259.
164. Dreisbach JA. *Lepr Rev,* 1952;23:101.
165. Mortimer EA Jr. *Pediatrics,* 1977;60:780.
166. Loughnan PM. *J Pediatr,* 1978;92:1019.
167. Levy M, Granit L, Laufer N. *N Engl J Med,* 1977;297:789.
168. Okada M, Inoue H, Nakamura T, et al. *N Engl J Med,* 1985;312:992.
169. Zylber-Katz E, Linder N, Granit L, et al. *Eur J Clin Pharmacol,* 1986;30:359.

170. MacKintosh D, Buchanan N. *Br J Clin Pharmacol*, 1985;19:856.

171. Hoppu K, Neuvonen PJ, Korte T. *Br J Clin Pharmacol*, 1986;21:533.

172. Hofmeyr GJ, van Idlekinge B. *Lancet*, 1983;1:647.

173. Jorboe CH, Cook LN, Malesic I, et al. *J Clin Pharmacol*, 1981;21:405.

174. Redman CW, Kelly JG, Cooper WD. *Eur J Clin Pharmacol*, 1990;38:99.

175. Matsuda S. *Biol Res Pregnancy*, 1984;5:57.

176. Nilsson S, Nygren KG, Johansson EDB. *Am J Obstet Gynecol*, 1978;132:653.

177. Koup JR, Rose JQ, Cohen ME. *Epilepsia*, 1978;19:535.

178. Steer PL, Biddle CJ, Marley WS, et al. *Can J Anaesth*, 1992;39:231-235.

179. McQuinn RL, Pisani A, Wafa S, et al. *Clin Pharmacol Ther*, 1990;48:262-267.

180. Wagner X, Jouglard J, Moulin M, et al. *Am Heart J*, 1990;119:700-702.

181. Buchanan RA, Eaton CJ, Koeff ST, et al. *Curr Ther Res*, 1969;11:533.

182. Mattern J, Mayer PR. *Am J Ophthalmol*, 1990;109:598-599.

183. Retief EF, Heyns ADuP, Oosthuizen M, et al. *Am J Med Sci*, 1979;277:281.

184. Bell RAF, Dale IM. *Arthritis Rheum*, 1976;19:1374.

185. Blau SP. *Arthritis Rheum*, 1973;16:777.

186. Gottlieb NL. *Arthritis Rheum*, 1974;17:1057.

187. Ostensen M, Skavdal K, Myklebust G, et al. *Eur J Clin Pharmacol*, 1986;316:251.

188. Bennett PN, Humphries SJ, Osborne JP, et al. *Br J Clin Pharmacol*, 1990;29:777-779.

189. Cote CJ, Kenepp NB, Reed SB, et al. *Br J Anaesth*, 1976;48:541.

190. Liedholm H, Wahlin-Boll E, Hanson A, et al. *Eur J Clin Pharmacol*, 1982;21:417.

191. Ostensen M, Brown ND, Chiang PK, et al. *Eur J Clin Pharmacol*, 1985;28:357.

192. Nation RL, Hackett LP, Dusci LJ, et al. *Br J Clin Pharmacol*, 1984;17:368.

193. Townsend RJ, Benedetti T, Erickson SH, et al. *Drug Intell Clin Pharm*, 1982;16:482.

194. Townsend RJ, Benedetti TJ, Erickson SH, et al. *Am J Obstet Gynecol*, 1984;149:184.

195. Eeg-Olofsson O, Malmros I, Elwin CE, et al. *Lancet*, 1978;2:215.

196. Fairhead FW. *Lancet*, 1978;2:576.

197. Lebedevs TH, Wojnar-Horton RE, Yapp P, et al. *Br J Clin Pharmacol*, 1991;32:751-754.

198. Postellon DC, Aronow R. *JAMA*, 1982;247:463.

199. Holmdahl KH. *Acta Radiol*, 1955;45:305.

200. Berlin CM Jr, Lee C. *Fed Proc*, 1979;38:426.

201. Dyggve HV, Dam H, Sondergaard E. *Acta Obstet Gynecol Scand*, 1956;35:440.

202. Kries RV, Shearer M, McCarthy PT, et al. *Pediatr Res*, 1987;22:513.

203. Wischnik A, Manth SM, Lloyd J, et al. *Eur J Clin Pharmacol*, 1989:36:521-524.

204. Lunell HO, Kulas J, Rane A. *Eur J Clin Pharmacol*, 1985;28:597.

205. Atkinson H, Bogg EJ. *J Pediatr*, 1990;116:156.

206. Diaz S, Herreros C, Juez G, et al. *Contraception*, 1985:32:53-74.

207. Shaaban MM, Odlind V, Salem HT, et al. *Contraception*, 1986;33:357-363.

208. Shikary ZK, Betrabet SS, Patel ZM, et al. *Contraception*, 1987;35:477-486.

209. McCann MF, Moggia AV, Higgins JE, et al. *Contraception*, 1989;40:635-648.

210. Zeisler JA, Gaarder TD, DeMesquita SA. *Drug Intell Clin Pharm*, 1986;20:691.

211. Nikodem VC, Hofmeyr GJ. *Eur J Clin Pharmacol*, 1992;42:695-696.

212. Cruikshank DP, Varner MW, Pitkin RM. *Am J Obstet Gynecol*, 1982;143:685.

213. Buchanan RA, Eaton CJ, Koeff ST, et al. *Curr Ther Res Clin Exp*, 1968;10:592.

214. Blinick G, Inturrisi CE, Jerez E, et al. *Am J Obstet Gynecol*, 1975;121:617.

215. Blinick G, Wallach RC, Jerez E, et al. *Am J Obstet Gynecol*, 1976;125:135.

216. Cooper DS, Bode HH, Nath B, et al. *J Clin Endocrinol Metab*, 1984;58:473.

217. Campbell AD, Coles FK, Eubank LLK, et al. *J Pharmacol Exp Ther*, 1961;131:18.

218. White WB, Andreoli JW, Cohn RD. *Clin Pharmacol Ther*, 1985;37:387.

219. Shore MF. *Can Pharm J*, 1970;103:358.

220. Ilett KF, Hackett LP. *Br J Radiol*, 1981;54:537.

221. Lownes HE, Ives TJ. *Am J Obstet Gynecol*, 1987;157:446.

222. Valdivieso A, Valdes G, Spiro TE, et al. *Ann Intern Med*, 1985;102:135.

223. Terwilliger WG, Hatcher RA. *Surg Gynecol Obstet*, 1934;58:823.

224. Robieux I, Koren G, Vandenbergh H, et al. *J Toxicol Clin Toxicol*, 1990;28:365-370.

225. Miller RD, Keegan KA, Thrupp LD, et al. *Am J Obstet Gynecol*, 1984;148:348.

226. Devlin RG, Duchin KL, Fleiss, PM. *Br J Clin Pharmacol*, 1981;12:393.

227. Belton EM, Jones RV. *Lancet*, 1965;2:691.

Appendix References *Continued*

228. Jamali P, Tam YK, Stevens RD. *Drug Intell Clin Pharm*, 1982;16.
229. Liu DTY, Savage JM, Donnell D. *Br J Clin Pharmacol*, 1987;23:99.
230. Ehrenkranz RA, Ackerman BA, Hulse JD. *J Pediatr*, 1989;114:478-480.
231. Varsano I, Fischl J, Tikvah P, et al. *J Pediatr*, 1973;82:886.
232. Laumas KR, Malkani PK, Bhatnagar S, et al. *Am J Obstet Gynecol*, 1967;98:411.
233. Pincus G, Bialy G, Layne DS, et al. *Nature*, 1966;212:924.
234. Olsson B, Bolme P, Dahlstrom B, et al. *Eur J Clin Pharmacol*, 1986;30:213.
235. Sioufi A, Hillion D, Lumbroso P, et al. *Br J Clin Pharmacol*, 1984;18:453.
236. Fidler J, Smith V, DeSwiet M. *Br J Obstet Gynaecol*, 1983;90:961.
237. Leuxner E, Pulver R. *MMW*, 1956;98:84.
238. Mirkin B. *J Pediatr*, 1971;78:329.
239. Ostensen M. *Eur J Clin Pharmacol*, 1983;25:829.
240. McKenzie SA, Selley JA, Agnew JE. *Arch Dis Child*, 1975;50:894.
241. Katz FH, Duncan BR. *N Engl J Med*, 1975;293:1154.
242. Pittard WB III, Glazier H. *J Pediatr*, 1983;102:631.
243. Diaz S, Jackanicz TM, Herreros C, et al. *Contraception*, 1985;32:603.
244. Kunka RL, Venkataramanan R, Stern RM, et al. *Clin Pharmacol Ther*, 1984;35:675.
245. Levitan AA, Manion JC. *Am J Cardiol*, 1973;32:247.
246. Karlberg B, Lundberg D, Aberg H. *Acta Pharmacol Toxicol*, 1974;34:222.
247. Bauer JH, Pape B, Zajicek J, et al. *Am J Cardiol*, 1979;43:860.
248. Kampmann JP, Johansen K, Hansen JM, et al. *Lancet*, 1980;1:736.
249. Findlay JWA, Butz RF, Sailstad JM, et al. *Br J Clin Pharmacol*, 1984;18:901.
250. Hardell L-I, Lindstom B, Lonnerholm G, et al. *Br J Clin Pharmacol*, 1982;14:656.
251. Clyde DF, Shute GT, Press J. *J Trop Med Hyg*, 1956; 59:277.
252. Hill LM, Malkasian GD Jr. *Obstet Gynecol*, 1979;54:366.
253. Horning MG, Stillwell WG, Nowlin J, et al. *Mod Probl Paediatr*, 1975;15:73.
254. Werthmann MW, Krees SV. *Med Ann DC*, 1973;42:4.
255. Hackett LP, Wojnar-Horton RE, Dusci LJ, et al. *Br J Clin Pharmacol*, 1990;29:277-278.
256. Phelps DL, Karim A. *J Pharm Sci*, 1977;66:1203.
257. Foulds G, Miller RD, Knirsch AK, et al. *Clin Pharmacol Ther*, 1985;38:692.
258. Jarnerot G, Into-Malmberg MB. *Scand J Gastroenterol*, 1979;14:869.
259. Berlin CM Jr, Yaffe SJ. *Dev Pharmacol Ther*, 1980;1:31.
260. Kauffman RE, O'Brien C, Gilford P. *J Pediatr*, 1980;97:839.
261. Chaiken P, Chasin M, Kennedy B, et al. *J Clin Pharmacol*, 1983;23:385.
262. Lindberberg C, Boreus LO, DeChateau P, et al. *Eur J Respir Dis*, 1984;65:87.
263. *Br Med J*, 1969;4:791.
264. Posner AC, Prigot A, Konicoff NG. *Antibiotics Annual, 1954-1955*, 1955:594.
265. Yurchak AM, Jusko WJ. *Pediatrics*, 1976;57:518.
266. Anderson LW, Qvist T, Hertz J, et al. *Acta Anaesthesiol Scand*, 1987;31:30.
267. Williams RH, Kay GA, Jandorf BJ. *J Clin Invest*, 1944;23:613.
268. Von Kobyletzki D, Dalhoff A, Lindemayer H, et al. *Infection*, 1983;11:144.
269. Moiel RH, Ryan JR, *Clin Pediatr*, 1967;6:480.
270. Sagranes R, Waller ES, Goehrs HR. *Drug Intell Clin Pharm*, 1985;19:55.
271. Arnauld R. *Ouest Med*, 1972;25:959.
272. Miller RD, Salter AJ. *Hellenic Soc Chemother*, 1974;1:687.
273. Alexander FW. *Arch Dis Child*, 1979;54:240.
274. Von Unruh GE, Froescher W, Hoffman F, et al. *Ther Drug Monit*, 1984;6:272.
275. Anderson P, Bondesson UP, Mattiasson I, et al. *Eur J Clin Pharmacol*, 1987;31:625.
276. Orme ML'E, Lewis PJ. *Br Med J*, 1977;1:1564.
277. Pons G, Francoual C, Guillet P, et al. *Eur J Clin Pharmacol*, 1989;37:245-248.
278. Wild CP, Pionneau FA, Montesano R, et al. *Int J Cancer*, 1987;40:328.
279. Maxwell SM, Apeagyei F, de Vries HR, et al. *J Toxicol Toxin Rev*, 1989;8:19-29.
280. Zarba A, Wild CP, Hall AJ, et al. *Carcinogenesis*, 1992;13:891-894.
281. Steglink LD, Filer LJ Jr, Baker BL. *J Nutr*, 1979;109:2173.
282. Mangurten HH, Kaye CI. *J Pediatr*, 1982;100:596.
283. Radisch B, Luck W, Nau H. *Toxicol Lett*, 1987;36:147.

284. Miyazaki T, Akiyama K, Kaneko S, et al. *Bull Environ Contam Toxicol*, 1980;25:518.
285. Resman BH, Blumenthal HP, Jusko WJ. *J Pediatr*, 1977;91:477.
286. Wolff MS. *Am J Ind Med*, 1983;4:259.
287. Egan H, Goulding R, Roburn J, et al. *Br Med J*, 1965;2:66.
288. Quinby GE, Armstrong JF, Durham WF. *Nature*, 1965;207:726.
289. Bakken AF, Seip M. *Acta Paediatr Scand*, 1976;65:535.
290. Adamovic VM, Sokic B, Smiljanski MJ. *Bull Environ Contam Toxicol*, 1978;20:280.
291. Savage EP, Keefe TJ, Tessari JD, et al. *Am J Epidemiol*, 1981;113:413.
292. Wilson DJ, Locker DJ, Ritzen CA, et al. *AJDC*, 1973;125:814.
293. Bouwman H, Becker PJ, Cooppan RM, et al. *Bull World Health Organ*, 1992;70:241-250.
294. Emanuel B, Schoenfeld A. *J Pediatr*, 1961;58:263.
295. Simpson WJ, Tuba J. *J Oral Med*, 1968;23:104.
296. Esala S, Vuori E, Helle A. *Br J Nutr*, 1982;48:201.
297. Dreyfus-See G. *Rev Med Interne*, 1934;51:198.
298. Ando M, Hirano S, Itoh Y. *Arch Toxicol*, 1985;56:195.
299. West RW, Wilson DJ, Schaffner W. *Bull Environ Contam Toxicol*, 1975;13:167.
300. Rabinowitz M, Leviton A, Needelman H. *Arch Environ Health*, 1985;40:283.
301. Sternowsky JH, Wessolowski R. *Arch Toxicol*, 1985;57:41.
302. Koos BJ, Longo LD. *Am J Obstet Gynecol*, 1976;126:390.
303. Amin-Zaki L, Elhassani S, Majeed MA, et al. *J Pediatr*, 1974;85:81.
304. Pitkin RM, Bahns JA, Filer LA Jr, et al. *Proc Soc Exp Biol Med*, 1976;151:565.
305. Stegink LD, Filer LJ Jr, Baker GL. *Proc Soc Exp Biol Med*, 1972;140:836.
306. Miller RW. *J Pediatr*, 1977;90:510.
307. Rogan WJ, Bogniewska A, Damstra T. *N Engl J Med*, 1980;302:1450.
308. Wickizer TM, Brilliant LB, Copeland R, et al. *Am J Public Health*, 1981;71:132.
309. Brilliant LB, Van Amburg G, Isbister J, et al. *Lancet*, 1978;2:643.
310. Wickizer TM, Brilliant LB. *Pediatrics*, 1981;68:411-415.
311. Bagnell PC, Ellenberg HA. *Can Med Assoc J*, 1977;117:1047.
312. Higginbottom MC, Sweetman L, Nyhan WL. *N Engl J Med*, 1978;299:317.

POST-TEST

For questions 1 to 16, choose the best answer.

1. The breastmilk of women with cystic fibrosis and hyperlipoproteinemia may have a change in
   A. milk protein composition.
   B. milk glucose level.
   C. milk fat composition.
   D. There is no alteration.

2. A woman with diabetes mellitus may have delayed lactogenesis when
   A. serum glucose levels are within normal ranges.
   B. she is taking NPH insulin.
   C. serum citrate levels are high.
   D. serum glucose levels are not within normal ranges.

3. Which is true of the bone mineral density of well-nourished nonadolescent women living in the United States?
   A. There is increased bone density during pregnancy and lactation
   B. There is decreased bone density during pregnancy and increased bone density during lactation.
   C. There is decreased bone density during pregnancy and lactation but density is recovered after weaning.
   D. There is increased bone density during pregnancy and decreased bone density during lactation.

4. Which condition affecting the infant may be of concern to women with silicone breast implants?
   A. Iron deficiency anemia
   B. Atypical connective tissue disease
   C. Multiple sclerosis
   D. Atopic eczema

5. A mother with cytomegalovirus (CMV) could breastfeed
   A. a premature infant with low levels of antibodies.
   B. a full-term healthy infant.
   C. an immunocompromised infant.
   D. A mother with CMV should not breastfeed.

6. To what extent can a woman with phenylketonuria breastfeed her infant?
   A. She can totally breastfeed.
   B. She can partially breastfeed.
   C. She cannot breastfeed.

7. The disorder associated with lactation failure is
   A. galactosemia.
   B. phenylketonuria.
   C. Sheehan's syndrome.
   D. hyperlipoproteinemia.

8. There is a reduction in linoleic acid in the breastmilk of mothers with

    A. phenylketonuria.
    B. diabetes mellitus.
    C. galactosemia.
    D. cystic fibrosis.

9. Which is true of a lactating woman with diabetes mellitus?

    A. There is an increased risk of mastitis and Candida infection.
    B. There is an alteration of the fatty acid content of the breastmilk.
    C. There is an alteration of the amino acid content of the breastmilk.
    D. There is a decrease in the protein content of the breastmilk.

10. Which statement best defines galactorrhea?

    A. A metabolic disturbance of galactose
    B. Presence of galactose in stools
    C. Secretion of fluid containing lactose and fat independent of pregnancy
    D. Presence of galactose in urine

11. An immunnoglobulin and vaccine has been developed for

    A. cytomegalovirus.
    B. hepatitis C.
    C. hepatitis B.
    D. Epstein-Barr virus.

12. Which statement is true for the HIV seropositive woman?

    A. The HIV seropositive woman should breastfeed in developed and developing countries.
    B. The HIV seropositive woman should breastfeed only if she lives in a developed country.
    C. The HIV seropositive woman should breastfeed only if she lives in a developing country.
    D. The HIV seropositive woman should not breastfeed at all.

13. Which contraceptives are recommended to use during lactation?

    A. Condoms
    B. Norplant
    C. Estrogen-containing birth control pills
    D. A and B

14. A woman using the Lactational Amenorrhea Method should not

    A. limit breastfeeding sessions.
    B. breastfeed at night.
    C. delay introduction of supplements.

15. Bromocriptine will _____ lactation; metoclopramide will _____ milk production.

    A. inhibit; inhibit
    B. stimulate; inhibit
    C. inhibit; stimulate
    D. stimulate; stimulate

16. _____ will not transfer readily into human milk.
    A. Compounds having low-molecular weight
    B. Compounds whose milk-to-plasma ratio is less than 1
    C. Compounds that have high lipid solubility
    D. Compounds that are nonionized at a maternal pH of 7.4

For questions 17 to 20, identify the best answer from the following key:

A. Breastfeeding is contraindicated.

B. Breastfeeding is allowed.

17. Inactive herpes simplex virus

18. Hepatitis B

19. HIV-1 seropositive living in a developing country

20. HIV-1 seropositive living in a developed country

SECTION B

Infant Health Issues

Robin McRoberts, MS, RD/LD
Rebecca F. Black, MS, RD/LD, IBCLC
Richard A. Simpson, DMD
Bryn Hamilton, RD/LD, IBCLC

LEARNING OBJECTIVES

At the completion of this section, the learner will be able to do the following:

1. Describe techniques for maintaining the infant's thermal regulation.
2. Discuss the prevention and treatment of newborn hypoglycemia.
3. Differentiate among the types of jaundice and discuss care for the breast-feeding infant who has hyperbilirubinemia.
4. Cite the research on infections in breast- versus bottle-feeding populations.
5. Recognize symptoms of growth deficit, or failure to thrive, and cite three interventions.
6. State biochemical guidelines for the assessment of iron deficiency anemia.
7. Discuss the factors that contribute to optimal infant oral health care.

OUTLINE

I. Clinical Conditions That Cause Concern During the Neonatal Period

    A. Thermal regulation

    B. Neonatal hypoglycemia

    C. Neonatal hyperbilirubinemia
       1. Development of hyperbilirubinemia
       2. Physiologic jaundice
       3. Pathologic jaundice

4. Breastfeeding jaundice
5. Breastmilk jaundice (late-onset jaundice)

II. Infant Infections and Breastfeeding

   A. Morbidity and mortality rates

   B. Sepsis

   C. Respiratory illness

   D. Botulism

   E. Urinary tract infections

   F. Gastroenteritis and diarrhea

   G. Otitis media

   H. Miscellaneous other infections, diseases

III. Infant Oral Health Care

   A. Oral hygiene for the breastfeeding infant

   B. Fluoride administration and supplementation

   C. Dental caries and nutrition

   D. Breastfeeding and dental caries

   E. Teething

   F. Nonnutritive sucking

   G. Injury prevention

   H. The first dental exam

IV. Conditions of Nutritional Concern

   A. Failure to thrive—growth deficit
      1. Evaluation for FTT—growth deficit
      2. Diagnosis of breastfed infants' FTT—growth deficit
      3. Maternal problems that can cause FTT—growth deficit
      4. Infant problems that can cause FTT—growth deficit
      5. Preparation of a nutrition care plan

   B. Iron-deficiency anemia
      1. Screening
      2. Preventing iron deficiency anemia
      3. Supplementation guidelines
      4. Differential diagnosis

   C. Adverse reactions to foods
      1. Breastfeeding's role in preventing atopic disease
      2. Maternal diet modifications

   D. Phenylketonuria

PRE-TEST

For questions 1 to 5, choose the best answer.

1. When compared to an adult, infants have a much narrower range of external temperatures to which they can adapt without suffering cold stress for all of the following reasons except

    A. large surface area in proportion to mass.
    B. less subcutaneous fat for the provision of thermal insulation.
    C. less ability to control skin blood flow.
    D. lower energy requirement per unit of weight.

2. A cool delivery room environment combined with low relative humidity will _____ heat loss in the neonate by the process of _____.

    A. encourage; convection
    B. discourage; convection
    C. encourage; evaporation
    D. discourage; evaporation

3. Interventions to prevent the neonate's heat loss include all of the following except

    A. swaddling.
    B. drying of the infant.
    C. skin-to-skin care.
    D. intravenous fluids.

4. Situations that place an infant at risk for hypoglycemia include all of the following except

    A. hypothermia, sepsis, shock, and asphyxia.
    B. maternal diabetes.
    C. small for gestation age.
    D. gradual discontinuation of intravenous fluids.

5. Jaundice that occurs because of inadequate nursing sessions, resulting in a reduced intake of breastmilk, is called

    A. breastmilk jaundice.
    B. breastfeeding jaundice.
    C. pathologic jaundice.
    D. hemolytic jaundice.

For questions 6 to 10, choose the best answer from the following key:
    A. Brown fat
    B. Rh incompatibility
    C. Smoking
    D. Platelet-activating factor
    E. Inositol

6. May reduce respiratory distress syndrome in preterm infants.

7. Causes the mother to produce antibodies against fetal red blood cells.

8. Believed to be involved in the development of certain inflammatory bowel diseases.

9. Metabolized to create heat in nonshivering thermogenesis.

10. Increases the risk of respiratory disease.

For questions 11 to 20, choose the best answer.

11. A child's first dental exam should be scheduled
    A. after his or her third birthday.
    B. when the child first experiences a toothache.
    C. when the parent first sees or suspects a cavity.
    D. within six months of the eruption of the first tooth.

12. For dental caries to develop, the following factor(s) must be present:
    A. a susceptible host (the tooth).
    B. bacteria that can cause tooth decay.
    C. time.
    D. fermentable carbohydrates.
    E. All of the above

13. If a family's water supply is not fluoridated, fluoride supplementation for children is not necessary as long as the teeth are being brushed with flouridated toothpaste.
    A. True
    B. False

14. The use of phototherapy, a radiant heat warmer, or presence of an ostomy in a preterm infant increases
    A. calorie needs.
    B. protein needs.
    C. calorie and protein needs.
    D. fluid needs.

15. Altered levels of polyunsaturated fatty acids have been found in the milk of mothers whose infants have
    A. diabetes.
    B. atopic eczema.
    C. an allergy to soy.
    D. hyperlipidemia.

16. The serum ferritin level is a useful guide to the level of _____ iron and the serum transferrin receptor is a sensitive index of _____ iron need.
    A. cellular; storage
    B. storage; circulating
    C. storage; cellular
    D. circulating; storage

17. _____ will not influence maternal milk production negatively.
    A. Maternal fatigue and stress
    B. Retained placental fragments
    C. Maternal smoking
    D. Excessive kcalories

18. The creamatocrit gives a measure of the percentage of "cream," which may be helpful in determining the etiology of growth deficit in an exclusively breast-fed infant because
    A. there is a linear relationship between the fat and energy content of the milk.
    B. the creamatocrit can identify abnormalities of fat absorption.

C. the creamatocrit will be abnormally high in the milk of mothers whose infants experience growth deficit.

D. it is indicative of a mother's operational milk-ejection reflex.

19. The iron needs of the exclusively breastfed, full-term infant are adequate

A. through the first year of life.

B. until 9 months of age.

C. until 2 months of age.

D. until 6 months of age.

20. Select the most appropriate guidance to give expectant parents with a strong history of food allergies.

A. The mother should avoid all allergenic foods during pregnancy and lactation.

B. The infant should receive only hypoallergenic formula as allergens will be in the mother's milk.

C. The mother should avoid allergenic foods during lactation.

D. The infant should not receive colostrum as it is high in allergenic proteins.

Introduction

This section discusses infant health issues including clinical conditions that cause concern during the neonatal period. Some of these conditions are thermal regulation, neonatal hypoglycemia, and neonatal hyperbilirubinemia. The association between the protective benefit of breastfeeding and the reduced occurrence and severity of infant infections is briefly discussed. See Module 1, *The Support of Breastfeeding*, Chapter 2, for a more in-depth exploration of breastfeeding advantages. Optimal infant oral health care begins in infancy and guidelines for care are outlined in this section. Also discussed is the role of breastfeeding in the occurrence or prevention of caries.

Growth deficit, iron deficiency anemia, and adverse reactions to foods in infants are reasons for concern for healthgivers around the world. Breastfeeding's role in improving outcome in many of these conditions is examined in the following dialogue. The infant with a neurologic problem, physical defect (cleft palate or lip), or genetic problem (Down syndrome) is discussed in Chapter 3 of this module.

Clinical Conditions That Cause Concern During the Neonatal Period

THERMAL REGULATION

The axillary temperature of the newborn ranges from 36.5°C to 37°C (97.6°F–98.6°F). For a healthy full-term infant, the temperature should stabilize within 10 hours of birth. Temperatures below 36.1°C may indicate the environment is too cold and that the infant is subject to cold stress; an axillary temperature greater than 37.2°C (99°F) can result from an environment that is too warm, dehydration, or infection and sepsis.

Humans are homoiotherms (warm blooded) and are able to maintain a constant core body temperature regardless of a fairly wide range of environmental temperatures. For infants the range of external temperatures to which they can adapt without suffering cold stress is narrower than that for adults (Hey & Scopes, 1993). The newborn has a large surface area in proportion to mass, less subcutaneous fat for the provision of thermal insulation, and a relatively lessened ability to control skin blood flow. These conditions increase the potential for heat loss. Newborns also differ from adults in mechanisms of thermogenesis, or heat production. The neutral environmental temperature zone of the newborn is 32°C to 34°C (89.6°F–93.2°F) as compared with the adult's neutral zone of 26°C to 28°C (78.7°F–82.4°F). In this range, an individual is able to maintain a normal internal temperature with minimal metabolism and oxygen consumption for heat production. When environmental temperatures drop below this range, a metabolic response to cold is needed to replace heat loss and this range represents the thermal range of minimal stress (Hey & Scopes, 1993).

For the neonate, heat transfer can occur in four ways: evaporation, radiation, convection, and conduction. Heat transfer then depends on the temperature of the air and walls of the environment, the air movement, and water vapor pressure—humidity. A cool delivery room environment, combined with low relative humidity, encourages heat loss by evaporation. Drying the newborn at birth is a means to minimize evaporative heat loss. Radiant loss of heat involves the transfer of heat to cooler objects in the environment and can be minimized by providing skin-to-skin contact with the mother with an outside cover over the infant, swaddling of the infant in warm blankets, and the use of radiant warmers. The air speed in the delivery room contributes to convection heat loss in the newborn. Swaddling and infant warmers can help prevent this type of heat loss. Conductive heat loss requires the neonate to come into direct contact with cooler objects. Warm mattresses and contact with the mother can prevent this type of heat loss.

Thermogenesis and heat retention are achieved through mechanisms such as non-shivering thermogenesis, muscular activity, and positional changes. Vasomotor control allows the newborn to retain heat. In nonshivering thermogenesis, the newborn increases heat production by increasing the metabolic rate and rate of oxygen consumption. Brown fat is metabolized to create the needed heat. Infants are born with brown fat cells, which make up 2% to 6% of the total body weight of the newborn (Klaus & Fanaroff, 1993). Brown fat is found at the nape of the neck, posterior to the sternum, surrounding the kidneys and adrenal area, and in the perineal areas, and it is available for weeks after birth. Rich in mitochondria and fat vacuoles with an abundant blood and sympathetic nerve supply, brown fat reacts to cold stress in the following way:

- norepinephrine stimulates brown fat metabolism by activating lipoprotein lipase,
- lipoprotein lipase breaks down fat to form triglycerides,
- triglycerides are hydrolyzed to glycerol and free fatty acids, and
- a heat-producing reaction occurs.

When newborns are exposed to cold they become restless and have an increased muscular activity. Flexion in the newborn is a way to decrease the amount of skin surface exposed to cold and to conserve heat. It is believed that the newborn does change position and increase muscular activity during periods of cold stress (Hey & Scopes, 1993). The newborn also constricts the skin's blood vessels, which is a mechanism to retain heat and help to maintain core body temperatures. But the newborn has less subcutaneous fat for thermal insulation, so this mechanism alone will not maintain core body temperature.

There does not appear to be a single environmental temperature best for all sizes and conditions of newborns. The preterm infant will usually need a warmer environment than the term infant. There can be severe problems when a newborn is exposed to environmental temperatures above or below her or his neutral temperature zone. Cold stress leading to cold injury may result in metabolic acidosis, a decrease in arterial oxygen blood level, and hypoglycemia (Klaus & Fanaroff, 1993). Hyperthermia can develop rapidly, and although infants have more sweat glands per unit of body weight than adults, the response of each gland is one-third that of an adult's. Thus sweating is not an effective mechanism for lowering the newborn's temperature. Heat stress will increase metabolic rate and respirations and serious overheating can cause cerebral damage from dehydration, heat stroke, or even death (Hey & Scopes, 1993). Fluctuations in the environmental temperature can also contribute to apnea in the newborn (Klaus & Fanaroff, 1993).

NEONATAL HYPOGLYCEMIA

Hypoglycemia is defined as an abnormally low blood glucose level. Serum glucose levels below 35 mg/dL during the first 72 hours are considered low for the term neonate. In a preterm neonate, levels less than 25 mg/dL during the first 72 hours of life are considered evidence of hypoglycemia. For any neonate, after 72 hours of life levels below 45 mg/dL are considered to indicate hypoglycemia is present (Behrman & Vaughan, 1991). In maternal diabetes, hypoglycemia is reported to occur in 75% of newborns but only 1% of 1,000 live births otherwise.

Other infants at risk for hypoglycemia are infants who have suffered intra-uterine growth retardation (IUGR), usually labeled small for gestational age (SGA). There have been several reports of high serum concentration of gluconeogenic precursors in SGA infants, which suggests that the hypoglycemia may be caused by dysfunctioning gluconeogenic enzymes such as pyruvate carboxylase and phosphoenol pyruvate carboxykinase (Haymond et al., 1974; Lindblad, 1970; Mestyan et al., 1975). Defects are also present in fatty acid oxidation as evidenced by serum free fatty acid concentrations being lower in hypoglycemic SGA infants when compared to normoglycemic SGA and appropriate for gestational age (AGA) control groups (de Leeuw & de Vries, 1976; Harris, 1974; Keele & Kay, 1966; Schultz et al., 1976). Preterm neonates have decreased stores of glycogen and immature hepatic enzymes necessary for gluconeogenesis and are also at greater risk for hypoglycemia. Infants experiencing hypothermia, sepsis, shock, and asphyxia may also have hypoglycemia. Other conditions that may predispose an infant to hypoglycemia are abrupt discontinuation of intravenous fluids, incorrect positioning of umbilical catheters, and certain medications. Table 2B–1 summarizes various causes of hypoglycemia.

The neonate requires large amounts of energy during the birth process. The metabolism of glucose is an important source of energy. After birth, the infant loses the maternal supply of glucose. Neonatal hypoglycemia may be expressed by a weak cry, apnea, cyanosis, hypothermia, irritability, lethargy, feeding problems, and tremors or seizures (Torrence, 1985). Some neonates may have low-level hypoglycemia and yet not exhibit symptoms. Confirmation of hypoglycemia should be done by determining serum glucose levels. To obtain a drop of blood for glucose assessment, many use the widely available glucose oxidase reagent sticks. The test is quick but abnormal results should be confirmed by laboratory analysis. Recently the validity of using glucose oxidase reagent sticks has been questioned (Cornblath et al., 1990).

Guidelines for monitoring newborn serum levels vary widely from hospital to hospital. Recommendations from nursing textbooks state that infants at risk for hypoglycemia should have an initial check during the first hour of life, then one

Table 2B–1   Causes of Hypoglycemia

Causes Resulting in Diminished Hepatic Glucose Output	Causes Resulting in Increased Peripheral Uptake of Glucose	Miscellaneous Causes
Diminished glycogen stores in liver	Pancreatic islet cell tumor	Idiopathic transient hypoglycemia
Immaturity	Pancreatic islet cell hyperplasia	Central nervous system diseases or
Intrauterine malnutrition, small-for-date infant	Nesidioblastoma	anomalies
Postnatal starvation	Maternal diabetes	Salicylate poisoning
Hypothermia; asphyxia	Erythroblastosis	Idiopathic hypoglycemia of childhood
Chronic diarrhea	Beckwith's syndrome or the "infant giant"	Ketotic hypoglycemia
Hepatocellular disease	Hereditary tyrosinemia	Cardiac malformations (especially hypoplastic left heart syndrome)
Glycogen synthetase deficiency	Other hyperinsulinemic or possible hyperinsulinemic states	Tumors
Monosaccharide intolerance	Maternal tolbutamide ingestion	Neonatal sepsis
Defective glucose release or defective new glucose formation in liver	Abrupt cessation of intravenous glucose infusion	
Liver glycogen disease (especially Type I or glucose-6-phosphatase deficiency)	Maple syrup urine disease	
Galactosemia	Methylmalonic acidemia	
Hereditary fructose intolerance	Leucine sensitivity	
Fructose-1, 6-diphosphate deficiency		
Pyruvate carboxylase or phosphoenol-pyruvate carboxy-kinase deficiencies		
Growth hormone deficiency		
Adrenocortical insufficiency		

Source: Barness, LA (Ed.) (1993). *Pediatric Nutrition Handbook,* p. 246. Elk Grove Village, IL: AAP. Used with permission of the American Academy of Pediatrics.

every 2 hours for the first 8 hours of life, and every 4 to 6 hours thereafter until the infant is 24 hours old. Neonates who are able to feed orally should be put to the breast within the first hour after delivery. When the neonate cannot be fed orally, intravenous glucose infusions should be started. The amount of glucose in the infusion is based on the weight of the neonate and the severity of hypoglycemic symptoms. For symptomatic hypoglycemia, a 2- to 4-mL/kg bolus infusion of 10% glucose should be given immediately (Behrman & Vaughan, 1991). A glucose infusion of 8 mg/kg per minute is recommended for continuous intravenous therapy (Behrman & Vaughan, 1991). Site care is very important because the glucose solution may cause tissue burning and sloughing (Oehler, 1981). The neonate's condition must be watched carefully once intravenous glucose has been initiated, with the goal of weaning to maintenance of glucose levels through feedings.

In the infant of the mother with diabetes, hypoglycemia occurs early and is proportional to the mother's level of hyperglycemia at delivery. Cord blood glucose and micro sugars at one-half and one hour of age are monitored to determine the potential for hypoglycemia based on the curve of glucose disappearance (Lawrence, 1994). Provided the mother is able, lactation should be established quickly with close monitoring so that glucose can be managed by breastfeeding.

NEONATAL HYPERBILIRUBINEMIA

No matter what the feeding preference is, clinical jaundice occurs in 80% of all newborns (Osborn, 1986) and 50% of all full-term newborns become visibly jaundiced during the first week of life (Maisels, 1982). Full-term breastfed infants are more likely to develop hyperbilirubinemia than their formula-fed counterparts (Maisels et al., 1986; Schneider, 1986). A majority of breastfed infants will be treated for hyperbilirubinemia (Eggert et al., 1985; Maisels & Krung, 1992), and it is more common in Asian and Native American infants (Lawrence, 1994).

Development of Hyperbilirubinemia

In utero, as fetal red blood cells break down and form bilirubin, the maternal hepatic and intestinal systems clear the fetal blood of excess bilirubin. After delivery, the infant has a surplus of red blood cells, or polycythemia. As these red blood cells break down, there is a rise in serum bilirubin levels to a peak of approximately 6.0 mg/dL on day 3. This declines to approximately 2 to 3 mg/dL by day 6. By days 11 through 14, the normal adult level of 1.0 mg/dL is usually obtained (Lawrence, 1989). Bilirubin molecules are insoluble in water and bind to albumin for transport to the liver. Hepatocytes attach the albumin–bilirubin complex to glucuronide. This conjugated bilirubin is water soluble and can be cleared from the bloodstream (Wilkerson, 1988).

Once conjugated, the bilirubin is excreted from the liver into bile and transported to the intestine. Meconium has high concentrations of bilirubin, which is responsible for its dark color. As meconium is passed by the infant, the bilirubin is removed from the body. At serum levels greater than 5.0 mg/dL, bilirubin will be deposited in the fatty subcutaneous tissue yielding a yellow tint. Any interruption of this cycle can lead to the bilirubin being reabsorbed into the infant's system, causing hyperbilirubinemia. (See Figure 2B–1.)

Figure 2B-1

Graphic explanation of bilirubin metabolism.

Source: Adapted from Sherwen, LN, Scoloveno, MA, Weingarten, CT (1995). *Nursing Care of the Childbearing Family,* p. 1068. Norwalk, CT: Appleton & Lange. Reprinted with permission.

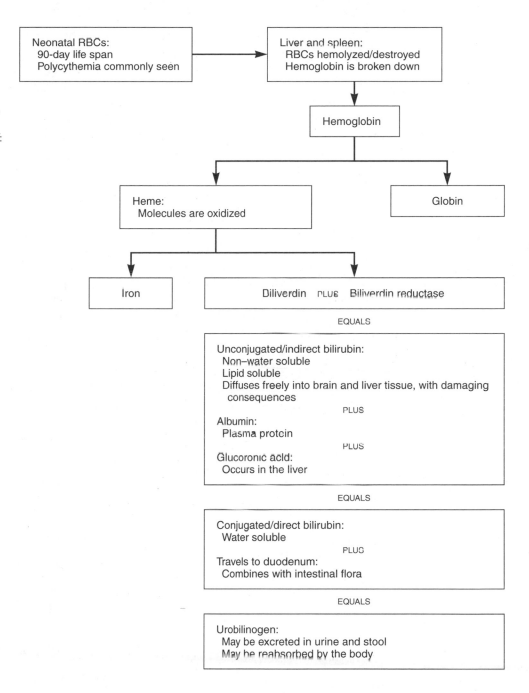

Bilirubin has been shown to be a potent antioxidant in vitro (Stocker et al., 1987; Stocker et al., 1990) and in vivo (Dennery et al., 1992). Stocker and associates (1990) showed that bilirubin prevents oxidation of linoleic acid in vitro. In animal models, jaundiced rats had significantly less lipid peroxidation in the blood after exposure to hyperoxia than the nonjaundiced rats and a decreased hyperoxia-induced lung edema (Dennery et al., 1992). In a small group of preterm infants, higher bilirubin levels were associated with a lower incidence of oxygen radical-mediated injury (Hegyi et al., 1994).

Kernicterus, or bilirubin encephalopathy, is damage to the brain caused by bilirubin. As serum levels rise, excess is stored in cells. Bilirubin is toxic to tissues. Term infants without hemolysis are at low risk for developing kernicterus. Bilirubin concentration and production rate must overwhelm the capacity of the body to keep it from reaching toxic levels in the brain in order to cause kernicterus. Factors that put an infant at higher risk for kernicterus when bilirubin levels are greater than 20 mg/dL include sepsis, hypoxia, acidosis, prematurity, and hemolysis. The likelihood of developing kernicterus appears to be a function of concentration and duration of bilirubin exposure (Brodersen & Stern, 1990). As with many vitamins, it appears there may be a window of opportunity where bilirubin is protective, beyond which it becomes detrimental.

Physiologic Jaundice

Physiologic jaundice is not caused by breastfeeding and is part of a normal process. Yet the incidence of physiologic jaundice could be related to mismanagement of breastfeeding (delayed initial feeds, water supplementation). Physiologic jaundice usually occurs after two to three days of life. Bilirubin levels peak at 5 mg/dL to 10 mg/dL by day 3 to 5 and decrease to 2 mg/dL by day 7 (Wilkerson, 1988). It is associated with polycythemia.

Other factors causing high red blood cell count include perinatal hypoxia and trauma. Delayed cord clamping at birth can predispose the newborn to polycythemia and hyperbilirubinemia. If the infant's liver is immature, it may inhibit the normal bilirubin transport system. Since the newborn's intestinal tract is sterile, it lacks the enzymes to assist bilirubin conversion and excretion. Intestinal reabsorption of bilirubin is the major cause of physiologic jaundice (Wilkerson, 1988). Water supplements will not enhance the clearance of bilirubin. The bowel is the primary excretion site of bilirubin and the kidneys only excrete it when the bowel is overloaded (de Carvalho et al., 1981). Discontinuation of breastfeeding is not a treatment for physiologic jaundice.

Pathologic Jaundice

Pathologic jaundice is caused by blood incompatibilities between the mother and infant and may cause red blood cell lysis. The infant may be jaundiced within 24 hours of birth and serum levels rise quickly (Auerbach & Gartner, 1987).

Erythroblastosis fetalis is a hemolytic disease of the newborn characterized by anemia, jaundice, enlargement of the liver and spleen, and generalized edema. It can occur when there is an incompatibility between the Rh blood groups of the mother and fetus—erythroblastosis fetalis occurs when an Rh-negative mother is pregnant with an Rh-positive fetus. The mixing of maternal and fetal blood causes a reaction and the mother's body produces antibodies against the fetal red blood cells that carry the Rh-positive antigen. These antibodies cross the placental barrier and cause lysis of the infant's red blood cells. The hemolytic anemia is life threatening for the infant. Today, this is not often seen because of monitoring and the development of RhoGam (Dunn et al., 1988).

ABO incompatibility occurs when there is an incompatibility between the major blood groups (A, B, AB, O) of the mother and the fetus. A Coombs test of the cord blood tests for the presence of antibodies and hemolysis (Newman & Maisels, 1992). Table 2B–2 shows a comparison of ABO incompatibility and Rh incompatibility.

Table 2B–2 Comparison of ABO Incompatibility and RH Incompatibility

	ABO Incompatibility	Rh Incompatibility
Definition	Incompatibility between the major blood groups (A, B, AB, O) of the mother and the fetus. When the fetal blood mixes with the maternal blood, a reaction occurs, causing the fetal RBCs to be destroyed.	Incompatibility between the Rh blood groups of the mother and fetus. Occurs when an Rh– mother is pregnant with an Rh+ fetus. When maternal and fetal blood mix, a reaction is caused. The mother's body produces antibodies against the fetal RBCs that carry the Rh+ antigen (D). This causes the fetal RBCs to be destroyed through a process called immunization or sensitization. If a mixture of maternal and fetal blood cells occurs during labor, subsequent pregnancies with an Rh+ infant will be affected.
Incidence	Occurs in 20–25% of all pregnancies; in 10% of these cases, the newborn develops hemolytic disease.	Occurs in 9% of all pregnancies; 1 in 15 newborns of these pregnancies develops hemolytic disease.
Timing of signs and symptoms	After 24 hours of life; may develop during first pregnancy.	Often begins in utero; sensitization occurs during a first pregnancy, abortion, or blood transfusion; signs and symptoms generally appear in a subsequent pregnancy.
Common signs and symptoms	Jaundice related to hyperbilirubinemia.	Yellow amniotic fluid, umbilical cord, and vernix caseosa. Jaundice related to hyperbilirubinemia. Anemia. Enlarged liver and spleen. Petechiae and purpura. Possible cardiorespiratory collapse.
Laboratory tests	Weak to moderately positive Coombs' test. Bilirubin greater than 12 mg/dL in term newborn and greater than 15 mg/dL in preterm newborn.	Positive Coombs' test. Bilirubin greater than 12 mg/dL in term newborn and greater than 15 mg/dL in preterm newborn. Hemoglobin less than 13 g/dL or hematocrit less than 40%. Increased reticulocyte count.
Management	Phototherapy. Exchange transfusion in severe circumstances.	Phototherapy. Exchange transfusion. Administration of Rho(D) immune globulin to an Rh– mother at 28 weeks' gestation and after every pregnancy with an Rh+ fetus, whether the pregnancy reaches term or terminates in abortion.

Source: Sherwen, LN, Scoloveno, MA, Weingarten, CT (1995). *Nursing Care of the Childbearing Family*, p. 1211. Norwalk, CT: Appleton & Lange. Reprinted with permission.

Breastfeeding Jaundice

Breastfeeding jaundice is also referred to as inadequate nursing jaundice. It results from inadequate breastmilk volume. Infants have an above average weight loss after delivery and do not regain their birthweight by two weeks (Osborn, 1986). As a result of the inadequate volume of breastmilk ingested, infants become dehydrated and have less than six wet diapers a day. Urine is concentrated and dark in color. Stools are also infrequent and lack the characteristics of normal breastfed infant stools (yellow color, seedy consistency).

Breastfeeding jaundice is similar to physiologic jaundice but only occurs in breastfed infants. Breastfed infants are more likely to be jaundiced than formula-fed infants because they receive less calories initially, and they have a greater reabsorption of bilirubin through the small bowel (Alonso et al., 1991; Maisels & Newman, 1994). Breastfeeding jaundice appears after two to three days of life. Bilirubin peaks by the second or third day. Bilirubin levels gradually decrease but may remain elevated for as long as ten weeks. The rate of accumulation is less than 5 mg/dL per 24 hours but may peak at 15 mg/dL to 19 mg/dL. Higher bilirubin levels may be seen in premature or sick infants due to a smaller reserve of albumin for binding bilirubin.

An infant born at 37 weeks gestation has a four times greater risk of bilirubin greater than 13 mg/dL than an infant born at 40 weeks gestation. Breastfeeding jaundice occurs more frequently in primipara mothers and may be prevalent following a cesarean birth or anesthetic use (general or epidural) during delivery. Oxytocin and prostaglandin induction of labor and use of fluids of D_5W during labor may also increase the incidence of neonatal jaundice (Wilkerson, 1988). Breastfeeding should not be stopped for treatment of breastfeeding jaundice; instead, breastfeeding should be promoted and encouraged.

Treatment of Breastfeeding Jaundice

Encourage early feeds. Colostrum has a laxative effect and plays a role in excretion of meconium (de Carvalho et al., 1982). This helps reduce the rate of bilirubin reabsorption from the bowel. Infants who pass meconium in less than 12 hours after delivery are less jaundiced than infants who passed meconium more than 12 hours after delivery (Clarkson et al., 1984). Early feeds may increase stools; in turn, this will increase bilirubin excretion (de Carvalho, 1985).

Frequent Nursing Sessions   Mothers should be encouraged to breastfeed 10 to 12 times a day. Infants who breastfed an average of 10 times a day had lower serum concentration levels than those who nursed 6 times a day (6.5 mg/dL compared to 9.0 mg/dL) (de Carvalho et al., 1982). Frequent feeds help to increase the frequency and volume of stools, decreasing the serum bilirubin. On a comparison of stooling patterns between formula-fed and breastfed infants, formula-fed infants passed more stool, excreted more bilirubin, and had lower serum values than breastfed infants. When the stooling patterns of the breastfed infants were compared, infants with higher stool excretion followed the same pattern of increased bilirubin excretion and lower serum levels (de Carvalho, 1985). The length of time for each session is not as critical in determining serum bilirubin levels as is the number of feeds (de Carvalho et al., 1982).

Night feeding should be encouraged. Levels of prolactin increase during sleep, and with breast stimulation. Prolactin plays a role in the production of an adequate milk supply. Mature milk aids in a decrease of bilirubin levels (Lawrence, 1994). Nursing throughout the night also helps engorgement. Engorgement may lead to inadequate nursing sessions, in turn this may cause jaundice. If the infant will not nurse effectively for long periods of time, the nursing session should be divided between the two breasts. Mothers should be encouraged to use an electric pump to ensure emptying of the breasts and to promote milk production.

No Supplementation of Formula or Water   Supplements of formula or water are contraindicated for breastfeeding jaundice. Supplements decrease the volume of colostrum and breastmilk an infant will take during a nursing session. Supplementary feeds may lead to nipple confusion and a decrease in nursing. These factors contribute to engorgement and lack of self-confidence for the lactating woman. Water may prevent the infant from sensing hunger, which may lead to inadequate caloric intake and wasting. Studies have shown that supplements do not reduce serum bilirubin levels (de Carvalho et al., 1981).

Phototherapy   Phototherapy is initiated in full-term infants with no hemolysis when indirect serum bilirubin levels reach 12 mg/dL to 17 mg/dL and exchange transfusion is done if the level is 20 mg/dL or greater (Behrman & Vaughan, 1987). Newman and Maisels (1992) offer less rigid recommendations in treatment of hyperbilirubinemia. The following is a list of danger signs in a jaundiced infant:

- Family history of significant hemolytic disease
- Vomiting
- Lethargy
- Poor feeding
- Fever
- Dark urine
- Light stools

If one or more of these signs are seen, Newman and Maisels recommend aggressive evaluation and treatment. If no signs are identified, parents should be instructed about symptoms to watch for, but hospital discharge does not need to be delayed (Newman & Maisels, 1992). Early discharge and unrecognized hemolysis has led to the reappearance of cases of kernicterus in full-term infants (Maisels & Newman, 1994), so the importance of reviewing indicators of a problem with parents must be emphasized to personnel responsible for discharge instructions.

Breastfeeding should continue through phototherapy to ensure adequate caloric intake and hydration and to prevent engorgement. The mother should continue to nurse every two hours. Infants who receive phototherapy may be more difficult to feed and have a less effective suck. They may have to be stimulated during breastfeeding to keep them awake. Some ways to do this include the following:

- Unwrap the baby to cool off.
- Stimulate the soles of his or her feet or the top of the head.
- Do "baby sit up"—(rock the baby from back lying position to sitting several times).
- Put a cool cloth on the baby's forehead.
- Stroke the unwrapped baby, and/or massage the baby along his or her spine.

Breastmilk Jaundice (Late-Onset Jaundice)

Breastmilk jaundice is not seen in the neonatal period and occurs after the first week of life as physiologic jaundice reduces. Bilirubin levels peak at 10 to 15 days and may remain elevated for weeks. Approximately 2% to 4% of all full-term breastfeeding infants experience late onset jaundice (unconjugated bilirubin > 10 mg/dL) (Clarkson et al., 1984). For formula-fed infants, late onset jaundice is rarely seen (Clarkson et al., 1984). Infants with breastmilk jaundice thrive and gain weight. They have adequate urine output and stools. Breastmilk jaundice has not been shown to be deleterious to well newborns (Grunebaum et al., 1991).

Breastmilk jaundice can be diagnosed by interrupting nursing for at least 12 hours when bilirubin levels are > 16 mg/dL. Phototherapy should not be used when breastfeeding is stopped because it will cloud the diagnosis. Bilirubin levels decline during this period, often dropping in half within three days, but may increase gradually when breastfeeding is reinitiated. With a drop of 2 mg/dL or more after 12 hours without mother's milk, the diagnosis is confirmed. Bilirubin levels usually do not exceed the levels prior to the interruption. When bilirubin levels are more than 20 mg/dL, most physicians feel more comfortable if they have ruled out other causes of hyperbilirubinemia, especially if the infant was discharged very early from the hospital or birthing center. Thus, some doctors may hospitalize the infant for a complete bilirubin workup.

The cause of breastmilk jaundice is unknown. It has been associated with the steroid 5B-pregnane-3a, 20 B-diol—a breakdown product of progesterone and an isomer of pregnanediol which is present in the breastmilk (Brooten et al., 1985). This substance is not usually found in milk but is in the breastmilk of 10% of lactating women. It prevents the conjugation of bilirubin by inhibiting the hepatic enzyme glucuronyl transferase (Bevan & Holton, 1972). The glucuronide-inhibiting property may be related to elevated lipase activity in breastmilk. When lipase is elevated to abnormal levels, free fatty acid levels also become abnormally elevated. High levels of free fatty acids inhibit glucuronyl transferase, which is the enzyme necessary for the attachment of unconjugated bilirubin to glucuronide (Hargreaves, 1973). Unsaturated fatty acids and medium-chain saturated fatty acids are more inhibitory to glucuronyl transferase in vitro than saturated long-chain fatty acids (Bevan & Holton, 1972). Studies continue to determine the cause of breastmilk jaundice. These include the role of lipoprotein lipase, bile salt–stimulated lipase, and the role of free fatty acids and other lipases.

Treatment of Breastmilk Jaundice

Assessment must be completed to ensure that the jaundice is not caused by other physiologic disorders such as hemolytic disease, hypothyroidism, and glucose-6-phosphodehydrogenase (G6PD) deficiency. There have been no known cases of kernicterus caused by breastmilk jaundice. The recommendation is to keep serum bilirubin levels below 20 mg/dL. With continued breastfeeding, after a brief interruption (24 to 48 hours), there is a slow, steady decline in serum bilirubin levels over several weeks (Gartner & Arias, 1966). For most cases, interruption of breastfeeding is not necessary because the concentration of serum bilirubin will peak and then decline while the baby stays at the breast. It is important to ensure precautions are taken to keep the mother's milk supply adequate if breastfeeding is interrupted. If the physician believes supplementation is absolutely necessary, supplementation at the breast (after pumping) of pasteurized donor milk or formula with a nursing supplementer can be helpful in reducing serum bilirubin concentrations and keeping the breast stimulated. Phototherapy may be used with bilirubin levels between 15 mg to 20 mg except during breastmilk jaundice.

Figure 2B–2 shows the latest recommendations from the American Academy of Pediatrics for the treatment of hyperbilirubinemia. The algorithm individualizes treatment based on specific parameters exhibited by the infant (AAP, 1994).

Figure 2B–2

Algorithm: Management of hyperbilirubinemia in the healthy term infant.

Source: American Academy of Pediatrics, Provisional Committee for Quality Improvement and Subcommittee on Hyperbilirubinemia (1994). Practice parameter: Management of hyperbilirubinemia in the healthy term newborn. *Pediatrics*, 94 (4 pt 1):558-65 and *Pediatrics*, 95(3):458-61. Used with permission.

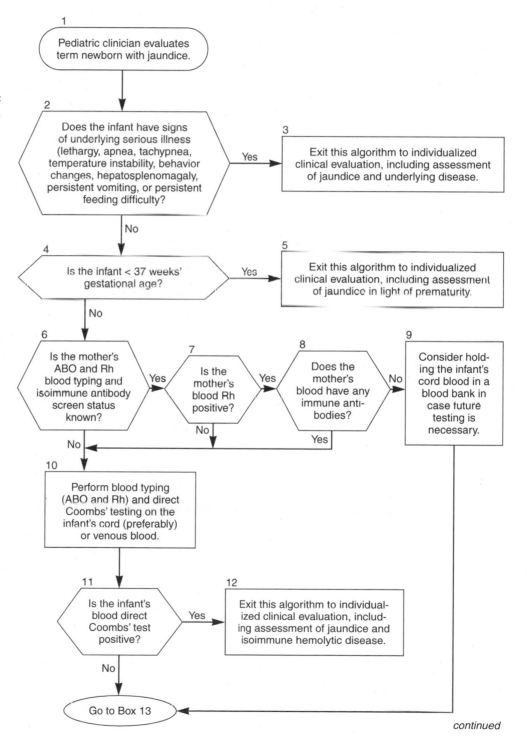

continued

Figure 2B–2 *continued*

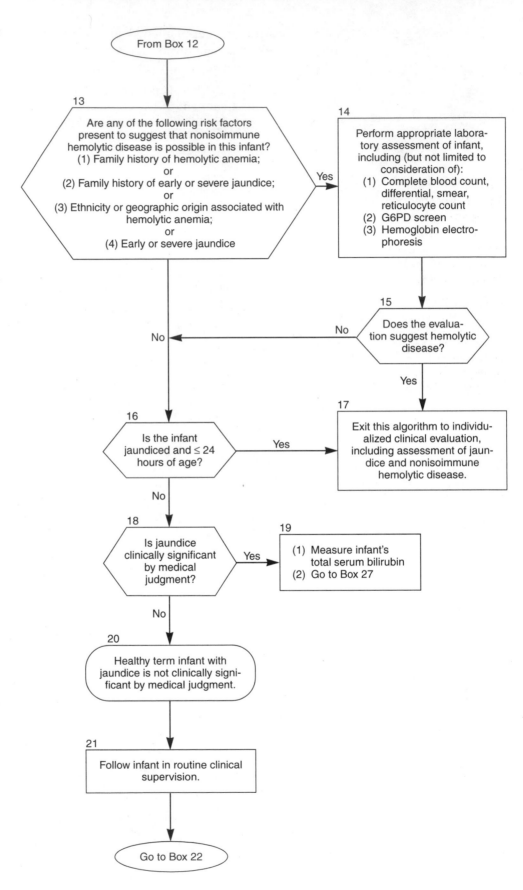

Figure 2B-2 *continued*

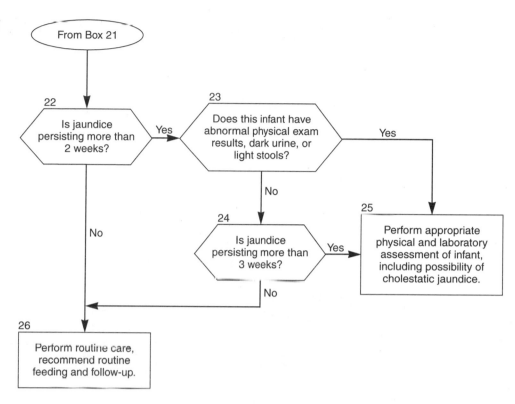

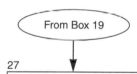

27

Management of Hyperbilirubinemia In the Healthy Term Newborn

| Age, hours | TSB* Level—mg/dL (µmol/L) | | | |
	Consider Phototherapy[+]	Phototherapy	Exchange Transfusion if Intensive Phototherapy Fails[++]	Exchange Transfusion and Intensive Phototherapy
≤ 24[§]	—	—	—	—
25–48	≥12 (170)	≥ 15 (260)	≥ 20 (340)	≥ 25 (430)
49–72	≥15 (260)	≥ 18 (310)	≥ 25 (430)	≥ 30 (510)
> 72	≥17 (290)	≥ 20 (340)	≥ 25 (430)	≥ 30 (510)

*TSB indicates total serum bilirubin.

[+]Phototherapy at these TSB levels is a clinical option, meaning that the intervention is available and may be used on the basis of individual clinical judgment.

[++]Intensive phototherapy should produce a decline of TSB of 1 to 2 mg/dL within 4 to 6 hours and the TSB level should continue to fall and remain below the threshold level for exchange transfusion. If this does not occur, it is considered a failure of phototherapy.

[§]Term infants who are clinically jaundiced at ≤ 24 hours old are not considered healthy and require further evaluation.

Infant Infections and Breastfeeding

MORBIDITY AND MORTALITY RATES

For every 1,000 formula-fed infants, 77 are hospitalized during the first four months of life while only 5 per 1,000 breastfed infants need to be hospitalized (Cunningham et al., 1991). Morbidity studies show that necrotizing enterocolitis, sepsis, and mortality are reduced when human milk is fed (Eibi et al., 1988; Lucas & Cole, 1990; Uraizee & Gross, 1989). The U.S. National Institute of Environmental Health Sciences estimates an extra 4 per 1,000 infants die each year in the United States because they are not breastfed (Rogan, 1989).

Habicht and associates (1986) found the relative mortality risk of not breastfeeding to be 2.67 and 5.20 for households with and without toilets. This translates into 47 and 153 deaths per 1,000 due to not breastfeeding. Mortality among artificially fed babies has been shown to be 3 to 5 times higher than for breastfed babies (Macedo, 1988). In developing countries, the highest infant mortality rate is during the first months of life (Khan et al., 1993). The major causes of death reported in the early period of life are septicemia and diarrhea.

The risk of neonatal septicemia has been reported to be 18 times higher among nonbreastfed than partially breastfed infants (Ashraf et al., 1993). The risk of dying from diarrhea is 23.5 times higher among nonbreastfed compared to exclusively breastfed infants in developing countries (Victoria et al., 1989). Theoretical calculations from a comprehensive worldwide review of morbidity and mortality studies suggest that breastfeeding can reduce diarrheal mortality by 25% during the first six months of life and by 8% to 9% during the first five years of life (Feachem & Koblinsky, 1984).

Hanson and Bergstrom (1990) postulate that infant mortality, birth rates, and breastfeeding are linked. The relationship between decreased child mortality rates and declining birth rates is multifactorial, with the evidence suggesting that decreasing infant mortality may lead to decreasing birth rates. They go on to state that breastfeeding leads to decreasing infant mortality, increased birth spacing, and decreased fertility. In a recent report, Hanson and colleagues (1994) reiterate the importance of early exclusive breastfeeding in decreasing infectious disease and death in children and in serving as a strong natural contraceptive, thus increasing the interval between births. The authors call for campaigns to promote breastfeeding worldwide and to encourage the Catholic church to promote breastfeeding as a natural contraceptive.

SEPSIS

Major protection against bacteremia-meningitis has been reported in industrial countries as well as in developing countries. In Atlanta, Georgia, the adjusted risk for bacteremia-meningitis is 12-fold for bottle-fed infants during the first six months (Cochi et al., 1986). In Finland, prolonged breastfeeding was found to protect against bacteremia-meningitis in children under five years with an odds ratio of 0.47 when controlling for day care, history of previous illness, and presence of siblings (Takala et al., 1989). In Pakistan, the risk of neonatal septicemia is 18 times higher among nonbreastfed than partially breastfed infants.

Formula feeding imposes an increased risk of *H. influenzae bacteremia* and meningitis to infants living in Finland (Takala et al., 1989). In New York and Connecticut, formula-fed infants had a 10-fold risk of hospitalization for bacterial infections and 4-fold risk of bacteremia and meningitis (Cunningham, Jelliffe, & Jelliffe, 1991).

RESPIRATORY ILLNESS

Bottle-fed infants have been shown to have sixfold the risk of respiratory illness compared with infants breastfed three or more months (Howie et al, 1990). The Beaudry and associates study (1995) showed a protective effect of breastfeeding on respiratory illness even after adjustment for infant age, socioeconomic class, maternal age, and cigarette consumption for a large cohort of 776 infants in Canada.

The prophylactic effect of breastfeeding helps fight the respiratory syncytial virus (Cunningham, 1992). Breastfeeding has also been found to be protective for serious *Hemophilus influenzae* (Hib) disease (Cochi et al., 1986) and acute lower-respiratory infection—pneumonia or bronchiolitis (Pisacane et al., 1994).

Hospitalization for respiratory infections is more frequent for formula-fed infants (Cunningham et al., 1991). Babies who were ever breastfed had half the hospitalizations for respiratory illness during early childhood than did formula-fed babies (Chen et al., 1988). Approximately twice as many formula-fed infants are shown to have episodes of acute chronic bronchitis (de Duran, 1991). The risk of death from lower-respiratory-tract infections is nearly four times higher for formula-fed infants living in urban environments of developing nations (Cunningham, 1992). Smoking and bottlefeeding act synergistically to raise the risk of serious respiratory illness by three- to fourfold (Chen et al., 1988).

Bronchiolitis parainfluenza virus has been found to be higher for infants never breastfed (Welliver et al., 1986) and less severe for infants breastfed at least one month (Porro et al., 1988). Inositol, a component of membrane phospholipids that enhances the synthesis and secretion of surfactant in immature lung tissue, is present in higher amounts in human milk than in formulas. Preterm colostrum is a rich source of inositol. Inositol significantly reduces the severity of a common occurrence in the neonatal intensive care unit (NICU)—the preterm infant with respiratory distress syndrome (RDS). Serum inositol levels have been shown to increase with preterm infants fed inositol-rich breastmilk in contrast to formula-fed preterm infants who show no rise in serum inositol levels (Pereira et al., 1990). The lack of inositol in formula places preterm infants consuming it at a higher risk for respiratory failure, bronchopulmonary dysplasia, and retinopathy if not supplemented early in life (Hallman et al., 1992).

BOTULISM

Infant botulism resulting in sudden death occurs only in formula-fed infants. Breastfeeding protects against fatal botulism (Cunningham, 1992). A nonfatal botulism has been identified in weaning breastfed infants (Istre et al., 1986; Spika et al., 1989). This is possibly due to alterations in gut flora during weaning (Cunningham, 1992).

URINARY TRACT INFECTIONS

Pisacane found the relative risk of a urinary tract infection while being breastfed during the first six months to be 0.38 in a study with 128 breastfed and 128 controls (formula-fed) (Pisacane et al., 1992). The urinary tract has mucosal tissue with the products of the secretory immune system "bathing" the area, which may explain how breastfeeding affords protection at a site removed from the gut.

GASTROENTERITIS AND DIARRHEA

Strong evidence for breastfeeding providing protection against gastroenteritis exists (Howie et al., 1990; Rogan et al., 1987). These benefits may be as a result of hygienic factors, specific immune factors (IgA), differences in bacterial flora (Duffy et al., 1986), nonspecific host factors (lactoferrin, epithelial receptor analogues) (Hanson et al., 1985), and/or the presence of milk mucins (Patton, 1994). The digestive system is colonized with nonpathogenic bacteria—*Bifido bacterium lactobacillus*—which reduces growth of *E. coli, Salmonella,* and *Shigella* and is responsible for the characteristic smell of breastfed infants' stools. High-iron infant formula tends to promote the development of clinical *salmonellosis,* while breastfeeding appears to be protective against *salmonellosis* (Haddock et al., 1991).

For rotavirus-positive gastroenteritis, the relative risk for exclusively breastfed infants was 0.27. For nonspecific gastroenteritis, the relative risk for infants exclusively breastfed four months or more was 0.29. For the infants receiving no breastmilk, there was a fivefold increased risk in moderate to severe illness. The attack rate for rotavirus–gastroenteritis was similiar between infants given any breastmilk compared to infants receiving none (Duffy et al., 1986). However, the severity of clinical symptoms, such as emesis, diarrhea, febrile seizures and dehydration, was significantly reduced in breastfed infants (Duffy et al., 1992).

Necrotizing enterocolitis (NEC) has been shown to be 6 to 10 times more common for formula-fed infants than for infants fed breastmilk exclusively and three times more common in infants fed formula and breastmilk. In infants < 30 weeks gestational age, NEC is 20 times more common in the formula-fed over the exclusively breastmilk-fed infant (Lucas & Cole, 1990). deCurtis and colleagues (1987) have also shown a beneficial effect of breastfeeding compared to formula feeding in the prevention of NEC in the human. Furukawa and associates (1993) have identified the presence of platelet-activating factor–acetylhydrolase in human milk (PAF-AH). PAF-AH is an enzyme that metabolizes platelet-activating factor—one of the most proinflammatory bowel agents (Esplugues & Whittle, 1989), and along with endotoxin and tumor necrosis factor-alpha (PAF) has been suggested to play a role in the development of NEC in the newborn (Caplan et al., 1990). PAF-AH is not present in bovine milk (Furukawa et al., 1993). PAF-AH in human milk survives at a low pH and is believed to be important in preventing the accumulation of PAF in the small intestine. More research will be needed to determine if this enzyme plays a significant role in preventing NEC.

Formula-fed infants have also been shown to have a higher rate of diarrhea. A three- to fivefold increased risk of diarrhea illness exists in formula-fed infants in industrial nations (Feachem & Koblinsky, 1984).

OTITIS MEDIA

Exclusive breastfeeding for four or more months has been shown to protect infants from single and recurrent episodes of otitis media (Duncan et al., 1993). Infants breastfed exclusively for four months have one-half the occurrence of otitis media compared to formula-fed infants. The risk of otitis media (Rogan et al, 1987) and lower-respiratory illness is doubled by not breastfeeding (Wright et al., 1989). Beaudry and associates (1995) observed a protective effect of breastfeeding for otitis media in a retrospective, cohort study that grouped together infants who were exclusively breastfed and those who received water or formula in addition to breastmilk.

It is unclear by what mechanisms or combinations this difference is seen. Contributors to the lower incidence of otitis media may be secretory IgA, prostaglandins (decreased inflammatory response), or positioning while breastfeeding, which may minimize pooling in the eustachian tube. Previous studies suggest the development of otitis media may be closely associated with nasopharyngeal colonization patterns of nontypeable *Haemophilus influenzae* (Faden et al., 1990; Faden et al., 1991).

Harabuchi and associates (1994) followed 68 human milk-fed children from birth to 12 months of age to assess the effect of human milk secretory IgA antibody to P_6, which is an outer membrane protein of nontypeable *Haemophilus influenzae* (a frequent cause of otitis media). The authors found the frequency of isolation of nontypeable *H. influenzae* was directly related to episodes of otitis media and that the level of human milk anti-P_6 secretory IgA antibody was inversely related to frequency of isolation of the organism. The authors suggest the protective effect of human milk against otitis media may be partly a result of inhibition of nasopharyngeal colonization with nontypeable *H. influenzae* by specific secretory IgA antibody (Harabuchi et al., 1994).

One of the most common illnesses in childhood is otitis media, with 62% of children having at least one episode during their first year of life. Formula feeding increases the risk, while four months of exclusive breastfeeding decreases the risk of single and recurrent otitis media. The duration of infections in infants who do contact the illness is decreased as well (Duncan et al., 1993; Fosarelli et al., 1985). Exclusive breastfeeding for more than six months resulted in one-third the infection rate observed in formula-fed infants during the first three years of life (Pukander et al., 1985). In 1990, it was reported that 30 million visits to the pediatrician for otitis media occur per year in the United States at a cost of $1 billion (Facione, 1990).

MISCELLANEOUS OTHER INFECTIONS, DISEASES

Breastfeeding has been found to decrease the risk of acute appendicitis (Pisacane et al., 1995), multiple sclerosis (Pisacane et al., 1994), inguinal hernia (Pisacane et al., 1995), and hypertrophic pyloric stenosis (Pisacane et al., 1996). Breastfeeding has been found in one case-control study to increase the risk for intussusception (the slipping of one part of an intestine into another part just below it) during infancy (Pisacane et al., 1993).

Infant Oral Health Care

As members of the early childhood health-care team, lactation consultants (LC) have a unique opportunity to educate, provide advice, and offer direction to the infant's parents regarding basic infant oral health care. Subjects, such as oral hygiene for the nursing infant, fluoride supplementation, dental caries (tooth decay), nutrition, teething, nonnutritive sucking, trauma prevention, and when to schedule the infant's first dental visit, ideally, should be introduced during prenatal classes. These subjects should then be readdressed throughout infancy by the primary care physician, the family dentist, and other health-care personnel. Unfortunately, this does not always occur, and all too often the first advice a parent receives regarding oral health care for the infant and toddler is from a dentist after a problem has developed.

The relationship established between a nursing mother and the LC is by its very nature informal, and often consists of more than one visit. Therefore, opportunity abounds to offer new parents early basic dental education and to direct them to their pediatrician, pediatric dentist, or family dentist when appropriate. Your counsel will be appreciated by the parents, and serves to further the cause of disease and pain prevention and the establishment of sound oral hygiene practices.

ORAL HYGIENE FOR THE BREASTFEEDING INFANT

Oral hygiene for any infant begins before birth, with the mother. An understanding by the mother of the importance of a healthy dentition and the need for daily hygiene and sound dietary practices is critical to the establishment of good habits in the home. Studies have shown a correlation between the oral microflora of the mother and that found in her infant (Berkowitz et al., 1981; Kohler & Bratthall, 1978; Rogers, 1981). Mothers with poor oral hygiene tend to have higher levels of disease-causing bacteria, fungi, and viruses. This undesirable imbalance could, by nature of their close contact, be transferred between the mother and her child.

Daily oral cleansing habits of children should begin when they are infants. The parents have the responsibility for this program, and it should be established even before the teeth begin to erupt. Daily cleaning of the infant's oral cavity, including the gums, cheeks, palate, and tongue, not only helps to ensure healthy soft tissues, but establishes a pattern of behavior in infancy that will become accepted and carry over into childhood. Initially, these cleanings should be with a soft cloth or moist gauze. Once the teeth have begun to erupt, around the age of 6 to 10 months, a gradual transition to a soft bristle toothbrush can occur.

Bacteria that form plaque and initiate dental caries have been shown to be present in the oral cavity soon after the eruption of the first tooth (Edwardsson & Mejare, 1978). This usually coincides with the introduction of other liquids (e.g., juices) and foods into the infant's diet. Therefore, daily mechanical removal of plaque is a critical step to early caries prevention. Ideally, this should be accomplished after each feeding. Since brushing may not always be convenient, a simple wiping of the teeth and soft tissues with a cloth will suffice after meals. Mechanical removal of plaque and debris is the goal, and this does not require toothpaste. A fluoridated toothpaste does provide an added preventive measure (topical fluoride) once teeth erupt, but it should be used sparingly due to the inability of the infant to expectorate.

Some additional helpful hints for home dental care for the infant include the following:

- Proper positioning for adequate visibility and accessibility
- Timing the cleaning so that it coincides with other established daily routines to decrease the chance for "forgetting," and to increase the chance for infant acceptance (e.g., after the evening bath)
- Encouraging the parent to become "creative," such as playing games while brushing, as the infant becomes older
- Reminding parents that, just like taking baths and going to bed, the child will have good days and bad days

The degree to which the parent pursues the issue will vary, but in the end, the parent must prevail. Finally, a pediatric dentist or family dentist can provide a more thorough discussion of home hygiene care.

FLUORIDE ADMINISTRATION AND SUPPLEMENTATION

Since 1965, there has been a marked reduction in the prevalence of caries in the United States and other countries (NIDR, 1979-80; NIDR, 1989-90). A major factor contributing to this significant public health success story appears to the increased accessibility to fluorides (beginning in infancy) as an inexpensive and highly effective preventive tool in the fight against this disease.

Fluoride becomes incorporated into the mineral structure of the tooth, and its presence appears to prevent dental caries by: (1) increasing the tooth's resistance to acid dissolution, (2) enhancing the process of remineralization (in effect, reversing early carious lesions), and (3) reducing the potential of dental plaque that causes tooth decay. The benefits of fluorides can be acquired both systemically and topically. For infants and toddlers, the principal concern is that they receive an optimal level of systemic fluoride (Nowak & Crall, 1988).

The primary source of systemic fluoride is through naturally or artificially fluoridated drinking water. Fluoride consumed in this manner can safely reduce the incidence of caries by 40% to 50% in the primary dentition and by 50% to 65% in the permanent dentition (U.S. Department of Health, Education, and Welfare, 1979). The recommended fluoride concentration level for public drinking water is 0.6 to 1.0 parts per million (ppm).

Systemic fluoride supplementation, in the form of drops or chewable tablets, is recommended in cases in which adequate consumption of fluoridated water does not occur. Included in this category are (1) infants older than six months who derive all or most of their fluid intake from breastfeeding, (2) infants and children living in nonfluoridated communities or in communities with less than optimum levels of fluoride in the water supply (< 0.6 ppm), and (3) cases where the family utilizes bottled water or home-filtration systems for their primary source of water for drinking and cooking.

Topical fluoride, primarily that found in toothpastes, offers additional protection against tooth decay. However, infants and toddlers are not capable of expectorating and the topical fluoride soon becomes systemic because it is swallowed. The knowledge that this occurs, as well as the recent rise in incidence of dental fluorosis (staining of the permanent teeth) has brought about a reexamination of recommendations regarding flouride concentrations in toothpastes, frequency of toothpaste utilization, and levels of prescribed fluoride supplementation (Burt, 1992; Levy, 1994). In the future, it is likely that "children's-strength" fluoridated toothpastes will be available. Furthermore, dentists and physicians have recently received new guidelines for fluoride supplementation.

The ADA Council on Dental Therapeutics, the American Academy of Pediatric Dentistry (AAPD), and the American Academy of Pediatrics (AAP) have adopted a newly adjusted dosage schedule for dietary fluoride supplementation. This new schedule postpones prescribing of fluorides for infants in nonfluoridated communities until six months of age, reduces the dosage strength for each age group, and reduces the minimum recommended water fluoride level from 0.7 ppm to 0.6 ppm. The adjusted schedule should help to maximize benefits while reducing the incidence of dental fluorosis (AAPD, 1994-95; AAP, Committee on Nutrition, 1995).

Fluoride will continue to play a vital role in dental caries prevention, and its use should be encouraged. When young children are concerned, however, the following are commonsense guidelines for infants and toddlers:

- Use toothpaste sparingly—"pea size" or smaller amount.
- Use toothpaste no more than once or twice a day.
- Supervise preschool-age children when they brush.
- Avoid use of fluoride mouth rinses until age 5 or 6, when the child can demonstrate mastery of rinsing and expectoration.
- New parents should seek advice from their pediatric dentist or pediatrician regarding the need for supplementation.

DENTAL CARIES AND NUTRITION

Dental caries is a complex disease of the teeth that is multifactorial in nature, and leads to the destruction of the inorganic and organic components of the tooth. Put into simplified terms, there are four requirements for this process to occur (Adair, 1988):

1. A susceptible host (the tooth)
2. The presence of bacteria (primarily *Streptococcus mutans*)
3. A substrate (fermentable carbohydrates)
4. Time

The presence of susceptible teeth is a constant. Susceptibility of these teeth to decay, however, can be reduced by absorption of systemic fluoride during tooth formation, and by frequent exposure to topical fluoride sources after eruption into the oral cavity. Additional preventive measures, such as professionally applied sealants on posterior teeth, can also significantly reduce caries susceptibility.

Dental plaque is that often invisible, sticky substance that adheres to the tooth, consisting primarily of bacteria and food debris, held together by polysaccharide chains. As carbohydrates are consumed by the human host, the bacteria (primarily *streptococcus mutans*) metabolize this substrate and the resultant by-product is acid. As acid levels within plaque increase, the pH level at the tooth surface decreases and demineralization occurs. This is the beginning of tooth decay. Long-term exposure to mature plaque and low pH levels can also lead to gum disease.

Regular and thorough cleaning of the teeth and oral cavity can reduce the levels of bacteria available to form plaque, as well as the degree of maturation of the bacterial colonies in plaque. Frequent cleaning can also reduce the time that a particular substrate is available to the bacteria, and the amount of time the plaque has to act on that substrate. The result is more elevated pH levels, less demineralization, and healthier hard and soft tissues.

The presence of *Streptococcus mutans* in the mothers is a risk factor for the development of caries in both breastfed and formula-fed infants. The presence of *Streptococcus mutans* in the mother's mouth has been correlated with primary oral infection by *Streptococcus mutans* in the infant's mouth (Berkowitz, Turner, & Green, 1981; Köhler, Bratthall, & Krasse, 1983). Also, studies have shown that the establishment of *Streptococcus mutans* in the infant or child can be delayed by caries-preventive measures by the mother (Köhler, Bratthall, & Krasse, 1983; Köhler, Andreen, & Jonsson, 1984).

An obvious critical requirement for the development of dental disease is the substrate. Much is still to be learned about the potential for various substances to promote tooth decay (the substance's cariogenicity). However, three factors seem to play a significant role: (1) adhesiveness, (2) solubility, and (3) percentage of available fermentable carbohydrates. An additional critical factor is the frequency with which cariogenic substances are consumed.

Foods that are difficult to solubilize or that adhere to the teeth and soft tissues are difficult to clear from the mouth and are available for fermentation for longer periods of time. This results in a drop in the pH to a level that promotes bacterial growth and demineralization (Stephan, 1940). Foods high in fermentable carbohydrates can rapidly alter the oral environment and lead to increased acid levels. Many of these high-carbohydrate substances are also naturally acidic (fruit juices, carbonated beverages), which only serves to potentiate an already destructive process.

BREASTFEEDING AND DENTAL CARIES

The relationship between nighttime bottle feedings and the use of the bottle beyond 12 months of age with a devastating dental caries pattern known as Baby Bottle Tooth Decay (BBTD) is well-documented in the literature (Kroll & Stone, 1967; Ripa, 1988; Shelton, 1977). This caries syndrome has a distinctive clinical presentation, consisting primarily of destruction of the smooth surfaces of the upper incisors followed by various surfaces of the upper and lower molars (McDonald & Avery, 1983; Ripa, 1988; Rule, 1982). An association between breastfeeding and dental caries has not been as clearly established.

Several authors have suggested that this disease pattern can occur, albeit at a much lower incidence, in breastfed children. These proposals have been based primarily on a few case reports (Brams & Maleney, 1983; Gardner et al., 1977; Kotlow, 1977), studies demonstrating the cariogenicity potential of lactose (Roberts et al.,

1983), and the relative high percentage of lactose (7%) found in human milk (Darke, 1976; Rugg-Gunn et al., 1985). Suppositions have also been made in many of these articles about the relative high frequency of breastfeedings, especially at night, and the possibility of "pooling" of the milk around the teeth similar to that found during bottle feeding. Abbey (1979), however, doubts that breastmilk stagnates on or around the teeth during or after breastfeeding, citing deglutition research and cineradiographic studies evaluating the feeding cycle and the infantile swallow; and there are currently no in vivo studies clearly demonstrating pH drops in the presence of breastmilk to levels low enough, and for a long enough period of time, to cause significant demineralization of enamel.

The majority of case studies, although raising significant questions about the possibility of extensive caries development in some children who participate in prolonged, ad lib, and nighttime breastfeeding beyond 12 months of age, failed to adequately investigate other dietary factors, oral hygiene habits at home, or the availability and frequency of exposure to fluorides (Brams & Maleney, 1983; Gardner et al., 1977; Kotlow, 1977).

A recent investigation of prolonged, on-demand breastfeeding and dental caries in Ireland was carried out for 107 children (59 weaned; 48 nursing) breastfed on demand for at least two years. The following information was evaluated: dental examination for caries, enamel hypoplasia, and opacities; saliva samples from infants and mothers (N = 48) who were still breastfeeding for *Streptococcus mutans* analysis; and 25 mL of nocturnal breastmilk samples (N = 25) for lactose analysis. The study found four factors significantly associated with high incidence of caries:

1. Defective enamel
2. Maternal stress and/or bereavement during pregnancy
3. Reduced intake of dairy products during pregnancy (retrospective maternal dietary recall)
4. Medically diagnosed maternal illness during pregnancy associated with antibiotic use.

There was a trend for dental caries to be associated with *Streptococcus mutans* in both the child's and mother's mouth but it was not significant (Torney, 1995).

Further studies investigating the relationship of breastfeeding habits and dental caries are needed, and any study should include the preceding external variables as well as other factors—possible inherited susceptibility, oral microflora profiles, and antibody levels.

An additional argument proposed recently to dispute any connection between dental caries and breastfeeding is the research on dental caries in deciduous (first) teeth in skulls that are at least 200 years old (Bentzen, 1929; Höjgaard, 1980; Keene, 1986; Moore & Corbett, 1971, 1973; Pedersen, 1938) and in skulls from children living in traditional cultures (Campbell & Gray, 1936; Campbell, 1938a,b; Nicholls, 1914; Pedersen, 1938; Sampson, 1932). These studies show very low rates of dental caries in populations in which breastfeeding was the normal way to feed infants.

The nutritional and immunologic advantages of breastfeeding are well-documented, and the AAPD endorses the position of the American Academy of Pediatrics on the promotion of breastfeeding (AAPD, 1997–1998). Mothers should be supported in their efforts to breastfeed, but they should not become complacent to the possibility of the development of dental disease in their children as teeth erupt and the diet becomes more complex.

TEETHING

Eruption of the primary teeth begins at 6 to 10 months of age. By 12 months, the 8 incisors are usually present, and by 2 to 2½ years of age, all 20 primary teeth have erupted. Sequence and timing vary between individuals and genders, with girls slightly ahead of boys.

Teething is a normal physiologic process and significant problems or complication are the exception. Restlessness, irritability, and excessive drooling are not uncommon, however. Mild swelling and/or bruising of the alveolar soft tissue directly over an erupting tooth may also be seen, but lancing of these tissues is generally not indicated. In some cases, systemic manifestations, such as a rise in temperature, rashes, or gastrointestinal disturbances, have been attributed to teething (Carpenter, 1978; Honig, 1975), but care must be taken to avoid scapegoating teething while missing an underlying illness (e.g., otitis media). If systemic symptoms persist for more than 24 hours, or if the infant's or child's condition progressively deteriorates, a physician should be consulted.

Relief of teething discomfort can usually be accomplished with gum massage, and with teething rings or cool washcloths to chew on and apply pressure. Teething rings should not be frozen because tissue burns may occur. Over-the-counter topical anesthetics are not recommended because the duration of benefit is limited (6–8 minutes), toxicity can develop with overuse, and the gag reflex could be temporarily suppressed. When medication appears necessary, acetaminophen may be considered after consultation with a physician or dentist.

For some breastfeeding mothers, their first experience with infant teething can be an uncomfortable one. The infant quickly learns that chewing provides relief for sore gums. If biting and nipple soreness occur, the mother should be encouraged and informed that this is only transient. Furthermore, since the tongue covers the lower teeth while nursing, chewing of the nipple is an indication that the infant is no longer feeding and other forms of relief mentioned earlier can be offered.

NONNUTRITIVE SUCKING

Nonnutritive sucking is a normal part of neonatal development, and its prevalence in infancy is almost universal (Christensen & Fields, 1994). The influence of breastfeeding and nonnutritive sucking at the breast on the incidence and duration of other forms of sucking is unclear. Numerous studies and articles on this complex subject have been conflicting and inconclusive (Finochi, 1992). Many LCs object to the use of this term when applied to feeding at the breast since the breast is never emptied during the lactation period and the term implies that no nutrients are delivered.

Present even before birth, the need for nonnutritive sucking appears to reach a peak by seven months of age, and then usually decreases with the development of other sensory and motor activities (Brazelton, 1956). When digit or pacifier sucking is present and persists beyond infancy, or increases after weaning, there is often a corresponding rise in concern among parents or other caregivers. Parental or professional intervention at an early age should be discouraged, however, because most children spontaneously discontinue this behavior by two to four years of age (Nowak et al., 1986; Traisman & Traisman, 1958).

The effects of nonnutritive sucking on the primary dentition are usually minor and most self-correct if the habit is discontinued before the primary incisors begin to exfoliate. Early evaluation and monitoring of the existing habit by a dentist, the developing dentition, and the gradual maturation of the swallow mechanics is important, however. This period of "watchful waiting" (Christensen & Fields, 1988) offers opportunities for the dentist to observe significant changes, provide encouragement and advice, and plan age-appropriate intervention and treatment when indicated.

INJURY PREVENTION

During the first three years of life, injuries to the face, jaws, teeth, and other oral structures are not uncommon. Life-threatening injuries, such as asphyxiation, can also easily occur by way of the oral cavity. A great many of these injuries are preventable. Discussing age-appropriate injury prevention with parents and other caregivers is an important part of comprehensive pediatric health care, and this should be accomplished at every opportunity by each member of the health-care team. The following are some simple guidelines the LC can offer to parents to help reduce the chance of injury to the oral and perioral structures of infants and toddlers:

- Never warm expressed breastmilk in the microwave because "hot spots" can scald the oral cavity and esophagus.
- Never tie a pacifier around an infant's neck with a ribbon or string.
- Keep small objects that can be aspirated or swallowed out of the child's reach.
- Always use a child restraint appropriate for the child's age and weight when traveling in an automobile.
- Use cabinet latches and keep harmful chemicals out of reach.
- Adjust temperature settings on hot water heaters to no higher than 140°F.
- Never allow an infant or toddler access to areas of the room where electrical cords are present; severely disfiguring injuries can occur when a child chews or bites an electrical cord.
- As the child begins to learn to walk, do not use a walker.
- Remove low-level furniture, especially coffee tables, from the home until the youngest child is at least four years of age.
- Do not allow the child to walk with objects in his or her mouth.
- Do not leave a child unattended near stairs, and use sturdy safety gates at the top of stairs whenever possible.
- Nail down or remove loose carpeting.
- Always be safety conscious and use common sense when small children are around.

For more information on child safety and injury prevention, contact the American Academy of Pediatric Dentistry or the American Academy of Pediatrics (see Chapter 3, Resources).

THE FIRST DENTAL EXAM

Whether by habit or tradition, the prevailing recommendation for when to schedule a child's first dental exam has been after the third birthday. With our ever-expanding knowledge of growth and development, oral and dental diseases and their prevention, behavior-management techniques, and the need for early intervention, there has been a recent shift in the traditional schools of thought as they pertain to the youngest age groups.

The American Academy of Pediatric Dentistry now recommends: "oral examination and preventive health education within six (6) months of the eruption of the first primary tooth and no later than 12 months of age" (AAPD, 1997–1998). This early dental visit is primarily intended to evaluate the infant's current oral health status, assess various risk factors for oral disease, educate the parents regarding the development of dental disease and its prevention, and to make recommendations pertaining to the need for future visits.

A health questionnaire should be completed and the dentist and his or her staff need to evaluate the child and discuss a variety of topics, including oral hygiene, injury prevention, dietary habits, nonnutritive sucking, fluorides, growth and development, and the prevention and treatment of dental disease. Anticipatory guidance will be given specific to each family's needs and risk factors, with additional information or appropriate referral being offered as indicated.

The majority of health-care professionals now recognize that the prevention and treatment of dental disease plays an important role in achieving optimum physical health and self-esteem in a child. Through prenatal and postnatal counseling from each member of the pediatric health-care team, early administration of fluorides, and a dental exam by 12 months of age, great strides can continue to be made in the prevention of dental disease.

Conditions of Nutritional Concern

FAILURE TO THRIVE—GROWTH DEFICIT

Failure to thrive (FTT) can occur in any infant, although poverty is the single greatest risk factor. It occurs in approximately 10% of the pediatric population and accounts for approximately 1% to 5% of the hospital pediatric admissions (Hufton & Dates, 1977; Peterson et al., 1984). FTT can occur at any age. The newer term for FTT is *growth deficit*. It is defined as weight and/or height below the third percentile for age based on standardized growth charts, weight for height below the fifth percentile, or a fall-off of growth velocity of two major percentiles (Berkowitz & Sklaren, 1984; Kristiansson & Fallstom, 1987).

Lawrence's (1994) definition of failure to thrive is: "When the infant continues to lose weight after 10 days of life, does not regain birth weight by 3 weeks of age, or gains at a rate below the tenth percentile for weight gain beyond 1 month of age." The long-term effects of this problem include growth deficits through the school-aged years, disorders in personality, and cognitive defects (Berkowitz & Sklaren, 1984; Kristiansson & Fallstom, 1987). Follow-up on children three years after documented FTT has found that they continue to suffer from significant health problems (Singer, 1986).

Evaluation for FTT—Growth Deficit

The health-care provider must determine if the growth deficit has a social or medical etiology; these may be difficult to separate. Many questions need to be answered during this period. Care must be taken to avoid placing blame on the caregiver. Components of a thorough investigation include medical, nutritional, social, developmental, and physical assessments (see Table 2B–3).

Table 2B–3   Components of Failure-to-Thrive—Growth-Deficit—Assessment

Nutritional	Medical	Physical
Weaning history	Prenatal history	Review of systems examination
Feeding milestones	Family history	Metabolic examination
Context of meals—style	Neonatal history	Temperature
Independence	Infancy history	Respiration rate
Feeding observation		Blood pressure
Food frequency (24-hour recall)		Fluid balance
Anthropometric assessment		Heart rate
		Electrolyte

Developmental	Social
Screening evaluation	Multiproblem family
Temperamental assessment	Social isolation
	Unplanned or difficult pregnancy
	History of loss and/or violence
	Availability of food

FTT is classified as organic (if a diagnosable physical condition is present to cause the growth retardation) or nonorganic (80% of the cases) (Berkowitz & Sklaren, 1984). Medical conditions most commonly causing organic FTT are gastrointestinal disorders (gastroesophageal reflux, chronic diarrhea, malabsorption, bowel malformations), central nervous system (CNS) problems (cerebral palsy, microcephaly, and asphyxia), cardiac lesions, pulmonary disease, and endocrinopathies (Berkowitz & Sklaren, 1984; Peterson et al., 1984). Nonorganic FTT is labeled transactional or interactional and is felt to be caused by several variables such as the parent's history (their childhood experiences, health, and emotional status), the child (neurological status, temperament), the interaction between the child and the family, and the level of stress and support in the environment and family situation (Altemeier et al., 1985; Casey, 1987; Casey et al., 1984).

In actuality, the two types of FTT overlap, as there are emotional risks to the child failing to thrive secondary to an organic cause and medical risks for the child with nonorganic FTT due to malnutrition (Bithony & Newberger, 1987; Casey et al., 1984; Peterson et al., 1984). Malnutrition is the presenting medical problem often and can cause irritability, disturbances in temperament, and difficulty in feeding. Several types of nutritional inadequacies have been identified: adequate amounts of food to support normal growth in normal infants are offered but are not accepted by the infant; large amounts of food are lost through vomiting and regurgitation; excessive fecal losses of nutrients and unusually high energy requirements occur; or an insufficient amount of food is offered to the infants (Fomon, 1974). The reasons for an infant to refuse food may be an unnatural sucking and swallowing mechanism (seen especially in preterm infants), nasal obstruction, a small jaw, cleft palate or lip, or a large tongue. When the infant–mother interaction is disturbed the child may refuse food.

Treatment should be based on the results of the assessment. In one case, treatment may be as simple as the provision of growth hormone, but in another, intense medical, family, and nutritional intervention may be needed. The physician should evaluate the child and take a complete medical history, family and prenatal history, developmental assessment, clinical evaluation, anthropometric measurements, nutritional history, social situational analysis, behavioral and interactional qualities, and biochemical tests (Peterson et al., 1984). Hospitalization may be necessary to complete the evaluation. Biochemical tests should include a complete blood count, serum electrolytes and acid-base status, urinalysis, lead levels, serum glucose, serum protein, BUN, and liver function. Stools should be checked for pH level, stool-reducing substance, fat, parasites, and eosinophils (Rudolph, 1985). Skeletal age determination can help in some cases (Steele, 1986). Table 2B–3 summarizes the components of an evaluation for FTT and Table 2B–4 shows the components in more detail.

Diagnosis of Breastfed Infants' FTT—Growth Deficit

Breastfeeding infants' FTT can occur because of maternal and/or infant causes. Poor production and poor milk-ejection reflex are commonly a result of illness, fatigue, psychological and pharmacologic factors, and dietary reasons. Poor intake and excessive losses by the infant occur for various reasons. Figure 2B–3 is a diagnostic flow chart for FTT.

Table 2B–4   Detailed Components of the Evaluation for FTT—Growth Deficit

MEDICAL, FAMILY, PRENATAL HISTORY

- Hospitalizations, medications, frequent illnesses, accidents, pica or lead ingestion
- Family situation—disruptions in the family, number of family members, level of concern of parents, amount of time child spends out of the home
- Growth patterns of parents and other siblings, inherited or familial diseases (such as Down syndrome, thyroid insufficiency, microcephaly), slow development in other family members
- Infections during pregnancy; use of drugs, alcohol, and cigarettes; difficult pregnancy or labor; premature birth; gestational age and low Apgar scores; medical or feeding problems in perinatal period

DEVELOPMENTAL AND CLINICAL ASSESSMENT

- Record of developmental milestones
- Current rating of development on Denver Development Screening test or similar tool
- Parent's perception of how child compares with other children of his or her age developmentally
- Signs of malnutrition (muscle wasting, thin arms and legs, protuberant abdomen, thin skin with decreased subcutaneous skin, hollow look to the face)
- Indicators of possible neglect (untreated diaper rash, dirty clothes, or poor hygiene), possible abuse (bruises; evidence of unusual scarring; evidence of injured skeleton; frequent, unexplained accidents)

BEHAVIORAL AND INTERACTIONAL QUALITIES

- Infants with FTT are often jittery, irritable, and fussy (Showers et al., 1986)
- Behaviors exhibited by infants with FTT include flexed hips and knees, expressionless faces, abnormal gaze, general inactivity, and lack of physical response to a stimulus (Powell et al., 1987), reduced vocalizations by mother and infant (Berkowitz & Senter, 1987), delays in oral–motor performance/less ability to communicate needs during a feeding session (Mathiesen et al., 1989)
- Decreased responsiveness of the mother to the infant's cues has been found in FTT infants (Casey et al., 1984; Fosson & Wilson, 1987)

ANTHROPOMETRIC ASSESSMENT

- Weight and length or height—Decreases reflect an ongoing malnourished state
- Weight and age—Wasting. This is the first to decrease if malnourished and is a predictor of mortality/morbidity.
- Length and age—Stunting. This is a predictor of chronic poor nutrition.
- Arm circumference and triceps skinfold measurement—Can be used to determine midarm muscle circumference and arm fat area (Frisancho, 1981). Below 5% indicates depletion of fat store and muscle protein.
- Head circumference—Use NCHS standards. Reflects caloric intake or medical problem.

NUTRITION AND FEEDING PATTERN

- Present intake, changes in intake, food likes and dislikes, problems surrounding the feeding situation, 7-day food diaries
- Estimation of amount of breastmilk per day; formula and how prepared; position of infant during feedings; estimated losses from regurgitation, vomiting, and urinary output
- Feeding observation—length of a total feed, emotional context of feeding, interaction between caregiver and child or infant, use of feeding devices, maladaptive feeding behaviors (gagging, choking, holding of the breath, pica, vomiting at sight of food, rumination, refusal of food)

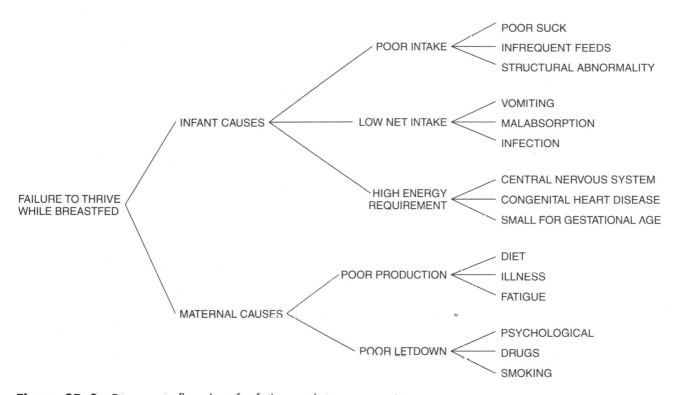

Figure 2B-3   Diagnostic flowchart for failure to thrive.
Source. Lawrence, P. (1994) *Breastfeeding—A Guide for the Medical Profession*, p. 368. St. Louis: Mosby. Reprinted with permission.

Maternal Problems That Can Cause FTT—Growth Deficit

Some maternal problems that cause FTT—growth deficit include anatomic causes, low milk production causes, style of nursing, and the fat content of the milk.

Anatomic causes that result in low milk production include insufficient glandular tissue, retaining placental fragments, breast reduction surgery, Sheehan's syndrome, and untreated thyroid hormone deficiency. Low milk production by mothers can be caused by poor caloric intake, illness, use of drugs (including some OTC ones), smoking, fatigue, and excessive alcohol intake. The style of nursing is not usually an issue for infants who are thriving but in growth deficit, caloric density is the goal and switch nursing may decrease fat intake per feeding.

Anatomic Causes

Lactation failure caused by insufficient glandular tissue in the presence of symmetry of breasts and normal prolactin levels has been described (Neifert et al., 1985; Niefert & Seacat, 1987). Retained placental fragments can be detected by questioning breast changes and patterns of lochia in postpartum women. Breast-reduction surgeries that cut nerve pathways can block the signaling of the hypothalamus and pituitary gland to secrete lactogenic hormones. Sheehan's syndrome causes an infarct of the pituitary due to excessive blood losses and hypotension and results in lactation failure.

Low Milk Production

Woolridge (1995) proposes the schema in Table 2B–5 to classify low milk supply. Diets, maternal illness, fatigue, and poor release of milk can all contribute to poor

Table 2B–5 Low Milk Supply Schema

Pathophysiological	Physiological	Behavioral	Iatrogenic
• Milk output < 150 g/ 24 hr • Etiology—? thyroid deficiency, retained placenta, Sheehan's syndrome	• Milk output of 150–350 g/24 hr • No identifiable origin • Unresponsive to therapeutic agents	• Milk output < 450 g/ 24 hr • Induced by infant self-limiting intake at an inappropriate level • Outcome of behavioral coping strategy in response to aversive stimuli • Output > 350 g/24 hr— may respond to pharmacotherapeutic agents	• Milk output < 450 g/ 24 hr • Increased milk output at an earlier stage • Now dropped and cannot get back up • Output > 350 g/24 hr— may respond to pharmacotherapeutic agents

production of milk. Marginal diet in Western cultures, particularly caloric deficits, has been shown to decrease milk production. The level of 1,800 kcalories (kcal) has been reported as an energy threshold for lactation below which milk production is affected negatively (Dewey et al., 1991). Brewer's yeast and herbal teas such as Fenugreek and mother's milk teas have been used as nutritional supplements and reported anecdotally to be successful in increasing the milk supply.

Infections that may be common in postpartum women include urinary tract infections, endometritis, or upper-respiratory infection, which may cause problems with milk production. Thyroid disease in the mother may also influence milk production (Lawrence, 1994). Fatigue can be devastating to lactation, especially during the first month postpartum while the breastmilk supply is being established. The infant's and/or the family's demands and work, school, or other responsibilities may lead to a lack of sleep and fatigue.

Smoking can interfere with the MER. A clear relationship between smoking and the amount of milk produced has been shown (Hopkinson et al., 1992). Moderate to heavy drinking by lactating women is believed to interfere with oxytocin release based on animal models. Flavor changes in the milk after drinking have been reported to decrease infant intake during a feeding (Lawton, 1985; Mennella & Beauchamp, 1991). Delays in motor activity at one year have been reported in the children of women who drink heavily (Little et al., 1989).

Medications may interfere with prolactin (L-dopa and ergot preparations) or oxytocin release, and OTC antihistamines may reduce milk volume. Estrogen-containing oral contraceptives lower milk volume as well. Psychological inhibition can occur and may be obvious, such as in the case of a disapproving partner, or subtle, such as an unusual routine or disruption in the community environment (a building project begun in the neighborhood, a violent or frightening incident, and so on).

The report of a 5% Insufficient Milk Syndrome was discussed in the popular media in the mid-1990s (Gorman, 1994; Heller, 1994; Helliker, 1994; Kanagaratnam, 1994; Khan, 1994; Priest, 1994; *Providence Journal-Bulletin*, 1994a,b). This claim has sent clinicians looking in the literature for reported cases, clinical trials, or letters to the editor to validate the claim of a 5% incidence rate for Insufficient Milk Syndrome. It has been found that there is a complete lack of research verification for that percentage but one commentary speculates on the subject (Neifert, 1987).

There have also been numerous reports from the biocultural perspective of the anthropologists (Greiner, 1981; Greiner, Van Esterik & Latham, 1981; Gussler & Briesemeister, 1980, 1981) about the Insufficient Milk Syndrome. Research documenting low milk supply is limited but includes the report on reasons for weaning from the Dunedin Multidisciplinary Child Development Study (Hood et al., 1978) and the report on breast surgery, appearance, and pregnancy-induced breast changes on lactation sufficiency as measured by infant weight gain (Neifert, 1990). Most clinicians do not believe the Insufficient Milk Syndrome rate is as high as 5%.

Style of Nursing

The switch-nursing technique has been recommended to build milk supplies, but according to Lawrence (1994), this interrupts the release of fat and the production of fat-rich hindmilk. Feeding on one breast per feeding may increase the percent of calories taken from fat and thereby influence infant weight gain. A creamatocrit check before and after may be useful for determining the success of the intervention, although this is not practical in most clinical settings. The use of a baby scale, which can calculate weight before and after a feeding, can help the clinician determine if the switch-nursing technique is detrimental to the optimal delivery of milk volume but cannot tell the clinician if the caloric delivery is better, because fat calories may be lower using the switch-nursing technique.

Creamatocrits

Testing human milk for macronutrient levels outside of the context of clinical research is generally not necessary. There is one quick and fairly accurate measurement that may be helpful, especially when problem solving for a breastfeeding infant's FTT—growth deficit—or in feeding preterm infants when optimal provision of energy is desired. This test measures the percentage of cream, or "creamatocrit," found to be useful because there is a linear relationship between fat and energy content (Lucas et al., 1978). Use of the following formulas has been suggested to determine fat and kcal in conjunction with the creamatocrit measurement:

$$\text{Fat (g/L)} = \frac{(\text{creamatocrit [\%]} - 0.59)}{0.146}$$

$$\text{kcal} = 290 + (66.8 \times \text{creamatocrit [\%]})$$

The following additional formulas for calculating the fat–energy content of milk using a creamatocrit measurement have been published by Silprasert and associates (1986):

$$\text{Fat (g/L)} = (6.24 \times \text{creamatocrit [\%]}) - 3.08$$
$$[r = 0.98, \text{ 95\% confidence limit} = \pm 4.39 \text{ g/L}]$$

$$\text{kcal/dL} = (5.57 \times \text{creamatocrit [\%]} + 45.13$$
$$[r = 0.92, \text{ 95\% confidence limit} = \pm 12.61 \text{ kcal/dL}]$$

Several studies have been done to validate the method. Energy values calculated by creamatocrit were more accurate when compared to energy values from percentage of carbon (using a bomb calorimeter) when fresh or fresh-frozen samples were used rather than pooled, pasteurized milk samples (Smith et al., 1985). Lemons and associates (1980) actually measured the total fat and caloric content of milk and validated the creamatocrit method, which also showed that freezing or pasteurization has no effect on the creamatocrit.

Lawrence (1994) lists the following special cautions to take when using the creamatocrit test:

- The sample should be representative of the 24-hour day and be well mixed.
- Sampling should include complete pumpings from one breast and not spot samples.
- The tube should be three-quarters full and sealed at one end.
- The sample should be centrifuged for 15 minutes in a standard tabletop centrifuge.
- If there is a small layer of liquid fat on top, it should be included.
- The tube should be kept vertical.
- The measurement should be taken within one hour of centrifugation.

Michaelsen and colleagues (1990) have described the use of a simple and rapid infrared analysis of creamatocrit by milk banks. Correlations between results using this method and standard reference methods were reported by these authors. Of 224 women (2,554 collections of milk), the mean protein content was 9 g/L and the mean fat content was 39 g/L. This method has implications for milk banks because they can screen for high-protein or high-fat milk, and they can "create" higher-energy content milk or higher-protein-content milk by milk-sample pooling, which can be used for very low-birth-weight infants; small for gestational age; or other infants who need additional calories, fat, or protein.

Infant Problems That Can Cause FTT—Growth Deficit

Conditions that can cause infant FTT while exclusively breastfeeding include poor intake, low net intake, and high energy requirements. Causes of poor intake are poor suck, infrequent or inadequate feeds, and structural abnormalities. Vomiting and diarrhea, malabsorption, and infection result in low net intake. Infants with neurologic problems, congenital heart disease, and SGA have high energy requirements. Underlying physical problems can impact on feeding as well as on utilization of energy and energy needs. With the increasing growth of family-centered care in which the infant is hospitalized for only a short period of time or is maintained in the same room with the mother, the risk of not identifying feeding problems increases.

Close follow-up of breastfed infants is essential, especially in parts of the Western world where the norm is to bottle feed. The question of whether the breastfed child shows signs of growth deficit is multifactorial and the LC should refer any breastfeeding dyad that has not been evaluated by a physician to a pediatrician or family practice physician.

Babies at particular risk for FTT include SGA infants, infants with metabolic disorders, infants with jaundice, infants with vomiting and diarrhea, infants with infections, infants with signs of dehydration and hypernatremia, and infants with increased metabolic rates (high energy requirements).

Small-for-Gestational-Age Infants

Infants are born small for gestational age for many reasons, including placental insufficiency, maternal disease, toxemia, excessive maternal smoking, poor maternal nutritional status, and intrauterine infections such as toxoplasmosis. They are small at birth despite being full-term. They have a large nutritional deficit and require calories that are similar to the needs of the infant who is an appropriate weight for gestation. Thus, for SGA infants, caloric requirements are not based on actual weight but on optimal weight. Frequent feedings, including night feedings, are necessary. If the infant is not gaining weight at the desired rate and the mother has an ample milk supply, the mother can manually or mechanically express her hindmilk after feedings and give it to the infant by using a nursing supplementer, feeding tube, or dropper.

Because SGA infants may have an inability to suck effectively at first, aggressive management is important during the early postpartum period and close monitoring should be scheduled. Should supplementation be necessary due to the mother's insufficient milk supply (because of poor stimulation to the breast at feeding), the amount of supplement should be monitored and gradually decreased as the mother's milk supply increases. The nutrient density or composition of the milk can be altered by nutritional engineering (i.e., the addition of modular supplements). The use of a feeding supplementer is recommended so that the infant can be maintained at the breast. In the case of a poor maternal milk supply, the supplement to use will need to be formula.

Some clinicians choose to use one of the 24- or 27-kcal/oz. formulas but, if cost or availability is an issue, a 20-kcal/oz. formula can be fortified with 0.5 cc of oil (corn, canola, MCT, Microlipid, and so on) per 30 cc of formula, which will bring the formula to a 24-kcal/oz. density. This would be appropriate for a short-term situation while the maternal milk supply increases. If an infant weighs less than 2,000 g and is on full breastfeeds but is not gaining appropriately, it may be best to use a human milk fortifier or protein modular component added to hindmilk. Certainly, in either of these cases, the mother should be referred to an experienced infant feeding nutritionist who preferably is an LC, and a physician should supervise the infant's care.

Infant Metabolic Disorders

Screening for metabolic disorders is mandated by law in most states and should include screening for galactosemia, phenylketonuria, maple syrup urine disease, urea cycle disorders, and thyroid disorders. The alteration in metabolic functioning most often involves deficient enzyme activity and, for most infants, is inherited as an autosomal recessive trait. The maternal metabolism provides the enzyme activity for the fetus, so these disorders may not be evident until after birth. An untreated, severe case can cause irreversible brain damage (AAP, 1992). Galactosemia is discussed under Contraindications to Breastfeeding in Section A of this module.

Infant Vomiting and Diarrhea

Vomiting is often the presenting symptom for more serious medical problems involving the gastrointestinal tract such as pyloric stenosis and other metabolic disorders. It is usually not common for breastfed infants, although some spitting up after feeds is not unusual, and should not be of concern unless the infant's weight gain is compromised or aspiration is a concern. Causes of vomiting that may be a result of breastfeeding include overfeeding, maternal diet of foods that the infant may be allergic to, or overconsumption of foods that adversely affect flavor.

Gastroesophageal reflux is a commonly diagnosed vomiting disorder, and the recommended management includes adding cereal to the infant's diet. This can be detrimental to the breastfeeding dyad because it requires the mother to pump her milk and feed via bottle. For many mothers, the reflux can be handled by elevating the infant for a sufficient period of time after feedings, provided the infant continues to gain weight appropriately. Except in the more severe cases, reflux is more of a laundry problem than a feeding problem.

Breastfeeding mothers often use the term *diarrhea* to describe breastfeeding stools; this is particularly the case for mothers who have never been exposed to a breastfed infant before or have not been prepared to expect the differences in the stools of the breast- and formula-fed infant. Diarrhea is actually uncommon in well, breastfed infants although maternal consumption of cathartics may contribute to looser stools. Diarrhea can be secretory or osmotic in pathophysiology. When a food substance that is usually absorbed is not or is malabsorbed, an osmotic load in the distal small intestine and colon can result in osmotic diarrhea and subsequent increased nutrient losses. The most commonly malabsorbed nutrient is carbohydrate.

Examples of causes of osmotic diarrhea include laxative preparations (e.g., lactulose and milk of magnesia), lactase deficiency, congenital sucrase-isomaltase deficiency, hypermotility disorders (such as in irritable colon of infancy and the diffuse mucosal injury found in infections), inflammatory bowel disease, or celiac disease (Moutos, 1996). When feeding is halted, osmotic diarrhea stops.

Secretory diarrhea, on the other hand, is not related to food intake and is caused by pathogens such as enterotoxigenic *E. coli*, cholera, or hormone (vasoactive intestinal polypeptide)-secreting tumors—ganglioneuroma, the oversecretion of gastrin as seen in Zollinger-Ellison syndrome, or congenital chloridorrhea (congenital disorder of electrolyte transport) (Moutos, 1996). When diarrhea is present for less than two weeks, it is considered acute and its cause is usually viral (rotavirus), bacterial (*Shigella, Salmonella, Campylobacter,* and so on), or protozoal (*Giardia*).

Hydration and electrolyte replacement are the first priority. After an infant is rehydrated, breastfeeding should continue during diarrhea because breastmilk contains many anti-infective factors and maintains a small amount of milk passing through the intestine at a time, which allows the intestine time to absorb the nutrients. If an infant is not breastfed, the use of oral rehydration solutions is encouraged. Only in intractable vomiting, severe dehydration, high stool output, or carbohydrate malabsorption would rehydration by intravenous fluids be necessary.

Chronic diarrhea in infants is most often caused by cow's milk and soy protein intolerance, protracted infectious enteritis, microvillus inclusion disease, autoimmune enteropathy, Hirschsprung's disease, congenital transport defects, and nutrient malabsorption (Moutos, 1996). Contrary to what is believed by many mothers, the use of high-carbohydrate foods and beverages, such as tea, apple juice, gelatin desserts, powdered drink mixes, and so on, may exacerbate diarrhea. Instead, low-carbohydrate, high-fat foods are indicated. Any prolonged incidence of diarrhea should be evaluated for the underlying etiology because growth will continue to suffer if the cause of the diarrhea is not identified and treated. Chronic diarrhea can lead to mucosal injury and malabsorption that results in malnutrition.

Infants with Infections

Chronic and acute infections may deter growth in an otherwise healthy infant taking in adequate kcalories. The possibility of gastrointestinal and/or urinary tract infections should be considered when the presence of respiratory and ear infections has been eliminated. Chronic viral infections, such as cytomegalovirus and hepatitis, can also cause growth faltering.

Infants with High Energy Requirements

Infants with congenital heart disease, preterm infants, and infants who are unable to maintain adequate body temperature may have increased energy requirements. Infants who appear hyperactive, and who startle easily and sleep poorly, may have neurologic disorders; or when this has been ruled out, a hyperactive infant may be breastfeeding from a mother who is taking in too much caffeine. The half-life of caffeine increases in the neonate so that an accumulation may make the infant symptomatic. The limited use of caffeine is recommended, and for some infants, it may be optimal for mothers to forgo caffeine-containing beverages completely.

Infants with Signs of Dehydration and Hypernatremia

Cases of dehydration and hypernatremia in exclusively breastfed infants have been publicized in the lay press recently, causing much discussion and controversy. It may be that poor breastfeeding management is to blame for the majority of these cases. Nevertheless, the LC must know how to identify signs of dehydration and make an immediate referral for treatment (see Tables 2B–6 and 2B–7). An assessment of the degree of dehydration usually can be made quickly by looking at skin turgor and tone. Electrolyte levels may be depressed. High breastmilk sodium levels may need to be ruled out and this can be done by measuring milk electrolyte levels and infant urine levels (Lawrence, 1994). Each breast should be sampled separately before and after feeding and the samples from a single breast mixed. Lethargy and inadequate stooling and urine output are common signs of dehydration. Elevated serum BUN, creatinine, and hematocrit are present as a result of fluid volume depletion. The urinary specific gravity is also increased. Hypernatremic dehydration is an emergency requiring hospitalization; cardiovascular collapse with hypothermia and hypoglycemia can occur if untreated.

For breastfed infants with severe dehydration, hypernatremia is reported to occur in one-half of them (Roddey et al., 1981; Rowland et al., 1982). Several cases of elevated milk sodium have been reported. Whether elevated milk sodium causes insufficient milk or is an effect of insufficient milk is not known. It is known that sodium levels are higher in weaning milk and in women who are not lactating during the postpartum period (both are states of breast involution). Maternal dietary intake does not influence the passage of sodium into breastmilk because sodium entry into milk is a controlled mechanism not influenced by maternal serum levels (Ereman et al., 1987).

Preparation of a Nutrition Care Plan

The nutritional management of the infant or child with FTT must be carefully planned to consider all the social and medical variables influencing the nutritional status. The plan should include a nutritional evaluation at periodic intervals; long-term monitoring of the progress of growth; and instruction to the family about the exact amounts, types, and preparation of food to provide adequate calories and protein to allow for catch-up growth. Growth charts should be used to establish growth patterns, but recognizing that these growth grids are based on healthy, full-term infants who were formula-fed is important. Each grid measures nutritional deficiencies in different ways. The stages of malnutrition and clinical indicators of malnutrition are summarized in Tables 2B–8 and 2B–9, and factors that contribute to nutrition and feeding difficulties are summarized in Table 2B–10.

Table 2B–6   Assessment of Diarrhea Patients for Dehydration

FIRST, ASSESS YOUR PATIENT FOR DEHYDRATION.

	A	B	C
1. LOOK AT:			
CONDITION	Well, alert	•Restless, irritable•	•Lethargic or unconscious; floppy•
EYES[1]	Normal	Sunken	Very sunken and dry
TEARS	Present	Absent	Absent
MOUTH and TONGUE[2]	Moist	Dry	Very dry
THIRST	Drinks normally, not thirsty	•Thirsty, drinks eagerly•	•Drinks poorly or not able to drink•
2. FEEL: SKIN PINCH[3]	Goes back quickly	•Goes back slowly•	Goes back very slowly
3. DECIDE:	The patient has NO SIGNS OF DEHYDRATION	If the patient has two or more signs, including at least one •sign•, there is SOME DEHYDRATION	If the patient has two or more signs, including at least one •sign•, there is SEVERE DEHYDRATION
4. TREAT:	Use Treatment Plan A	Weigh the patient, if possible, and use Treatment Plan B	Weigh the patient and use Treatment Plan C URGENTLY

TREATMENT PLAN A

To treat diarrhea at home:

1. Give more fluids than usual to prevent dehydration.
2. Give child adequate food to prevent malnutrition.
3. Reexamine within three days for repeated vomiting, watery stools, marked thirst, eating or drinking poorly, fever, blood in stool.

TREATMENT PLAN B

To treat dehydration:
Approximate amount of oral rehydrating solution (90 mg Na/L) to give first 4 hr:

Wt (kg)	<5	5–7.9	8–10.9	11–15.9	16–29.9	30+
mL	200–400	400–600	600–800	800–1200	1200–2200	2200–4000

TREATMENT PLAN C

To treat dehydration quickly:

1. Start IV fluids immediately (100 cc/kg).
2. Ringer's lactate or normal saline.
3. Reassess every 1–2 hr.
4. After 3–6 hr, reassess and institute plan A, B, C.

[1]In some infants and children the eyes normally appear somewhat sunken. It is helpful to ask the mother if the child's eyes are normal or more sunken than usual.

[2]Dryness of the mouth and tongue can also be palpated with a clean finger. The mouth may always be dry in a child who habitually breathes through the mouth. The mouth may be wet in a dehydrated patient owing to recent vomiting or drinking.

[3]The skin pinch is less useful in infants or children with marasmus (severe wasting) or kwashiorkor (severe undernutrition with oedema), or obese children.

Source: Adapted from WHO/CDD/Ser 80. Geneva, Switzerland: World Health Organization, 1990. Barness, LA (Ed.) (1993). *Pediatric Nutrition Handbook*, p. 426. Elk Grove Village, IL: AAP. Used with permission of American Academy of Pediatrics.

Table 2B-7 Recommendations for the Use of Oral Solutions for Treating Pediatric Patients with Gastrointestinal Fluid Losses

	Rehydration Solution	Maintenance Solution
Purpose	Treatment of acute dehydration (extracellular volume contraction)	Prevention of dehydration caused by diarrhea or maintenance of hydration after treatment of dehydration
Sodium	75–90 mEq/L	40–60 mEq/L
Potassium	20 mEq/L	20 mEq/L
Anions	20–30% of anions as base (acetate, lactate, citrate, or bicarbonate) and the remainder as chloride	20% to 30% of anions as base (acetate, lactate, citrate, or bicarbonate) and the remainder as chloride
Carbohydrate	Glucose: 2.0–2.5% (110–140 mM/L)	Glucose: 2.0–2.5% (110–140 mM/L)
Administration	Volume given to equal estimated fluid deficit: usually 40–50 mL/kg to be given over about 4 hr; reevaluate clinical status and therapy after 3–4 hr	Daily volume should not exceed 150 mL/kg per 24 hr; if additional fluid is needed to satisfy thirst, a low-solute fluid such as water or human milk should be used

Source: Barness, LA (Ed.) (1993). *Pediatric Nutrition Handbook,* p. 221. Elk Grove Village, IL: AAP. Used with permission of American Academy of Pediatrics.

Table 2B-8 Assessing the Stages of Malnutrition

Stage	Weight and Age	Height and Age	Weight and Height
Normal	> 90% median	> 95% median	> 90% median
Mild malnutrition	75–90% median	90–95% median	81–90% median
Moderate malnutrition	60–74% median	85–89% median	70–80% median
Severe malnutrition	< 60% median	< 85% median	< 70% median

Source: Frank, DA, Silva, M, Needleman, R (1993). Failure to thrive: Mystery, myth and method. *Contemporary Pediatrics,* 10:114. Reprinted with permission.

Table 2B-9 Clinical Indicators of Malnutrition

- Abnormality of fat metabolism
- B vitamin deficiencies
- Cheliosis
- Chronic dry skin and/or eczema
- Dermatitis, diarrhea, growth deficit
- Edema, hair loss
- Iron deficiency
- Protein deficiency
- Spoon nails
- Vitamin E deficiency
- Zinc deficiency

To develop the nutrition care plan, consideration of all the data gathered in the assessment is imperative. When calculating needs for the infant or young child with growth deficit, use the calories for weight age as a guide. This can be done by determining at what age the present weight would be at the 50th percentile on the growth chart. The recommended values for the weight age are used to calculate the calories and protein needs and can be used to estimate catch-up growth requirements.

Treatment requires that caloric needs for catch-up growth be provided by the plan. *Catch-up* growth occurs when an infant is on a caloric level adequate to provide a growth velocity for age that is one-and-one-half times the norm. Calorie and protein requirements by age are listed in Chapter 1 of this module. To estimate catch-

Table 2B–10 Factors That Contribute to Nutrition and Feeding Difficulties

Factors	Nutrition and Feeding Difficulties
Prolonged exclusive breastfeeding	Deficit in developmental process of eating

Gastrointestinal tract abnormalities
   Esophageal atresia
   Tracheo-esophageal fistula
   Diaphragmatic hernia
   Pyloric stenosis
	Vomiting and/or aspiration

Mechanical factors
   Macroglossia
   Cleft lip
   Fusion of gums
   Tumors of mouth or gums
   Temporomandibular ankylosis or hypoplasia
	Interfere with sucking

Congenital abnormalities of the nose, mouth, and jaw
   Chonal atresia
   Cleft lip and palate
   Micrognathia and glossoptosis
   Postintubation dysphagia
   Palatal paralysis
   Pharyngeal tumors
   Pharyngeal diverticula
   Familial dysautomia
	Feeding difficulties
	Disorders of swallowing

Malabsorption
   Immaturity
   Congenital or acquired disaccharidase deficiency
   Monosaccharide malabsorption
   Milk allergy
   Cystic fibrosis
   Celiac disease
   Protein–calorie malnutrition
   Congenital immunological deficiency
   Hirschsprung's disease
   Acrodermatitis enteropathica (zinc) deficiency
   Necrotizing enterocolitisis
   Biliary atresia, neonatal hepatitis
	Diarrhea or steatorrhea from excess fecal losses

Low-birth-weight infants	Increased kcal requirements
Maternal anesthesia or analgesia	Absent or diminished suck
Anoxia or hypoxia	Absent or diminished suck
Prematurity	Absent or diminished suck Feeding difficulties
Trisomy 21	Absent or diminished suck
Trisomy 13–15	Absent or diminished suck
Hypothyroidism	Decreased kcal requirements

Neuromuscular abnormalities
   Kernicterus
   Werdnig-Hoffman disease
   Neonatal myasthenia gravis
   Congenital muscular dystrophy
	Absent or diminished suck
	Feeding difficulties

Infections of the central nervous system
   Toxoplasmosis
   Cytomegalovirus
   Bacterial meningitis
	Absent or diminished suck

up growth requirements see Table 2B-11. These guidelines are used to estimate catch-up growth requirements; precise individual needs will vary and be mediated by medical status and diagnosis. Table 2B–12 shows guidelines to follow when working with the infant who is breastfed and experiencing a growth deficit and for feeding the toddler who is not gaining appropriately.

To be more aware of medical problems that may alter your care plan, a discussion with the physician is a good idea. For example, if an infant has renal involvement, you may need to restrict the phosphorus, sodium, potassium, and fluid and increase the percentage of kcalories from fat. Once you determine needed macronutrients, determine fluid needs. Again, a thorough recognition of the medical basis for failure to thrive is essential. If the infant has a cardiac problem in which a volume overload is a concern, you may have to increase the density of the breastmilk or other feeding to meet the infant's needs while recognizing that fortification will lower the available free water. Whenever modular supplements are added, the free water in cc per kg decreases.

Once you have determined the volume you can feed the infant, calculate the nutrient contribution of that volume of breastmilk and compare it to the needs calculated for weight for age. The difference in caloric and protein needs for catch-up growth and the calories and protein being delivered during current feedings can then be quantified. These steps will help you to know how much to add to feedings to meet that need.

Fortification of Human Milk

Fortification of human milk can be done using hindmilk and oils for fat; human milk additives for protein, sodium, chloride, and kcalories; modular carbohydrate and protein products; 20-, 24-, and 27-kcal/oz. formulas, and special metabolic formulas. What and how much to use depends on each infant as previously dis-

---

Table 2B-11   Estimating Catch-up Growth Requirements

$$\text{Catch-up Growth Requirement (kcal/kg/day)} = \frac{\text{Calories Required for Weight and Age (kcal/kg/day)}}{\text{Actual Weight (kg)}} \times \text{Ideal Weight for Age (kg)}$$

1. Plot the child's height and weight on the NCHS growth charts or breastfeeding growth chart.
2. Determine at what age the present weight would be at the 50th percentile (weight age).
3. Determine recommended calories for weight age.
4. Determine the ideal weight (50th percentile) for the child's present age.
5. Multiply the value obtained in (3) by the value obtained in (4).
6. Divide the value obtained in (5) by actual weight.

Estimated protein requirements during catch-up growth can be calculated similarly:

$$\text{Protein Requirement (g/kg)} = \frac{\text{Protein Required for Weight and Age (g/kg)}}{\text{Actual Weight (kg)}} \times \text{Ideal Weight for Age (kg)}$$

Source: Rathbun, JM, Peterson, KE (1987). Nutrition in failure to thrive. In: Grand, RJ, Sutphen, JL, Dietz, WH (Eds.), *Pediatric Nutrition*, p. 638. Boston: Butterworth. Adapted from Petersen, KE, Washington, JS, Rathbun, J. Team management of failure to thrive. *J Am Diet Assoc* 1984; 84:810-15. Reprinted with permission of authors.

Table 2B-12 Guidelines for Feeding Management During Growth Deficit

ASSISTING THE BREASTFED INFANT WITH GROWTH DEFICIT

1. Refer to physician for medical problems and to establish joint roles in caring for mother–infant dyad.
2. Correct dehydration, electrolyte disturbances.
3. Assess breastfeeding technique and frequency.
4. Determine adequacy of milk transfer utilizing test weighing of infant if available.
5. Rule out abnormalities or conditions in mother that influence milk volume or milk composition negatively.
6. Measure and analyze human milk fat concentrations (optional).
7. Perform oral–motor assessment on infant if needed. Consult with occupational therapy, speech therapy, or physical therapy specialist.
8. Determine need for supplementation and/or fortification of breastmilk feeding based on growth deficit alone (kcal supplementation) and/or nutritional lab abnormality such as low albumin or low prealbumin (protein supplementation).
9. Develop a feeding plan and instruct the mother.
10. Work with physician to determine need for pharmacotherapeutic agents to increase the maternal milk supply.
11. Monitor, evaluate, and adjust plan at regular intervals.
12. Maintain documentation of intervention and outcomes.
13. Send report to primary care provider.

FEEDING GUIDELINES FOR POSTINFANCY

1. Plan meals and snacks at scheduled times.
2. Eat often, not constantly. Offer food every two to three hours.
3. Place child in appropriate position to eat. Make sure child can reach food easily.
4. Allow child to self-feed.
5. Don't force-feed, bribe, or cajole.
6. Offer solids first.
7. Add gravy, margarine, grated cheese, and other high-calorie foods to dishes. Monitor for steatorrhea, which may indicate fat malabsorption.
8. Limit intake of beverages. Do not encourage fluid consumption within an hour of eating.
9. Use modular supplements to increase the nutrient density of the food, if necessary.
10. Monitor, evaluate, and adjust plan at regular intervals.
11. Maintain documentation of intervention and outcomes.
12. Send report to primary care provider.

cussed. A pediatric registered dietitian who is skilled in "feeding engineering" can work closely with the LC on the delivery method.

When working with breastfeeding mothers, a test pumping of 12 hours to several days can give you information on the potential amount of human milk that will be available for fortification. Tailoring the milk can be done by adding most of the protein supplement, if protein deficiency is evident and renal function allows, to the first 50% of the anticipated feeding and then adding the other modular supplements (fats and carbohydrates) in the amounts needed. To achieve increased kcalories, several options are available: feeding the hindmilk from the pool of milk samples at the beginning of the feeding, fortifying with carbohydrate and fat, or using higher calorie formulas as a supplement (24- to 27-kcal formulas).

Commonly used protein powders give 4 g of high biological value protein per scoop and carbohydrate powders provide 23 to 30 kcal/T. Regular oils and medium-chain triglyceride (MCT) oil provide 8.3 kcal/cc. Microlipid provides 4.5 kcal/cc.

When Supplementation Is Medically Necessary

Medical reasons for supplementation include severely ill babies, babies in need of surgery, very low-birth-weight infants, and infants with inborn errors of metabolism. Examples of a severely ill baby include one with severe dysmaturity accompanied by potentially severe hypoglycemia and the infant with acute water loss. When the infant is well, there are only a few maternal reasons to supplement including severe illness (psychosis, eclampsia, shock) or when a mother is taking medication contraindicated during breastfeeding (cytotoxic and radioactive drugs and antithyroid drugs other than propylthiourcil (WHO/UNICEF, 1992). Social reasons for supplementation include forced maternal–infant separation (geographic separation, arrest, child abduction).

IRON-DEFICIENCY ANEMIA

More is known about iron development than probably any mineral, yet iron needs during exclusive breastfeeding are not completely understood. Iron-deficiency anemia is one of the leading nutritional problems of infants, children, and women of childbearing age in the world. Guidelines for assessing anemia in the pregnant woman are outlined in Module 3, *The Science of Breastfeeding*, Chapter 2. The focus of the discussion here is on iron deficiency in the infant and child.

The iron content of newborn infants' blood averages about 75 mg/kg (Calvo et al., 1992), an amount that is adequate to maintain iron sufficiency for approximately six months of postnatal growth for term infants. For premature infants, however, total body iron is lower than it is for full-term infants, and iron deficiency can occur rapidly and continue into iron-deficiency anemia. Profound changes in iron metabolism and the rate of erythropoiesis occur after birth. At birth, most samples contain nucleated red blood cells and a reticulocyte count of approximately 4% to 5%. Accompanying this are elevated erythropoietin levels and erythroid hyperplasia in the bone marrow. This is felt to be a compensatory red blood cell production due to the decreased oxygen saturation of fetal blood. Hemoglobin concentrations vary with gestational age and, between the 38th and 40th week, increments of 1 g/dL to 3 g/dL are observed.

Other changes in erythropoiesis in the first week of life include a rapid fall of erythropoietin levels from the initial elevation to undetectable levels, a decline of red blood cell precursors in the bone marrow from 40% of nucleated elements at birth to 10%, a rapid decrease in reticulocytosis, and a loss of nucleated red blood cell precursors by two to three days of age. As a result of this, postnatal suppression of erythropoiesis and the expanding blood volume of the infant, a progressive decline in hemoglobin concentration starts by the end of the first week of life and reaches its nadir by 8 to 12 weeks of life (term newborn) and 4 to 7 weeks of life (premature infant). Hemoglobin concentrations as low as 9 g/dL (healthy term infant) and 7 g/dL to 8 g/dL (preterm infant) may result. Hemoglobin increases in the presence of adequate iron stores once active erythropoiesis resumes.

To meet the need of iron for growth and to replace normal losses, iron intake must supplement the body stores. Iron losses are small and constant except during periods of diarrhea during feedings of cow's milk (Bahna & Heiner, 1978) or during frequent drawing of blood such as in a hospital setting. In exclusively breastfed infants not receiving supplementary foods, iron supplementation is recommended at six months (AAP, 1993; IOM, 1991). Results from Saarinen and Siimes (1979) emphasize the composition of the whole diet in the absorption of dietary iron. An inhibitory effect by solid foods on the bioavailability of human milk iron has been postulated (Oski & Landaw, 1980; Saarinen and Siimes, 1979; Woodruff et al., 1977). Garry and associates (1981) contend that some breastfed infants might deplete their own iron reserves rapidly after six months unless supplemental iron is provided even when exclusively breastfed for six months.

Changes in the rate of iron incorporation occur around the fourth month of life. Whether these changes are attributable to the normal depletion of iron stores not balanced by an exogenous supply of iron or are a result of the early introduction of solids and a subsequent decrease in iron bioavailability from human milk has only recently been studied. Calvo and associates (1992) sought to address this question by following 25 infants who were breastfed exclusively for six months and were fed iron- and ascorbic acid–rich foods as supplemental foods (excluding iron-fortified products and known iron-absorption inhibitors). Also followed were 15 initially breastfed infants weaned to iron-fortified formula at two months of age. Results from this study report a negative iron balance, or total body iron (TBI), increment between four to six months for breastfed infants with a 27.8% prevalence of anemia for the breastfed group and 7.1% for the formula-fed group in the ninth month. Ferritin (storage iron) was absent in 27.8% of the breastfed group and none of the formula-fed group (Calvo et al., 1992). This recent work supports work by Pizarro and associates (1991) in which the prevalence of anemia at nine months of age in breastfed infants was 22.5% and 3.8% in infants fed iron-fortified formula.

The role and benefit of iron-fortified cereal has been questioned by Fomon (1987) because of its reliance on electrolytic iron, which may not have high bioavailability. To look at this question, Walter and associates (1993) used a field-trial approach with five groups (fortified cereal, unfortified formula; unfortified cereal, unfortified formula; unfortified cereal, fortified formula; breastfed, fortified cereal; and breastfed, unfortified cereal). Markers of iron nutritional status were completed through age 15 months or until hemoglobin values decreased below 10.5 g/dL. The percentages of infants removed from the study for low hemoglobin values and with two or more additional abnormal biochemical indices of iron were highest for the breastfed, unfortified cereal group (27%), followed by the unfortified formula, unfortified cereal (24%); breastfed, fortified cereal (13%); fortified cereal, unfortified formula (8%); with the lowest percentage of anemia present in the fortified formula, unfortified cereal (4%). Fewer formula-fed infants were excluded if they had received fortified formula or cereal than if neither fortified food had been provided.

In the breastfed group, the addition of fortified cereal with the addition of solid foods at four months decreased the number excluded for anemia at 8, 12, and 15 months. There were differences noted in the quantity of cereal taken by the groups, with the mean amount for formula-fed infants reaching 30 g per day within three weeks of their introduction and the mean amount in the breastfed group reaching 25 g per day but not until 7.5 months (3.5 months after cereal's introduction). It could be argued that a higher quantity of fortified cereal ingested from an earlier period by breastfed infants may more closely approximate the results found for the formula-fed infants fed either fortified formula or fortified cereal. The results of this study have implications for iron supplementation recommendations in that exclusively breastfed infants may be able to meet iron requirements beyond four to six months of age only when solid foods added during that time period are primarily iron-fortified infant cereals and large enough quantities are consistently consumed.

In a recent study of 30 infants who received no cow's milk, medicinal iron, or iron-enriched formula and cereal and were breastfed to their first birthday, 30% were anemic at one year of age. However, for the nonanemic infants, the duration of exclusive breastfeeding was significantly longer—6.5 months versus 5.5 months—and none of the infants who were exclusively breastfed for seven months or more were anemic, even though 43% of those who were breastfed for a shorter period of time were anemic. The infants exclusively breastfed for a prolonged period had good iron status at 12 and 24 months of age (Pisacane et al., 1995).

It is widely held that iron absorption and utilization are very low during the first two months of life. Opponents of early iron supplementation cite this as a reason not to supplement the exclusively breastfed infant before six months. However, Fomon and colleagues (1993) report that erythrocyte incorporation of ingested ^{58}Fe by 56-day-old breastfed infants is 20% of the dose they receive and 7% of the dose given to formula-fed infants, suggesting that breastfed infants may have a greater ability to absorb iron supplements than formula-fed infants. Additionally, the breastfed infant is capable of storing iron for later incorporation into erythrocytes as seen by a higher percentage of doses incorporated at 112 days than at 70 days.

Because iron status is believed to be low in the full-term, breastfed group by four to six months of age, and earlier in the preterm group, why not routinely supplement all breastfed infants at four months or earlier? Iron is a potent oxidative agent and its use increases the needs for antioxidant nutrients like vitamin E. For the preterm infant who has decreased stores of vitamin E, supplemental iron during the first month postnatal has been reported to predispose these infants to vitamin E deficiency (Dallman, 1988). For the preterm infant receiving human milk, this may not be a problem because human milk is particularly rich in vitamin E.

Excessive iron can also cause decreased absorption of other trace elements with similar absorption pathways, like zinc, copper, and manganese (Lonnerdal, 1989). Iron overload has also been implicated as a risk factor for coronary heart disease (Salonen et al., 1992), and there is an increased concern about the process of heart disease beginning in childhood (AAP, 1992). On the other hand, iron is an important component of many enzymes, which are involved in DNA synthesis; mitochondrial electron transport; catecholamine metabolism; maintenance of neurotransmitter levels; oxidative degradation of fatty acids; and the synthesis of monounsaturated and polyunsaturated fatty acids, plasmalogens, and prostaglandins.

Several studies have described the effects of iron undernutrition on brain growth and development during the preweaning period (Bedi, 1987; Lozoff & Brittenham, 1986; Webb & Oski, 1973). The brain depends on external sources of lipids (i.e., from the diet or hepatic synthesis). The myelin sheaths of the brain and spinal cord are 80% lipid. Lipid availability is dependent on iron nutriture. The effect of an iron deficiency on lipid metabolism could be disastrous during the myelination of the brain during infancy. In children deprived of iron, a decrease in learning capacity (IQ level) has been documented (Lozoff & Brittenham, 1986). A relationship between iron deficiency and cell-mediated immunity also has been reported

(Chandra, 1977). It has also been suggested that iron deficiency may cause altered behavior in infants (Walter et al., 1983) as measured on the Bayley Scales of Infant Development (Bayley, 1969).

If iron deficiency occurs during a critical period of brain growth, the resulting abnormalities may be irreversible. Youdim and Ben-Shacher (1987) reported that the earlier in life the nutritionally induced iron deficiency occurs, the more severe the consequences may be. Idjradinata and Pollitt (1993) found an increase in both mental and motor scores after four months of iron therapy for iron-deficient anemic infants. This contradicts other studies that showed little or no benefit of iron therapy in reversing lower test scores of infants (Lozoff, 1994).

Clearly, the controversy about when to begin supplementation with iron in the breastfed infant continues. Unfortunately, current screening mechanisms (hematocrit or hemoglobin) do not decline to abnormal levels until iron-deficiency anemia is evident, limiting the clinician's ability to recognize the breastfed infant at risk for anemia. Newer measurements, such as the transferrin receptor level that detects early iron deficiency at the cellular level, are still being tested but are promising screening tools.

Iron is transported to the cells by transferrin (80,000 dalton glycoprotein with two iron-binding domains and a half-life of eight days). Cell-surface transferrin receptors (transmembrane glycoprotein with two equal subunits of 94,000 MW and a half-life of approximately 60 hours) predominate on erythroid and placental cell surface and are found on all cell surfaces as well (Loh et al., 1980; Seligman et al., 1979; Wada et al., 1979). Diferric transferrin has a high affinity for cell-surface transferrin receptors (Huebers et al., 1981; Huebers et al., 1983). When the cell has sufficient accumulation of hemoglobin, the intact transferrin receptor is shed from the cell surface into the plasma.

Ferguson and associates (1992) reported that transferrin receptor density is directly related to the tissue's iron requirements and is a sensitive measure of iron-deficiency anemia. In addition, Ferguson (1992) showed that the transferrin receptor level in the anemia of chronic disease remained normal because of limited erythropoietin production, implying that it is reliable in differential diagnosis. Skikne and associates (1990) found serum transferrin receptor measurement to be of particular value in recent onset, mild iron deficiency. The clinical significance of the serum transferrin receptor as an early marker for iron deficiency in infants is yet to be reported but is promising.

Screening

Risk factors for the development of depleted iron stores include rapid growth, premature birth (see Table 2B–13), inadequate iron intake, and blood loss (can occur from feeding of cow's milk during the first six months of life and from blood drawing while in nurseries). Outpatient screening for iron-deficiency anemia is usually done at nine months for term infants and at three months for preterm infants. Screening is delayed if there is evidence of infection within the previous two weeks. Age and race guidelines should be followed in determining the cutoff values for diagnosis. There are differences present due to age, gender, ethnicity, stage of pregnancy, and puberty. For example, Hispanic populations have lower hemoglobins than Caucasian populations.

Confirmation of iron deficiency requires a minimum of three to four biochemical markers. No single measurement gives a reliable measure of iron deficiency in the

Table 2B–13
Iron and the Preterm Breastfeeding Infant (Age 0–12 mo)

Iron stores	Low
Iron intake	Low
Iron needs	High
Risk of deficiency	High

absence of anemia, which is most likely to be the case in the infant who may be receiving inadequate dietary iron. The measurements to detect iron deficiency and iron-deficiency anemia include hemoglobin or hematocrit, mean cell volume (MCV), serum iron and iron-binding capacity, and transferrin concentration (not affected by infection) and RBC erythrocyte protoporphyrin (indicates iron-deficiency anemia in a healthy individual but is also affected by lead poisoning and infection). Iron deficiency without anemia is a mild iron deficiency and the hemoglobin will be normal. In iron-deficiency anemia, the iron stores will be depleted and the hemoglobin will be low.

Moderate anemia is defined as a hemoglobin value of less than or equal to 10.0 g/dL and mild anemia is a hemoglobin value of 10.1 g/dL to 10.5 g/dL. MCV is decreased in iron deficiency or thalassemia minor. When the MCV is high in the presence of a low hemoglobin, other causes such as a folate or vitamin B_{12} deficiency should be identified. There is a decreased ratio of serum iron to iron-binding capacity because the latter is increased in iron deficiency. Serum ferritin allows evaluation of iron reserves. Low values are considered to be < 10 mcg L^{-1} for infants and children and < 12 mcg L^{-1} for adults. In the presence of anemia, ferritin levels are considered low if they are < 15 mcg L^{-1} in children and < 20 mcg L^{-1} in adults. A low hemoglobin in the presence of a ferritin level > 20 mcg L^{-1} indicates adequate iron stores and in the presence of normal erythropoiesis, should yield a rise in hemoglobin. The ability to discern early iron negative balance is important for the clinician (see Figure 2B–4). Current classifications of iron status are shown in Table 2B–14.

Preventing Iron-Deficiency Anemia

Prevention of iron deficiency should focus on education, enrichment, and fortification of the food supply as well as supplementation. Education should promote iron rich foods and teach parents about foods that affect iron absorption such as fiber (phytates) and calcium (see Table 2B–15).

Supplementation Guidelines

Supplementation guidelines for infants are controversial, especially for the preterm infant. For the human milk–fed infant, iron supplementation is recommended to begin between four and six months, depending on when solid foods are introduced into the infant's diet (AAP, 1993; IOM, 1991); however, controversy continues to surround this issue, especially since the recent publication by Pisacane and associates (1995) discussed in the previous narrative. Feeding iron-fortified formula to term infants if their mother does not breastfeed is recommended (AAP, 1993).

For the preterm infant, some argue for a delay in iron supplementation until eight weeks if the infant weighs < 1500 g while others routinely begin supplementation

Figure 2B–4

Progression from iron depletion to anemia.

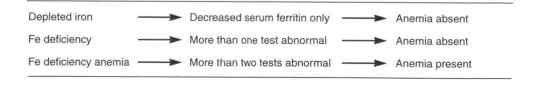

Table 2B–14 Iron Status Classifications

Iron Status	Laboratory Parameters
Iron deficiency with anemia	Hemoglobin level two standard deviation points below reference Two of three with abnormal levels: • MCV • Transferrin saturation • Free erythrocyte protoporphyrin
Iron deficiency without anemia	Hemoglobin normal Two of three with abnormal levels: • MCV • Transferrin saturation • Free erythrocyte protoporphyrin
Iron depletion	Low serum ferritin
Iron repletion	Normal hemoglobin
Iron sufficiency	Three normal iron measures

Table 2B–15 Iron Absorption Enhancers and Inhibitors

Enhancers	Inhibitors
Vitamin C	Phenolics
Cysteine	Phosphates, phytates
Lysine	Bran, lignin
Histidine	Proteins, egg
	Inorganic elements

Table 2B–16 Differences in Hemoglobin Iron of Preterm and Full-term Infants

	Birth	At One Year	Increase of
Preterm 1 kg	40 mg Fe	240 mg	200 mg
Full-term 3.5 kg	150 mg Fe	270 mg	120 mg

at two weeks of life. Arguments for early supplementation of the preterm infant are as follows (Thureen & Hay, 1993):

1. Iron stores are low in the very low-birth-weight preterm infant (see Table 2B–16).
2. There is some erythropoiesis occurring.
3. Liver can compensate for low iron stores but the brain cannot.
4. Early studies show developmental delays in infants with iron-deficiency anemia.
5. Even minimal effect on ferritin will be important in early weeks.
6. Use of erythropoietin may increase iron needs considerably.
7. Decreases need for transfusions.

Arguments for waiting to begin supplementation of the preterm infant are as follows (Thureen & Hay, 1993):

1. Iron deficiency is not a clinical problem in the first weeks of life.
2. Belief that iron supplementation has minimal effect on ferritin and none on hemoglobin due to decreased erythropoiesis.
3. There is an increased risk of free radical production due to the problems of prematurity such as retinopathy of prematurity, bronchopulmonary dysplasia, necrotizing enterocolitis.
4. Belief that nutritional immunity will be impaired because transferrin is saturated easily and there is a potential for free iron circulation.
5. High iron may affect zinc and copper absorption.

These concerns are theoretical because no detrimental effects of early iron supplementation have been proven at the levels given currently. Many question the value of ferritin in determining iron stores because of the intravariability of ferritin levels in each infant. Therefore, the risks of iron deficiency without anemia versus the potential toxicity of iron must be weighed.

Preterm Infants

Start ferrous sulfate at two weeks of age or when enteral feedings are tolerated at a dose of 2 mg/kg to 3 mg/kg per day to a maximum of 15 mg per day. Give vitamin E supplements also—often infants are on total parenteral nutrition (TPN) and receive vitamin E through this route. Vitamin E may not be necessary once the preterm infant begins taking breastmilk in significant quantities. If not started as discussed here, iron supplementation is definitely indicated by the time the infant's weight reaches about two kilograms or he or she goes home (Table 2B–16).

Full-Term Infants

Breastfed infants do not need to receive iron supplementation until solids are started. If iron-fortified cereal is the form of supplementation chosen, it should be offered two times per day so that about 1 mg/kg of body weight per day is provided. See the discussion that follows regarding delaying solids as a prophylaxis for iron-deficiency anemia.

Therapeutic Supplementation

When mild iron deficiency is detected, 3 mg/kg per day of iron as ferrous sulfate should be given for one month. For infants, this can be given as a single, before-breakfast dose to maximize absorption. Repeat laboratory tests should be done after one month. An increase of 1 g/dL of hemoglobin indicates a response and treatment should be continued for about four months to completely reverse anemia and restore iron stores (AAP, 1993).

Recent studies show that a weekly dose of supplemental iron is as effective as daily doses for children and adult women (Gross et al., 1994; Liu et al., 1994). Adherence to the treatment regime may be improved. There is also a decrease in gastrointestinal distress when a weekly dose of iron is given, which may also improve compliance. Iron absorption in the anemic patient is high (30–40%) early in the treatment period and decreases thereafter to 3% to 6%. A weekly dose seems to prevent the decreased absorption rate. Intestinal mucosal cells turn over every seven days, so the accumulation of iron in these cells is avoided. This iron accumulation is believed to be associated with gastrointestinal problems (Stephenson, 1995).

Differential Diagnosis

If a therapeutic trial with iron fails to correct anemia, a differential diagnosis must be made to distinguish iron-deficiency anemia from the anemia of chronic disease or infection, as well as other causes. Depressed serum ferritin levels (< 10 mcg/L) are seen in iron-deficiency anemia but are normal or elevated with infection and chronic disease. Lead poisoning and thalassemia minor can also cause microcytic anemia. In thalassemia minor, serum ferritin, transferrin saturation, and erythrocyte protoporphyrin are normal. In thalassemia major, erythrocyte protoporphyrin is very elevated and ferritin is high although hemoglobin decreases to below normal. In iron deficiency, erythrocyte protoporphyrin is somewhat elevated and in lead poisoning it is considerably elevated. When the mean cell volume is high in the presence of low hemoglobin, folate or vitamin B_{12} deficiency should be considered. Obviously, hemoglobin is not the only indicator that should be used to evaluate anemia.

Lactation consultants and WIC programs' personnel should be cautious about routinely recommending administering iron to patients with low hemoglobin. This is especially true for African American populations, because as many as 10% of this ethnic group's infants may have thalassemia major. A physician can best determine the cause of anemia.

ADVERSE REACTIONS TO FOODS

The main function of the immune system is to distinguish between self and non-self so that elements foreign to the body can be destroyed and tissues preserved. The immune response has T (thymus derived) and B (bone-marrow derived) lymphocytes and macrophages. When an antigen is introduced into the body, the B lymphocytes produce specific antibodies and the T cells begin the cell-mediated response. Regulatory T cells and macrophages direct both lymphocyte types.

Mucosal barriers in the intestinal tract protect self tissue from foreign antigens and include nonimmunologic and immunologic factors. Nonimmunoglobulin factors that protect the gastrointestinal tract include gastric acid, pancreatic and intestinal enzymes, the protein–phospholipid ratio of the microvillus, and the mucus coating of the microvillus. When the antigens penetrate the epithelial cells of the intestinal mucosa, they come into contact with lymphocytes and macrophages in the *lamnia propria*. This then signals the production of immunoglobulins A, E, G, and M (IgA, IgE, IgG, and IgM, respectively). The infant is susceptible to various antigens. In adults, secretory IgA (sIgA) is the major antibody of intestinal secretions. In the infant, there are relatively low concentrations of sIgA. The breastfed infant has an advantage over the formula-fed infant because the mother provides sIgA in her milk. For a discussion of how this occurs see Module 3, *The Science of Breastfeeding*, Chapter 2.

Adverse food reactions can be classified as food allergy (hypersensitivity) or food intolerance. Food allergy results from an antigen–antibody or antigen–cell interaction that has an adverse effect on the individual. Food intolerance results from nonimmunologic responses.

The combination of elevated concentration of IgE in cord blood and a family history of atopy has been proposed as a predictor of future allergic disease (Chandra et al., 1985; Magnusson, 1988). Until cord blood IgE becomes more available, the occurrence of IgE-mediated immediate reactions is often the first indication of an adverse food reaction (van Asperen et al., 1984).

Breastfeeding's Role in Preventing Atopic Disease

Breastfeeding has been found to protect the infant against possible adverse reactions to food antigens by three mechanisms (Taylor et al., 1973; Ziegler et al., 1986):

1. The size of the doses of foreign proteins that the infant is exposed to are minimized by breastfeeding.
2. Breastfeeding induces earlier maturation of the natural mucosal barrier against the entry of foreign proteins.
3. Breastfeeding provides passive protection against the entry of foreign proteins through the sIgA in human milk.

Breastfeeding has been shown to provide some protection against the early development of atopic disease (Businco et al., 1983; Chandra, 1979; Chandra et al., 1985, 1989; Hanson et al., 1984; Hattevig et al., 1989; Kajosaari & Saarinen, 1983; Matthew et al., 1977; Merrett et al., 1988; Saarinen et al., 1979; Sigurs et al., 1992; Wilson & Hamburger, 1988; Zeigler et al., 1986, 1989). Food allergies appear to be more frequent for formula-fed infants, with 7.4% of them developing cow's milk allergy and up to 50% being allergic to soy (Cunningham et al., 1991).

Although the practice of using casein hydrolysate formulas has been recommended for nonbreastfed infants at high risk for allergy, the American Academy of Pediatrics has stated that no published, well-controlled, double-blind studies exist to support the use of whey or casein hydrolysates for prophylactic treatment of infants with milk hypersensitivity (AAP, 1989). Anaphylactic reactions to both casein (Nutramigen, Alimentum, Pregestimil) and whey (Carnation Goodstart, Aifa-Re) hydrolysate formulas have been studied and results published (Businco et al., 1989; Ellis et al., 1991; Lifschitz et al., 1988; Saylor & Bahna, 1991; Schwartz & Amonette, 1991). See Table 2B–17 for some suggested strategies and mechanisms to prevent allergic diseases.

Maternal Diet Modifications for Breastfed Infants at Risk for Adverse Reactions to Food

Many reports have established that human milk contains a number of food antigens that are the result of the woman's diet (Cant et al., 1985; Clyne & Kulczycki, 1991; Cruz et al., 1981; Hanson et al., 1977; Jakobsson et al., 1985; Kilshaw & Cant, 1984; Kjellman & Johansson, 1979; Machtinger, 1989; van Asperen et al., 1984). Documentation of infants' adverse reactions to their mothers' milk also exists (Chandra, 1989; Chandra et al., 1989; Gerrard, 1979, 1984; Gerrard & Shenassa, 1983; Jakobsson & Lindberg, 1978; Lake et al., 1982; Machtinger, 1989; Machtinger & Moss, 1986; Matsumura et al., 1975; van Asperen et al., 1983; Warner, 1980).

For infants who are breastfed and exhibit allergy symptoms, an association has been found between low sIgA levels in maternal milk and high allergy symptom

Table 2B-17   Idealized Strategies and Mechanisms for the Prevention of Allergic Diseases in Infants

Strategy	Mechanism
Identify at-risk families	Document IgE reactivity in parents with history of allergic disorders or with existing atopic child.
Prevent postnatal sensitization to	
1. Food allergens	Begin maternal avoidance diet during lactation.
a. Transmitted through breastmilk	Withhold all nonbreastmilk foods except Nutramigen or Alimentum
b. Ingested by infant	for at least six months.
2. Environmental allergens	Encourage, instruct, and document avoidance of animals, mites, dust, and molds, as well as unnecessary medications.
Maximize immunologic competence	Encourage, instruct, and support breastfeeding for at least six months.
Minimize nonspecific enhancing factors	Discourage parental smoking; avoid viral illnesses; delay pertussis immunization.

Source: Modified from Hamburger, RN, Heller, S, Mellon, MH, et al. (1983). Current status of the clinical and immunologic consequences of a prototype allergic disease prevention program. *Ann Allergy*, 51:281. Reprinted with permission.

scores (Machtinger & Moss, 1986). Altered levels of polyunsaturated fatty acids have been found in the milk of mothers whose infants have atopic eczema (Manku et al., 1982; Wright & Bolton, 1989). Lower concentrations of a metabolite of linolenic acid (dihomo-gamma-linolenic acid) has been found in the milk (Morse et al., 1989) and the administration of gamma-linolenic acid (evening primrose oil is a good source) to the infant has been reported to alleviate the eczema (Biagi et al., 1988; Meigel et al., 1987; Morse et al., 1989).

The avoidance of major food antigens during pregnancy and lactation coupled with exclusive breastfeeding has been suggested as a means of decreasing atopic disease prevalence in infants believed to be at high risk for developing this problem (see Table 2B-17) (Chandra, 1987; Hamburger, 1984; Zeigler et al., 1986). Some believe that maternal avoidance of major food allergens while breastfeeding is helpful, but that avoidance during pregnancy is not supported by evidence (Fomon, 1993). This is based on reports that prenatal sensitization of the infant to food antigens occurs in less than 0.4% of cases (Zeigler et al., 1989). In one study, maternal avoidance of major food antigens during pregnancy was not shown to decrease the prevalence of atopic disease below that observed when the restrictions were imposed at the time of birth (Falth-Magnusson & Kjellman, 1987, 1992).

In another study, which measured cord blood IgE antibody levels to egg or milk in the infants born to atopic women, no differences were demonstrated between those whose mothers had or had not restricted their intake of these allergens (Lilja et al., 1988). Two studies (Chandra, 1987; Zeigler et al., 1989), which demonstrated a beneficial effect of maternal avoidance of major food allergens during pregnancy and lactation on the prevalence of atopic dermatitis in high-risk, breastfed infants, are believed to reflect only the influence of maternal dietary restrictions during lactation (Fomon, 1993). At least one major lactation reference recommends prenatal dietary modifications during pregnancy as well as lactation (Lawrence, 1994); however, the reference cited here was written prior to the publication of the other studies discussed.

Diet modification during lactation does appear warranted, however, for the high-risk family based on the reports cited here about food allergens in milk and documentation of reactions by infants. The most common allergens are found in cow's milk, soy milk, certain fruits and fruit juices (especially citrus ones, such as orange juice and tomatoes), and eggs and peanuts (Bock, 1987; Eastham, 1989; Gerrard et al., 1973; Jenkins et al., 1984; Kjellman et al., 1979; McDonald et al., 1984; Powell, 1978). Reactions to wheat and corn are less common. Tartrazine (FDC yellow no. 5) has also been suggested as an offender (Lawrence, 1994).

The mother's avoidance of the foods mentioned here should not present a deficiency of nutrients in the milk for the infant. The exception is that breastmilk is the major dietary source of vitamin D. Adequate exposure to sunlight or use of a liquid multivitamin containing vitamin D should be provided (some have tartrazine) because maternal diet does influence milk vitamin D levels. Mothers' diets should be supplemented with calcium from nondairy sources; the majority of studies documenting the adequacy of bone mineral density recovery after lactation are for populations that are well nourished with adequate intakes of calcium. See Section A of this chapter (under Osteoporosis) for a discussion of these studies.

PHENYLKETONURIA

Phenylketonuria (PKU) is the most common amino acid metabolic disorder. Due to a lack of the enzyme phenylalanine hydroxylase, phenylalanine builds up and becomes toxic. Serum levels of phenylalanine need to be controlled to between 120 μmol/L and 480 μmol/L to prevent toxic levels and the resulting mental retardation (Acosta, 1989; Acosta & Wentz, 1978).

Mothers can continue to breastfeed their infants with PKU, although extra care is required to ensure infant serum levels of phenylalanine remain within normal levels. Breastmilk has a phenylalanine content of 29 mg/100 mL to 64 mg/100 mL (Lawrence, 1989). Breastfeeding needs to be supplemented with phenylalanine-free formula to avoid the buildup of phenylalanine in the infant with this disorder. The length of nursing sessions and volume of supplements should be individualized for each infant.

Greve and colleagues (1994) found 7 to 9 breastfeeding sessions with supplements of phenylalanine-free formula within a 24-hour period supported normal blood levels and adequate weight gain. Blood levels were determined twice a week and weight checks were done weekly. Adjustments were made based on the results (Greve et al., 1994). When compared to infants receiving formula feeds, there was no difference in blood levels or length of time needed to achieve control.

Mothers should be instructed to express their milk, preferably with an electric pump, to maintain an adequate milk supply. The health-care team needs to provide support and encouragement to the lactating mother. The LC should work closely with the attending physician and dietitian to determine the amount of breastfeeding that can be combined with the specialized formula to maintain the infant's serum levels within a safe range.

POST-TEST

For questions 1 to 20, choose the best answer.

1. Infants have a narrower range of external temperatures that they can adapt to without suffering cold stress because of
   A. less subcutaneous fat for the provision of thermal regulation.
   B. lower energy requirement per unit of weight.
   C. less ability to control skin blood flow.
   D. A and B.
   E. A and C.

2. A _____ delivery room environment combined with low relative humidity will _____ heat loss in the neonate.
   A. cool; encourage
   B. cool; discourage
   C. warm; encourage
   D. warm; discourage

3. Heat loss prevention in the neonate can be accomplished by
   A. swaddling.
   B. drying the infant.
   C. skin-to-skin contact.
   D. all of the above.
   E. none of the above.

4. _____ does not increase the risk of hypoglycemia in an infant.
   A. Hypothermia
   B. Gradual discontinuation of intravenous fluids
   C. Maternal diabetes
   D. Sepsis

5. Jaundice that occurs from infrequent feedings at the breast is called
   A. breastmilk jaundice.
   B. breastfeeding jaundice.
   C. pathologic jaundice.
   D. hemolytic jaundice.

6. _____ may reduce respiratory distress syndrome in preterm infants.
   A. Antibiotic therapy
   B. Inositol
   C. High-volume ventilations

7. Rh incompatibility between mother and infant
   A. causes the mother to produce antibodies against fetal red blood cells.
   B. may cause jaundice in the infant.
   C. requires no additional treatment.
   D. A and B
   E. All of the above

8. _____ is believed to be involved in the development of certain inflammatory bowel diseases.

    A. ABO incompatibility
    B. Low protein intake
    C. Platelet activating factor
    D. High fat intake

9. _____ is used to create heat during nonshivering thermogenesis.

    A. White fat
    B. Yellow fat
    C. Brown fat

10. Identify the factor(s) that increase the risk of respiratory disease.

    A. Smoking
    B. Extreme prematurity
    C Use of ventilator
    D. A and B
    E. All of the above

11. A child should be taken for her or his first dental exam

    A. by the third birthday.
    B. within six months of the eruption of the first tooth.
    C. when the parent sees a cavity.
    D. immediately after mouth trauma.

12. Maternal causes of a breastfed infant's failure to thrive include all of the following except

    A. use of estrogen-containing birth control pills.
    B. use of switch-nursing techniques.
    C. metoclopramide therapy.
    D. maternal fatigue.

13. Fluoride supplements should be given when

    A. a child is using fluoridated toothpaste and the water supply is fluoridated.
    B. a child is using fluoridated toothpaste and the water supply is not fluoridated.
    C. infants breastfed exclusively are younger than six months old.

14. Fluid needs are increased when which factor(s) are present?

    A. Phototherapy
    B. Radiant heat warmer
    C. Ostomy
    D. A and B
    E. All of the above

15. Altered levels of polyunsaturated fatty acids have been found in the milk of mothers whose infants have

    A. atopic eczema.
    B. diabetes.
    C. an allergy to soy.
    D. hyperlipidemia.

16. The serum ferritin level is a useful guide to the level of _____ iron and the serum transferrin receptor is a sensitive index of _____ iron need.

    A. cellular; storage
    B. storage; cellular
    C. storage; circulating
    D. circulating; storage

17. All of the following influence maternal milk production except

    A. retained placental fragments.
    B. maternal smoking.
    C. excessive maternal caloric intake.
    D. maternal fatigue and stress.

18. A creamatocrit is used to

    A. measure the volume of expressed breastmilk.
    B. identify the fatty acid content of the milk.
    C. identify milk-ejection problems of the mother.
    D. measure the percentage of fat in the breastmilk.

19. Current recommendations for the exclusively breastfed, full-term infant are to start iron supplementation at

    A. one year of age.
    B. eight months of age.
    C. four to six months of age.
    D. two months of age.

20. Avoiding allergenic foods during lactation would be appropriate when

    A. the mother of the infant is experiencing reactions.
    B. the mother or another family member has a history of food allergies.
    C. the mother is breastfeeding a premature infant.
    D. the mother is expressing her breastmilk for her infant.

References

Abbey, LM (1979). Is breast feeding a likely cause of dental caries in young children? JADA, 98:21-23.

Acosta, PB (1989). *Ross Metabolic Formula System Nutrition Support Protocols*. Columbus, OH: Ross Laboratories.

Acosta, PB, Wentz, E (1978). *Management of Newborn Infants with PKU*. DHEW (HSA) Publication No. 79-5211. Washington, DC: U.S. Department of Health, Education and Welfare.

Adair, SM (1988). Epidemiology and mechanisms of dental diseases in children. In: Pinkham, JR (Ed.), *Pediatric Dentistry: Infancy Through Adolescence*, 1st ed. (pp. 9-22). Philadelphia: Saunders.

Adamopoulos, DA, Kapolla, N (1984). Prolactin concentration in milk and plasma of puerperal women and patients with galactorrhea. *J Endocrinol Invest*, 7:273.

Alford, C (1991). Breast milk transmission of cytomegalovirus (CMV) infection. In: Mestecky, J, Blair, C, Ogra, P (Eds.), *Immunology of Milk and the Neonate* (pp. 293-99). New York: Plenum Press.

Alonso, EM, Whitington, PF, Whitington, SH, Rivard, WA, Given, G (1991). Enterophepatic circulation of non-conjugated bilirubin in rats fed with human milk. *J Pediatr*, 118:425-530.

Altemeier, WA, III, O'Connor, SM, Sherrod, KB, Vietze, PM (1985). Prospective study of antecedents for nonorganic failure-to-thrive. *J Pediatr*, 106:360.

American Academy of Pediatric Dentistry (AAPD) (1997-1998). *Pediatric Dentistry, Special Issue Reference Manual*, 8:24.

AAPD (1994-1995). *Pediatric Dentistry, Special Issue. Reference Manual*, 5:7, 30-32.

American Academy of Pediatrics (AAP) (1992). National cholesterol education program. Report of the expert panel on blood cholesterol levels in children and adolescents. *Pediatrics*, 89(suppl):3(part 2):525-27.

AAP, Committee on Drugs (1994). Transfer of drugs and other chemicals into human milk. *Pediatrics*, 93(1):137-50.

AAP, Committee on Genetics (1992). New issues in newborn screening for phenylketonuria and congenital hypothyroidism. *Pediatrics*, 89:104-106.

AAP, Committee on Infectious Disease (1991). Report of the Committee, *Red Book*, 22 ed., Elk Grove Village, IL: AAP.

AAP, Committee on Infectious Diseases (1994). *1994 Red Book*, Elk Grove Village, IL: AAP, p. 239.

AAP, Committee on Nutrition (1989). Hypoallergenic infant formulas. *Pediatrics*, 83:1068-69.

AAP, Committee on Nutrition (1995). Fluoride supplementation for children: Interim policy recommendations. *Pediatrics*, 95(5):777.

AAP, Provisional Committee for Quality Improvement and Subcommittee on Hyperbilirubinemia (1994). Practice parameter: Management of hyperbilirubinemia in the healthy term newborn. *Pediatrics*, 94:558-65.

Andreasson, PA, Dias, F, Naucler, A, et al. (1993). A prospective study of vertical transmission of HIV-2 in Bissau, Guinea-Bissau. *AIDS*, 7:989-93.

Armstrong, JA (1991). Ultrastructure and significance of the lymphoid tissue lesions in HIV infection. In: Racz, P, Dijkstra, CD, Gluckman, JC (Eds.), *Accessory Cells in HIV and Other Retroviral Infections* (pp. 69-82). Basel, Switzerland: Karger.

Ashraf, RN, Jalil, F, Aperia, A, Lindblad, BS (1993). Additional water is not needed for healthy breast-fed babies in a hot climate. *Acta Paediatr*, 82(12):1107-11.

Auerbach, K, Gartner, LM (1987). Breastfeeding and human milk: Their association with jaundice in the neonate. *Clin Perinatol*, 14:89-107.

Backas, N (1994). OTC drugs and breastfeeding—Who makes the decision? *Medela Rental Round-Up*, 8(11):8-9.

Bahna, SL, Heiner, DC (1978). Cow's milk allergy: Pathogenesis, manifestations, diagnosis and management. *Adv Pediatr*, 31:1-27.

Baker, DH (1992). Cellular antioxidant status and human immunodeficiency virus replication. *Nutr Rev*, 50:15-18.

Barness, LA (Ed.) (1993). *Pediatric Nutrition Handbook*. Elk Grove Village, IL: AAP.

Bartlett, JG, Belitsos, PC, Sears, CL (1992). AIDS enteropathy. *Clin Infect Dis*, 15:726-35.

Bayley, N (1969). *Bayley Scales of Infant Development Manual*. New York: Psychological Corporation.

Beaudry, M, Dufour, R, Marcoux, S (1995). Relation between infant feeding and infections during the first six months of life. *J Pediatrics*, 126:(2)191-97.

Bedi, KS (1987). Lasting neuroanatomical changes following undernutrition during early life. In: Dobbing, J (Ed.), *Early Nutrition and Later Achievement* (pp. 1-36). London: Academic Press.

Beg, AA, Finco, TS, Nantermet, PV, Baldwin, AS (1993). Tumor necrosis factor and interleukin-1 lead to phosphorylation and loss of I kappa B alpha: a mechanism for NF-kappa B activation. *Mol Cell Biol*, 13(6):3301-10.

Bevan, BR, Holton, JB, Lathe, GH (1965). The effect of pregnanediol and pregnanediol glucuronide on bilirubin conjugation by rat liver slices. *Clin Sci*, 29:353-61.

Behrman, RE, Vaughan, VC (Eds.) (1987). *Nelson Textbook of Pediatrics*, 13th ed. Philadelphia: Saunders.

Behrman, RE, Vaughan, VC (Eds.) (1991). *Nelson Textbook of Pediatrics*, 14th ed. Philadelphia: Saunders.

Bejarano, MA, Zimmer, MA (1991). *Determination of low levels of silicones in human breast milk by the aqueous silanol functionality test*, Report Number I-0000-36332. Midland, MI: Dow Corning.

Bentzen, RC (1929). Dental conditions among the Mimbres people of South-Western United States previous to the year 600 AD. *Dental Cosmos*, LXXI:1068-73.

Berger, GMB, Spark, A, Vaillie, PM, Huskisson, J, Stockwell, G, van der Merwe, E (1983). Absence of serum-stimulated lipase activity and altered lipid content in milk from a patient with type I hyperlipoproteinaemia. *Pediatr Res*, 17(10):835-39.

Berger, LR (1981). When should one discourage breastfeeding? *Pediatrics*, 67:300.

Berkowitz, CD, Senter, SA (1987). Characteristics of mother–infant interactions in nonorganic failure to thrive. *J Fam Pract*, 25:377.

Berkowitz, CD, Sklaren, BC (1984). Environmental failure to thrive: the need for intervention. *Am Fam Physician*, 29:101.

Berkowitz, RJ, Turner, J, Green, P (1981). Maternal salivary levels of *Streptococcus mutans* and primary oral infection of infants. *Arch Oral Biol*, 26:147-49.

Berlin, CM, Jr (1981). Excretion of the methylaxanthines in human milk. *Semin Perinatol*, 5:389.

Berlin, CM, Jr (1995). Lecture presented at the International Lactation Consultant Association (ILCA) annual conference and meeting, Scottsdale, AZ.

Bevan, BR, Holton, JB (1972). Inhibition of bilirubin conjugation in rat liver slices by free fatty acids, with relevance to the problem of breast milk jaundice. *Clin Chem Acta*, 41:101-107.

Biagi, PL, Bordoni, A, Masi, M, Ricci, G, Fanelli, C, Patrizi, A, Ceccolino, E (1988). A long-term study of the use of evening primrose oil (Efamol) in atopic children. *Drugs Exp Clin Res*, 14:285-90.

Bithony, WG, Newberger, EH (1987). Child and family attributes of failure-to-thrive. *J Dev Behav Pediatr*, 8:32.

Bitman, J, Hamosh, M, Hamosh, P, Lutes, V, Neville, MC, Seacat, J, Wood, DL (1989). Milk composition of and volume during the onset of lactation in a diabetic mother. *Am J Clin Nutr*, 50:1364-69.

Bitman, J, Hamosh, M, Wood, DL, Freed, LM, Hamosh, P (1987). Lipid composition of milk from mothers with cystic fibrosis. *Pediatrics*, 80(6):927-32.

Blaauw, R, Albertse, EC, Beneke, T, et al. (1994). Risk factors for the development of osteoporosis in a South African population: a prospective analysis. *S Afr Med J*, 84(6):328-32.

Blau, H, Passwell, JH, Levanon, M, et al. (1983). Studies on human milk macrophages: Effect of activation on phagocytosis and secretion of prostaglandin E_2 and lysozyme. *Pediatr Res*, 17:241-45.

Bock, SA (1987). Prospective appraisal of complaints of adverse reactions to foods during children's first 3 years of life. *Pediatrics*, 79(5):683-88.

Boreus, LO, de Chateau, P, Lindberg, C, Nyberg, L (1982). Terbutaline in breast milk. *Br J Clin Pharmacol*, 13:731.

Brams, M, Maleney, J (1983). "Nursing Bottle Caries" in breast-fed children. *J Pediatrics*, 103:415-16.

Brazelton, TB (1956). Finger sucking in infancy. *Pediatrics*, 17:400.

Briggs, GR, Freeman, RK, Yaffe, SJ (1994). *Drugs in Pregnancy and Lactation*, 4th ed. Baltimore: Williams & Wilkins.

Bright, RA, Teng, LL, Moore, RM, Jr. (1993). National survey of self-reported breast implants: 1988 estimates. *J Long-Term Eff Med Implants*, 3:81-89.

Brodersen, R, Stern, L (1990). Deposition of bilirubin acid in the central nervous system—A hypothesis for the development of kernicterus. *Acta Paediatr Scand*, 79:12-19.

Brooten, D, et al. (1985). Breastmilk jaundice. *JOGNN*, 14:220-23.

Buimovici-Klein, E, Hite, RL, Byrne, T, et al. (1977). Isolation of rubella virus in milk after postpartum immunization. *J Pediatr*, 91:939-43.

Burkman, RT (1981). Association between intrauterine devices and pelvic inflammatory disease. *Obstet Gynecol*, 57:269-76.

Burt, BA (1992). The changing patterns of systemic fluoride intake. *J Dent Res*, 71(5):1228-37.

Businco, L, Cantani, A, Longhi, MA, et al. (1989). Anaphylactic reactions to a cow's milk whey protein hydrolysate (Alfa-Re, Nestlé) in infants with cow's milk allergy. *Ann Allergy*, 62:333-35.

Businco, L, Marchetti, F, Pellegrini, G, et al. (1983). Prevention of atopic disease in "at-risk newborns" by prolonged breastfeeding. *Ann Allergy*, 51:296.

Calvo, E, Galindo, AC, Aspres, NB (1992). Iron status in exclusively breast-fed infants. *Pediatrics*, 90:375-79.

Campbell, TD (1938a). Observations on the teeth of Australian Aborigines, Cockatoo Creek, Central Australia. *Aust J Dent*, XLII:41-47.

Campbell, TD (1938b). Observations on the teeth of Australian Aborigines, Mt. Liebig, Central Australia. *Aust J Dent*, XLII:85-89.

Campbell, TD, Gray, JH (1936). Observations on the teeth of Australian Aborigines. *Aust J Dent*, XL:290-95.

Cant, AJ, Bailes, JA, Marsden, RA (1985). Cow's milk, soya milk and goat's milk in a mother's diet causing eczema and diarrhea in her breast fed infant. *Acta Paediatr Scand*, 74:467-68.

Caplan, MS, Sun, X-M, Hsueh, W, Hageman, JR (1990). Role of platelet-activating factor and tumor necrosis factor-alpha in neonatal necrotizing enterocolitis. *J Pediatr*, 116:906-64.

Cardwell, P, Pharm, C, Hoey, C (1994). *Common over-the-counter drugs in breastfeeding.* Paper presented at the International Lactation Consultant Association annual meeting, Atlanta, GA.

Carpenter, JV (1978). The relationship between teething and systemic disturbances. *J Dent Child*, 45:381-84.

Casey, PH (1987). Failure-to-thrive: transitional perspective. *J Dev Behav Pediatr*, 8:37.

Casey, PH, Bradely, R, Wortham, B (1984). Social and nonsocial home environments of infants with nonorganic failure-to-thrive. *Pediatrics*, 73:384.

Centers for Disease Control and Prevention (CDC) (1985). Recommendations for assisting in the prevention of perinatal transmission of human-T-lymphotrophic virus type III/lymphadenopathy-associated virus and acquired immunodeficiency syndrome. *MMWR*, 34:721-26.

Chandra, RK (1977). Iron metabolism. CIBA Foundation symposium 51. Amsterdam: Elsevier.

Chandra, RK (1979). Prospective studies on the effect of breast feeding on incidence of infection and allergy. *Acta Paediatr Scand*, 68:691.

Chandra, RK (1987). Prevention of atopic disease: Environmental engineering utilizing antenatal antigen avoidance and breastfeeding. In: Goldman, AS, Atkinson, SA, Hanson, LA (Eds.), Human Lactation, Vol. 3: *The Effects of Human Milk on the Recipient Infants* (pp. 269-74). New York: Plenum Press.

Chandra, RK (1989). Maternal diet during pregnancy and lactation. In: Hamburger, RN (Ed.), *Food Intolerance in Infancy: Allergology, Immunology, and Gastroenterology* (pp. 23-26). New York: Raven Press.

Chandra, RK, Puri, S, Cheema, PS (1985). Predictive value of cord blood IgE in the development of atopic disease and role of breastfeeding in its prevention. *Clin Allergy*, 15:517-22.

Chandra, RK, Puri, S, Hamed, A (1989). Influence of maternal diet during lactation and use of formula feeds on development of atopic eczema in high-risk infants. *Br Med J*, 299:228-30.

Chen, Y, Shunzhang, Y, Wan-xian, L (1988). Artificial feeding and hospitalization in the first 18 months of life. *Pediatrics*, 81:58-62.

Christensen, JR, Fields, HW (1994). Non-nutritive sucking. In: Pinkham, JR (Ed.), *Pediatric Dentistry: Infancy through Adolescence*, 2nd ed. Philadelphia: Saunders.

Clarkson, JE, Cowan, JO, Herbison, GP, et al. (1984). Jaundice in full-term healthy neonates—A population study. *Aust Pediatr J*, 20:303-308.

Clyne, PS, Kulczycki, A (1991). Human breast milk contains bovine IgG. Relationship to infant colic? *Pediatrics*, 87:439-44.

Cochi, SL, Fleming, DW, Hightower, AW, Limpakarnjanarat, K, Facklam, RR, Smith, JD, Sikes, RK, Boome, CV (1986). Primary invasive *Haemophilus influenzae* type B disease: a population-based assessment of risk factors. *J Pediatr*, 108:887-96.

Conine, TA, Carty, E, Safarik, PM (1988). *Aids and Adaptations for Parents with Physical or Sensory Disabilities* (pp. 67-71). Vancouver, BC, Canada: University of British Columbia, School of Rehabilitative Medicine.

Cornblath, M, Schwartz, R, Aynsley-Green, A, Lloyd, JK (1990). Hypoglycemia in infancy: the need for a rational definition. *Pediatrics*, 85:834-37.

Croxatto, HB (1992). IUD mechanisms in action. In: *A New Look at IUD's—Advancing Contraceptive Choices.* March, New York: Wiley Liss.

Cruz, JR, Garcia, B, Urrutia, JJ, et al. (1981). Food antibodies in milk from Guatemalan women. *J Pediatr*, 99:600-602.

Cunningham, AS (1992). More on crib death and breastfeeding (letter). *J Hum Lact*, 8(1):7-8.

Cunningham, AS, Jelliffe, DB, Jelliffe, EF (1991). Breastfeeding and health in the 1980s: a global epidemiologic review. *J Pediatr*, 118(5):659-66.

Curtis, EM (1964). Oral contraceptive feminization of a normal male infant. *Obstet Gynecol*, 23:295.

Dallman, PR (1988). Nutritional anemia of infancy: Iron, folic acid and vitamin B$_{12}$. In: Tsang, RC, Nichols, BL (Eds.), *Nutrition During Infancy* (pp. 216-35). St. Louis: Mosby.

Darke, SJ (1976). Human milk versus cow's milk. *J Hum Nutr*, 30:233.

de Carvalho, M, Hall, M, Harvey, D (1981). Effects of water supplementation on physiologic jaundice in breast-fed babies. *Arch J Dis Child*, 135: 568-69.

de Carvalho, M, Klaus, M, et al. (1982). Frequency of breastfeeding and serum bilirubin concentration. *Am J Dis Child*, 136:737-38.

de Carvalho, M, Robertson, S, Klaus, M (1985). Fecal bilirubin excretion and serum bilirubin concentrations in breastfed and bottlefed infants. *J Pediatr*, 107:786-90.

deCurtis, M, Paone, C, Vetrano, G, Romano, C, Paludetto, R, Ciccimarra, F (1987). A case-control study of necrotizing enterocolitis occurring over 8 years in a neonatal intensive care unit. *Eur J Pediatr*, 146:398-400.

deGazelle, H, et al. (1983). Metoclopramide and breast milk. *Eur J Obstet Gynecol Reprod Biol*, 15:31-36.

de Jong-van den Berg, L, Mintzes, B (1995). Bromocriptine and lactation suppression: are the risks acceptable? *Pharmacy World Sci*, 17(4):93-95.

de Leeuw, R, de Vries, IJ (1976). Hypoglycemia in small-for-dates newborn infants. *Pediatrics*, 58(1):18-22.

de Martino, M, Tovo, PA, Tozzi, AE, et al. (1992). HIV-1 transmission through breast-milk: Appraisal of risk according to duration of feeding. *AIDS*, 6:991-97.

Dennery, PA, McDonagh, AF, Stevenson, DK (1992). In vivo role of bilirubin in neonatal antioxidant defenses (abstract). *Pediatr Res,* 31:A200.

Dewey, KG, Heinig, MJ, Nommsen, LA, Lonnerdal, B (1991). Maternal versus infant factors related to breast-milk intake and residual milk volume: the DARLING study. *Pediatrics,* 87(6):829-37.

Diaz, S, Cardenas, H, Brandeis, A, Miranda, P, Salvatierra, AM, Croxatto, HB (1992). Relative contributions of anovulation and luteal phase defect to the reduced pregnancy rate of breastfeeding women. *Fertil Steril,* 58(3):498-503.

Diaz, S, Croxatto, HB (1993). Contraception in lactating women. *Current Opin Obstet Gynecol,* 5(6):815-22.

Diaz, S, Seron-Ferre, M, Cardenas, H, Schiappacasse, V, Brandeis, A, Croxatto, HB (1989). Circadian variation of basal plasma prolactin, prolactin response to suckling and length of amenorrhea in nursing women. *J Clin Endocrinol Metab,* 68:946-55.

Diosi, P, Babusceac, L, Nevinglovschi, O, et al. (1967). Cytomegalovirus infection associated with pregnancy. *Lancet,* 1:1063-66.

Donnell, GN, Koch, R, Fishler, K, Ng, WG (1980). Clinical aspects of galactosemia. In: Burman, D, Holton, JB, Pennock, CA (Eds.), *Inherited Disorders of Carbohydrate Metabolism.* Lancaster, England: MTP.

Duffy, LC, Byers, TE, Riepenhoff-Talty, M, LaScolea, LJ, Zielezny, MA, Ogra, PL (1986). The effects of infant feeding on rotavirus-induced gastroenteritis: a prospective study. *Am J Pub Health,* 76:259-63.

Duffy, LC, Zielezny, MA, Dryja, D, Faden, H, Ogra, P (1992). Bifidobacterium colonization of human intestine: Cultivation and characterization of resident and ingestion strains. In: Picciano, MF, Lonnerdal, B (Eds.), *Mechanisms Regulating Lactation and Infant Nutrition Utilization* (pp. 383-87). New York: Wiley-Liss.

Duncan, B, Ey, J, Holberg, CJ, Wright, AL, Martinez, FD, Taussing, LM (1993). Exclusive breastfeeding for at least 4 months protects against otitis media. *Pediatrics,* 91(5): 867-72.

Dunkle, LM, Schmidt, RR, O'Connor, DM (1979). Neonatal herpes simplex infection possibly acquired via maternal breast milk. *Pediatrics,* 63:250.

Dunn, DT, Newell, ML, Ades, AE, et al. (1992). Risk of human immunodeficiency virus type I transmission through breastfeeding. *Lancet,* 340:585-88.

Dunn, P, Bhutani, V, Weiner, S, Ludomirski, A (1988). Care of the neonate with erythroblastosis fetalis. *JOGNN,* 17:382-86.

Dworsky, M, Yow, M, Stagno, S, et al. (1983). Cytomegalovirus infection of breast milk and transmission in infancy. *Pediatrics,* 72:295-99.

Eastham, EJ (1989). Regulation of the immune response. In: Middleton, E, Reed, CE, Ellis, EF, et al. (Eds.), *Allergy: Principles and Practice,* 3rd ed. (pp. 31-51). St. Louis: Mosby.

Edwardsson, S, Mejare, B (1978). *Streptococcus milleri* (Guthof) and *Streptococcus mutans* in the mouths of infants before and after tooth eruption. *Arch Oral Biol,* 23:811-814.

Eggert, LD, Pollary, RA, Folland, DS, Jung, AL (1985). Home phototherapy treatment of neonatal jaundice. *Pediatrics,* 76:579-84.

Ehrenkranz, RA, Ackerman, BA (1986). Metoclopramide effect on faltering milk production by mothers of premature infants. *Pediatrics,* 78:614-20.

Eibi, MM, Wolf, HM, Furnkranz, H, Rosenkranz, A (1988). Prevention of necrotizing enterocolitis in low-birth-weight infants by IgA–IgG feeding. *N Engl J Med,* 319: 1-7.

Eickman, FM (1992). Recurrent myocardial infarction in a postpartum patient receiving bromocriptine. *Clin Cardiol,* 15(10):781-83.

Ellis, MH, Short, JA, Heiner, DC (1991). Anaphylaxis after ingestion of a recently introduced whey protein formula. *J Pediatr,* 118:74-77.

Embree, J, Datta, P, Kreiss, J, et al. (1993). *Delayed seroconversion in infants born to HIV-1 seropositive mothers: Associated factors.* Paper presented at IXth International Conference on AIDS, Geneva.

Engelking, CW, Page-Lieberman, J (1986). *Maternal Diabetes and Diabetes in Young Children: Their Relationship to Breastfeeding.* Lactation Consultant Series. Wayne, NJ: Avery Publishing Group.

Ereman, RR, Lonnerdal, B, Dewey, KG (1987). Maternal sodium intake does not affect postprandial sodium concentrations in human milk. *J Nutr,* 117(6):1154-57.

Esplugues, JV, Whittle, BJ (1989). Gastric effects of PAF. *Methods Find Exp Clin Pharmacol,* 11(Suppl 1):61-66.

European Multicentre Study Group for Cabergoline in Lactation Inhibition (1991). Single-dose cabergoline versus bromocriptine in inhibition of puerperal lactation: randomised, double-blind, multicentre study. *BMJ* 302(6789):1367-71.

Facione, N (1990). Otitis media: An overview of acute and chronic disease. *Nurse Pract,* 15:11-22.

Faden, H, Stanievich, J, Brodsky, L, Bernstein, J, Ogra, PL (1990). Changes in nasopharyngeal flora during otitis media of childhood. *Pediatr Inf Dis J,* 9(9):623-26.

Faden, H, Waz, MJ, Bernstein, JM, Brodsky, L, Stanievich, J, Ogra, PL (1991). Nasopharyngeal flora in the first three years of life in normal and otitis-prone children. *Ann Otol Rhinol Laryngol,* 199(8):612-15.

Falth-Magnusson, K, Kjellman, N-IM (1987). Development of atopic disease in babies whose mothers were receiving exclusion diet during pregnancy—A randomized study. *J Allergy Clin Immunol,* 80:868-75.

Falth-Magnusson, K, Kjellman, N-IM (1992). Allergy prevention by maternal elimination diet during late pregnancy—A 5-year follow-up of a randomized study. *J Allergy Clin Immunol,* 89:709-13.

Feachem, RG, Koblinsky, MA (1984). Interventions for the control of diarrheal diseases among young children: promotion of breastfeeding. *Bull WHO,* 62:271-91.

Ferguson, B, Skikne, B, Simpson, K, Baynes, R, Cook, J (1992). Serum transferrin receptor distinguishes the anemia of chronic disease from iron deficiency anemia. *J Lab Clin Med,* 19:385-90.

Ferrari, C, Piscitelli, G, Crosignani, PG (1995). Cabergoline: a new drug for the treatment of hyperprolactinemia. *Human Reproduction*, 10(7):1647-52.

Ferris, AM, Dalidowitz, CK, Ingardia, CM, Reece, EA, Fumia, FD, Jensen, RG, Allen, LH (1988) Lactation outcome in insulin-dependent diabetic women. *J Am Diet Assoc*, 88:317-22.

Finochi, LL (1992). Breast feeding, bottle feeding and their impact on oral habits, a review of the literature. *Dental Hygiene*, 66:680-85.

Flick, JA (1994). Silicone implants and esophageal dysmotility: Are breastfed infants at risk? *JAMA*, 271:240-41.

Fomon, SJ (Ed.) (1974). *Infant Nutrition*. Philadelphia: Saunders.

Fomon, SJ (1987). Bioavailability of supplemental iron in commercially prepared dry infant cereals. *J Pediatr*, 110: 660-61.

Fomon, SJ (Ed.) (1993). *Nutrition of Normal Infants*. St. Louis: Mosby.

Fomon, SJ, Ziegler, EE, Nelson, SE (1993). Erythrocyte incorporation of ingested [58]Fe by 56-day-old breast-fed and formula-fed infants. *Pediatr Res*, 33:573-76.

Fosarelli, PP, DeAngelis, C, Winkelstein, J, Mellitis, ED (1985). Infectious illnesses in the first two years of life. *Pediatr Infec Dis J*, 4:153-59.

Fosson, A, Wilson, J (1987). Family interactions surrounding feeding of infants with nonorganic failure to thrive. *Clin Pediatr*, 26:518

Frank, DA, Silva, M, Needleman, R (1993). Failure to thrive: Mystery, myth and method. *Contemporary Pediatrics*, 10:114.

Frantz, AG, Wilson, JD (1985). Endocrine disorders of the breast. In: Wilson, JD, Foster, DW (Eds.), *Textbook of Endocrinology*, 7th ed. Philadelphia: Saunders.

Fraser, IS (1991). A review of the use of progestogen-only minipills for contraception during lactation. *Reproduction, Fertil Develop*, 3(3):245-54.

French Collaborative Study Group, The HIV Infection in Newborns (1994). Comparison of vertical human immunodeficiency virus type 2 and human immunodeficiency virus type 1 transmission in the French prospective cohort. *Pediatr Infect Dis J*, 13:502-506.

Frisancho, AR (1981). New norms of upper limb fat and muscle areas for assessment of nutritional status. *Am J Clin Nutr*, 34:25-40.

Furukawa, M, Narahara, H, Yasuda, K, Johnson, JM (1993). Presence of platelet-activating factor—Acetylhydrolase in milk. *J Lip Res*, 34:1603-09.

Gardner, DE, Norwood, JR, Eisenson, JE (1977). At-will breast feeding and dental caries: four case reports. *J Dent Child*, 44:186-91.

Gardner, DK (1987). Drug passage into breast milk: principles and concerns. *J Pediatr Perinatal Nutr*, 1:27-37.

Gardner, DK, Ruff, AJ (1995). Lecture presented at the La Leche League International conference, Chicago.

Garry, PJ, Owen, GM, Hooper, EM, Gilbert, BA (1981). Iron absorption from human milk and formula with and without iron supplementation. *Pediatr Res*, 15:822-28.

Gartner, LM, Arias, IM (1966). Studies of prolonged neonatal jaundice in the breastfed infant. *J Pediatr*, 68:54-66.

Gayle, HD, Gnaore, E, Adjorlolo, G, et al. (1992). HIV-1 and HIV-2 infection in children in Abidjan, Cote d'Ivoire. *J Acquir Immune Defic Syndr*, 5:513-17.

Gerrard, JW (1979). Allergy in breast-fed babies to ingredients in breast milk. *Ann Allergy*, 42:69-72.

Gerrard, JW (1984). Allergies in breastfed babies to foods ingested by the mother. *Clin Rev Allergy*, 2:143-49.

Gerrard, JW, MacKenzie, JWA, Goluboff, N, et al. (1973). Cow's milk allergy: prevalence and manifestations in an unselected series of newborns. *Acta Paediatr Scand*, 234:1-20.

Gerrard, JW, Shenassa, M (1983). Food allergy: two common types as seen in breast and formula fed babies. *Ann Allergy*, 50:375-79.

Gershon, AA (1990). Chickenpox, measles, mumps. In: Remington, JS, Klein, JO (Eds.), *Infectious Diseases of the Fetus and Newborn Infant*. Philadelphia: Saunders.

Gittleman, DK (1991). Bromocriptine associated with postpartum hypertension, seizures, and pituitary hemorrhage. *Gen Hosp Psy*, 13(4):278-80.

Glasier, A, McNeilly, AS, Baird, DT (1986). Induction of ovarian activity by pulsatile infusion of LHRH in women with lactational amenorrhoea. *Clin Endocrinol*, 24:243-52.

Glasier, A, McNeilly, AS, Howie, PW (1983). Fertility after childbirth: changes in serum gonadotrophin levels in breast and bottlefeeding women. *Clin Endocrinol*, 19: 493-501.

Goldfarb, J (1993). Breastfeeding, AIDS, and other infectious diseases. *Clin Perinatol*, 20:225-43.

Goldman, L (1995). *Medical Knowledge Self-Assessment Program 10—Rheumatology Section*. Philadelphia: American College of Physicians.

Gormon, C (1994). When breast-feeding fails. Low-milk syndrome poses a rare but frightening risk. *Time* (August 22), n:63.

Green, TP, Mirkin, BL, Peterson, PK, Sinaiko, AR, Ramsay, NK, O'Dea, RF (1984). Tobramycin serum level monitoring in young patients with normal renal function. *Clin Pharmacokinetics*, 9(5):457-68.

Greiner, T (1981). Responds to Gussler and Briesemeister's reply. *Med Anthropol*, 5:255-57.

Greiner, T, Van Esterik, P, Latham, MC (1981). The insufficient milk syndrome: an alternative explanation. *Med Anthropol*, 5:233-47.

Greve, LC, Wheeler, MD, Green-Burgeson, DK, Zorn, EM (1994). Breastfeeding in the management of the newborn with phenylketonuria: a practical approach to diet therapy. *J Amer Diet Assoc*, 94(3):305-309.

Gross, R, Schultink, W, Juliawati (1994). Treatment of anemia with weekly iron supplementation. *Lancet*, 344:821.

Gruenbaum, E, Amir, J, Merlob, P, et al. (1991). Breast milk jaundice: natural history, familial incidence and late neurodevelopmental outcome of the infant. *Eur J Pediatr*, 150:267-70.

Gupta, AP, Gupta, PK (1985). Metoclopramide as a lactogogune. *Clin Pediatr*, 24:269-72.

Gussler, JD, Briesemeister, LH (1980). The insufficient milk syndrome: a biocultural explanation. *Med Anthropol,* 4:145-74.

Gussler, JD, Briesemeister, LH (1981). Reply to Ted Greiner, Penny Van Esterik, and Michael C. Latham. *Med Anthropol,* 5:248-52.

Guthrie, DW, Guthrie, RA (1982). *Nursing Management of Diabetes Mellitus,* 2nd ed. St. Louis: Mosby.

Habicht, JP, DaVanzo, J, Butz, WP (1986). Does breastfeeding really save lives, or are apparent benefits due to biases? *Am J Epidem,* 123:279-90.

Hale, TH (1996). *Medications and Mothers' Milk,* 5th ed. Amarillo, TX: Pharmasoft Publishing.

Hamburger, RN (1984). Diagnosis of food allergies and intolerances in the study of prophylaxis and control groups in infants. *Ann Allergy,* 53:673-77.

Hamburger, RN, Heller, S, Mellon, MH, et al. (1983). Current status of the clinical and immunologic consequences of a prototype allergic disease prevention program, *Ann Allergy,* 51:281.

Hamosh, M, Bitman, J (1992). Human milk in disease: lipid composition. *Lipid,* 27:848-57.

Hamosh, M, Clary, TR, Chernick, SS, Scow, RO (1970). Lipoprotein lipase activity of adipose and mammary tissue and plasma triglyceride in pregnant and lactating rats. *Biochimica et Biophysica Acta,* 210:473-82.

Hanson, LA, Ahlstedt, S, Andersson, B, et al. (1984). The immune response of the mammary gland and its significance for the neonate. *Ann Allergy,* 53:576-81.

Hanson, LA, Ahlstedt, S, Carlsson, B, et al. (1977). Secretory IgA antibodies against cow's milk proteins in human milk and their possible effect in mixed feeding. *Int Arch Allergy Appl Immunol,* 54:457-62.

Hanson, LA, Ashraf, R, Zamar, S, Karlberg, J, Lindblad, BS, Jalil, F (1994). Breastfeeding is a natural contraceptive and prevents disease and death in infants, linking infant mortality and birth rates. *Acta Paediatr,* 83:3-6

Hanson, LA, Bergstrom, S (1990). The link between infant mortality and birth rates—The importance of breastfeeding as a common factor. *Acta Paediatr Scand,* 79:481-89.

Hanson, LA, Lindquist, B, Hofvander, Y, Zetterstrom, R (1985). Breastfeeding as a protection against gastroenteritis and other infections. *Acta Paediatr Scand,* 74:641-42.

Harabuchi, Y, Faden, H, Yamanaka, N, Duffy, L, Wolf, J, Krystofik, D (1994). Human milk secretory IgA antibody to nontypeable *Haemophilus influenzae:* possible protective effects against nasopharyngeal colonization. *J Pediatr,* 124:193-98.

Hargreaves, T (1973). Effect of fatty acids on bilirubin conjugation. *Arch Dis Child,* 48:446-49.

Harris, RJ (1974). Plasma nonesterified fatty acid and blood glucose levels in healthy and hypoxemic newborn infants. *J Pediatr,* 84(4):578-84.

Hattevig, G, Kjellman, B, Sigurs, N, et al. (1989). Effect of maternal avoidance of eggs, cow's milk and fish during lactation upon allergic manifestations in infants. *Clin Exp Allergy,* 19:27-32.

Hayes, K, Danks, DM, Givas, H, et al. (1972). Cytomegalovirus in human milk. *N Engl J Med,* 287:177-78.

Haymond, MW, Karl, IE, Pagliara, AS (1974). Ketotic hypoglycemia: An amino acid substrate limited disorder. *J Clin Endocrinol Metabol,* 38(4):521-30.

Hegyi, T, Goldie, E, Hiatt, M (1994). The protective role of bilirubin in oxygen-radical diseases of the preterm infant. *J Perinatol,* 14:296-300.

Heller, L (1994). When breast isn't best. *Redbook* (November), n:190.

Helliker, K (1994). Dying for milk. Some mothers, trying in vain to breast-feed, starve their infants. *Wall Street Journal* (July 22); LXXV (197):A1,A4.

Heneine, W, Woods, T, Green, D, et al. (1992). Detection of HTLV-II in breast milk of HTLV-II infected mothers. *Lancet,* 340:1157-58.

Hey, E, Scopes, JW (1993). Thermoregulation in the newborn. In: Avery, GB (Ed.), *Neonatology: Pathophysiology and Management of the Newborn,* 4th ed. Philadelphia: Lippincott.

Hill, RM, Craig, JP, Chaney, MD, Tennyson, LM, McCulley, LB (1977). Utilization of over-the-counter drugs during pregnancy. *Clin Obstet Gynecol,* 20:381.

Höjgaard, K (1980). Dentition on Um an-Nar (Trucial Oman) 2500 BC. *Scand J Dent Res,* 88:355-64.

Honig, JJ (1975). Teething—Are today's pediatricians using yesterday's notions? *J Pediatr,* 87:415-17.

Hood, LJ (1978). Breast feeding and some reasons for electing to wean the infant: a report from the Dunedin Multidisciplinary Child Development Study. *NZ Med J,* 621:273-76.

Hopkinson, JM, Schanler, RJ, Fraley, JK, Garza, C (1992). Milk production by mothers of premature infants: Influence of cigarette smoking. *Pediatrics,* 90(6):934-38.

Howie, PW, Forsyth, JS, Ogston, SA, Clark, A, Florey, C (1990). Protective effect of breastfeeding against infections. *Br Med J,* 300:11-16

Hreshchyshyn, MM, Hopkins, A, Zylstra, S, Anbar, M (1988). Associations of parity, breastfeeding, and birth control pills with lumbar spine and femoral neck bone densities. *Am J Obstet Gynecol,* 159:318-22.

Huebers, JS, Csiba, E, Josephson, B, Huebers, E, Finch, C (1981). Interaction of human diferric transferrin with reticulocytes. *Proc Nat Acad Sci USA,* 78:621-25.

Huebers, JS, Huebers, E, Csiba, E, Rummel, W, Finch, CA (1983). The significance of transferrin for intestinal iron absorption. *Blood,* 61:283-91.

Hufton, IW, Dates, K (1977). Nonorganic failure to thrive: a long-term follow-up. *Pediatrics,* 59-73.

Human Milk Banking Association of North America (HMBANA) (1994). Addendum 06137-0464, March 8.

Idjradinata, P, Pollitt, E (1993). Reversal of developmental delays in iron-deficient anemic infants treated with iron. *Lancet,* 341:1-4.

Institute of Medicine (IOM) (1991). *Nutrition During Lactation.* Washington, DC: National Academy of Sciences Press.

Isaacs, CE, Thormar, H, Pessolano, T (1986). Membrane-disruptive effect of human milk: inactivation of envelope viruses. *J Infect Dis,* 154:966-71.

Istre, GR, Compton, R, Novotny, T (1986). Infant botulism: three cases in a small town. *Am Dis Child*, 140:1013-14.

Jakobsson, I, Lindberg, T (1978). Cow's milk as a cause of infantile colic in breast-fed infants. *Lancet*, ii:437-39.

Jakobsson, I, Lindberg, T, Benediktsson, B, et al. (1985). Dietary bovine Beta lactoglobulin is transferred to human milk. *Acta Paediatr Scand*, 74:342-45.

Jenkins, HR, Pincott, JR, Soothill, JF, et al. (1984). Food allergy: the major cause of infantile colitis. *Arch Dis Child*, 59:326-29.

Kajosaari, M, Saarinen, UM (1983). Prophylaxis of atopic disease by six months' total solid food elimination. *Acta Paediatr Scand*, 72:411-14.

Kanagaratnam, T (1994). Insufficient Milk Syndrome. *American Baby* (November), n:60,64.

Katz, E, Adashi, EY (1990). Hyperprolactinemic disorders. *Clin Obstet Gynecol*, 33:622-39.

Kauppila, A, et al. (1981). A dose-response relation between improved lactation and Metoclopramide. *Lancet*, 1:1175-77.

Keele, DK, Kay, JL (1966). Plasma free fatty acid and blood sugar levels in newborn infants and their mothers. *Pediatrics*, 37(4):597-604.

Keene, HJ (1986). Dental caries prevalence in early Polynesians from the Hawaiian Islands. *J Dent Res*, 65:935-38.

Kennedy, K, Rivera, R, McNeelly, A, et al. (1989). Consensus statement on the use of breastfeeding as a family planning method. *Contraception*, 39:625-31.

Kennedy, K, Visness, C (1992). Contraceptive efficacy of lactational amenorrhoea. *Lancet*, 339:227-30.

Kent, GN, Price, RI, Gutteridge, DH, Allen, JR, Rosman, KJ, Smith, M, Bhagat, CI, Wilson, SG, Retallack, RW (1993). Effect of pregnancy and lactation on maternal bone mass and calcium metabolism. *Osteoporosis Int*, 3(suppl 1):44-47.

Khan, M (1994). Letters to the Editor: Breast-feeding education. *Time* (September), n:8.

Khan, SR, Jalil, F, Zaman, S, Lindblad, BS, Karlberg, J (1993). Early child health in Lahore, Pakistan: X. Mortality. *Acta Paediatr*, 82(suppl)390:109-17.

Kilshaw, PJ, Cant, AJ (1984). The passage of maternal dietary proteins into human breast milk. *Int Arch Allergy Appl Immunol*, 75:8-15.

Kinoshita, K, Hino, S, Amagasaki, T, et al. (1984). Demonstration of adult T-cell leukemia virus antigen in milk from three seropositive mothers. *Gann*, 75:103-105.

Kirshbaum, M (1990). The parent with a physical disability. In: Auvenshine, JM, Enriques, MG (Eds.), *Comprehensive Maternity Nursing: Perinatal and Women's Health*. Boston: Jones and Bartlett.

Kjellman, N-IM, Johansson, SGO (1979). Soy versus cow's milk in infants with a biparental history of topic disease: development of atopic disease and immunoglobulins from birth to 4 years of age. *Clin Allergy*, 9:347-58.

Klaus, M, Fanaroff, A (1993). *Care of the High-Risk Neonate*. Philadelphia: Saunders.

Klein, EB, Byrne, T, Cooper, LZ (1980). Neonatal rubella in a breast-fed infant after postpartum maternal infection. *J Pediatr*, 97:774-75.

Koch, R, Donnell, GN, Fishler, K, Ng, WG, Wenz, E (1982). Galactosemia. In: Kelly, VC (Ed.), *Pediatrics*. Philadelphia: Harper & Row.

Koetting, CA, Wardlaw, GM (1988). Wrist, spine, and hip bone density in women with variable histories of lactation. *Am J Clin Nutr*, 48:1479-81.

Köhler, B, Andreen, I (1994). Influence of caries-preventive measures in mothers on cariogenic bacteria and caries experience in their children. *Arch Oral Biol*, 39 (10):907-11.

Köhler, B, Bratthall, D (1978). Intrafamilial levels of *Streptococcus mutans* and some aspects of the bacterial transmission. *Scand J Dent Res*, 86:35-42.

Köhler, B, Bratthall, D, Krasse, B (1983).Preventive measures in mothers influence the establishment of the bacterium *Streptococcus mutans* in their infants. *Arch Oral Biol*, 28(3):225-31.

Kotlow, LA (1977). Breast feeding: a cause of dental caries in children. *J Dent Child*, 44:192-93.

Kristiansson, B, Fallstom, SP (1987). Growth at the age of 4 years subsequent to early failure to thrive. *Child Abuse Negl*, 11:35.

Kroll, RG, Stone, JH (1967). Nocturnal bottle-feeding as a contributory cause of rampant dental caries in the infant and young child. *J Dent Child*, 34:454-59.

Kulig, K, Moore, LL, Kirk, M, et al. (1991). Bromocriptine-associated headache: possible life-threatening sympathomimetic interaction. *Obstetr Gynecol*, 78(5, Pt 2): 941-43.

Kumagai, Y, Shiokawa, Y, Medsger, TA, Jr, Rodnan, GP (1984). Clinical spectrum of connective tissue disease after cosmetic surgery: observations on eighteen patients and a review of the Japanese literature. *Arthritis Rheum*, 27:1-12.

Kuwabara, K, Yakushiji, T, Watanabe, I, Yoshida, S, Koyama, K, Kunita, N (1979). Levels of polychlorinated biphenyls in blood of breast-fed children whose mothers are non-occupationally exposed to PCBs. *Bull Environ Contam Toxicol*, 21:458.

Labbok, MH (1989a). Breastfeeding and family planning programs: a vital complementarity. In: Baumslag, N (Ed.), *Breastfeeding: The Passport of Life* (pp. 48-55). NGO Committee on UNICEF (Working Group on Nutrition). Proceedings of December 10, 1988, meeting at UNICEF House, New York.

Labbok, MH (1989b). *Breastfeeding and Fertility: Mothers and Children Supplement* (p. 81). Washington, DC: American Public Health Association.

Labbok, MH, Cooney, K, Coly, S (1994). *Guidelines: Breastfeeding, Family Planning, and the Lactational Amenorrhea Method—LAM* (pp. 11-13). Washington, DC: Institute for Reproductive Health.

LaGrenade, L, Hanchard, B, Fletcher, V, et al. (1990). Infective dermatitis of Jamaican children: a marker for HTLV-I infection. *Lancet*, 336:1345-47.

Lake, AM, Whitington, PF, Hamilton, SR (1982). Dietary protein-induced colitis in breast-fed infants. *J Pediatr*, 101:906-10.

Landes, RD, Bass, JW, Millunchick, EW, et al. (1980). Neonatal rubella following postpartum maternal immunization. *J Pediatr*, 97:465-67.

Lawrence, R (1989). *Breastfeeding: A Guide for the Medical Profession*, 3rd ed. (p. 497). St Louis: Mosby.

Lawrence, R (1994). *Breastfeeding: A Guide for the Medical Profession*, 4th ed. (pp. 478-79, 589). St Louis: Mosby.

Lawton, ME (1985). Alcohol in breast milk. *Austr NZ J Obstet Gyn*, 25(1):71-73.

Lemons, JA, Schreiner, RL, Gresham, EL (1980). Simple method for determining the caloric and fat content of human milk. *Pediatrics*, 66:626.

Levine, JJ, Ilowite, NT (1994). Scleroderma-like esophageal disease in children breast-fed by mothers with silicone breast implants. *JAMA*, 271:213-16.

Levy, SM (1994). Review of fluoride exposures and ingestion. *Community Dent Oral Epidemiol*, 22(3):173-80.

Lewis, PJ, et al. (1980). Controlled trial of Metoclopramide and the initiation of breast feeding. *Br J Clin Pharmacol*, 9:217-19.

Lieberman, AB (1991). Pain relief in childbirth. *Lamaze Parents' Magazine*, 42-43.

Liedholm, H, Melander, A, Bitzen, PO, Helm, G, Lonnerholm, G, Mattiasson, I, Nilsson, B, Wahlin-Boll, E (1981). Accumulation of atenolol and metoprolol in breast milk. *Eur J Clin Pharmacol*, 20:229.

Lifschitz, CH, Hawkins, HK, Guerra, C, et al. (1988). Anaphylactic shock due to cow's milk protein hypersensitivity in a breastfed infant. *J Pediatr Gastroenterol Nutr*, 7:141-44.

Lilja, G, Dannaeus, A, Falth-Magnusson, K, et al. (1988). Immune response of the atopic woman and foetus: effects of high- and low-dose food allergen intake during late pregnancy. *Clin Allergy*, 18:131-42.

Lindblad, BS (1970). The venous plasma free amino acid levels during the first hours of life. I. After normal and short gestation and gestation complicated by hypertension, with special reference to the "small for dates" syndrome. *Acta Paediatr Scand*, 59(1):13-20.

Little, RE, Anderson, KW, Ervin, CH, Worthington-Roberts, B, Clarren, SK (1989). Maternal alcohol use during breast-feeding and infant mental and motor development at one year. *N Engl J Med*, 321:425.

Liu, XN, Kang, J, Zhao, L, Viteri, FE (1994). Weekly iron supplementation in Chinese preschool children is efficient and safe. *FASEB J*, 8(5):A922.

Liu, JH, Pack, KH (1988). Gonadotropin and prolactin secretion increases during sleep during the puerperium in nonlactating women. *J Clin Endocrinol Metab*, 66:839-45.

Loh, TT, Higuchi, DA, van Bockxmeer, FM, Smith, CH, Brown, EB (1980). Transferrin receptors on the human placental microvillus membrane. *J Clin Invest*, 65:1182-91.

Lönnerdal, B (1989). Food and dietary factors influencing levels and bioavailability of trace elements. In: Southgate, DAT, Johnson, IT, Fenwick, GR (Eds.), *Nutrient Availability: Chemical and Biological Aspects* (pp. 131-39). Cambridge, England: Royal Society of Chemistry.

Losonsky, GA, Gishaut, JM, Strussenberg, J, et al. (1982a). Effect of immunization against rubella on lactation products. 1. Development and characterization of specific immunologic reactivity in breast-milk. *J Infect Dis*, 145:654-60.

Losonsky, GA, Gishaut, JM, Strussenberg, J, et al. (1982b). Effect of immunization against rubella on lactation products. 2. Maternal–neonatal interactions. *J Infect Dis*, 14:666.

Lozoff, B (1994). Editor's Column: Iron deficiency and infant development. *J Pediatr*, 125:577-78.

Lozoff, B, Brittenham, G (1986). Behavioral aspects of iron deficiency. *Prog Hematol*, xiv:23-53.

Lucas, A, Cole, TJ (1990). Breast milk and neonatal necrotizing enterocolitis. *Lancet*, 336:1519-23.

Lucas, A, Gibbs, JAH, Lyster, RLJ, et al. (1978). Creamatocrit: simple clinical technique for estimating fat concentration and energy value of human milk. *Br Med J*, 1:1018.

Macedo, CG (1988). Infant mortality in the Americas. *PAHO Bull*, 22:303-12.

Machtinger, S (1989). Transfer of antigens via breast milk. In: Hamburger, RN (Ed.), *Food Intolerance in Infancy: Allergology, Immunology, and Gastroenterology* (pp. 23-36). New York: Raven Press.

Machtinger, S, Moss, R (1986). Cow's milk allergy in breast-fed infants: the role of allergen and maternal secretory IgA antibody. *J Allergy Clin Immunol*, 77:341-47.

Magnusson, CGM (1988). Cord serum IgE in relation to family history and as predictor of atopic disease in early infancy. *Allergy*, 43:241-51.

Maisels, MJ (1982). Jaundice in the newborn. *Pediatr Rev*, 3:305-19.

Maisels, MJ, Gifford, K, Antle, CE, et al. (1986). Normal serum bilirubin levels in the newborn and the effects of breastfeeding. *Pediatrics*, 78:837-43.

Maisels, MJ, Krung, E (1992). Risk of sepsis in newborn with severe hyperbilirubinemia. *Pediatrics*, 90:741-43.

Maisels, MJ, Newman, TB (1994). Kernicterus occurs in full-term healthy newborns without apparent hemolysis. *Pediatr Res*, 35:239A.

Mandell, H, Berant, M (1985). Oral contraceptives and breastfeeding: haematological effects on the infant. *Arch Dis Child*, 60:971-80.

Manku, MS, Horrobin, DF, Morse, N, Kyte, N, Kyte, V, Jenkins, K, Wright, S, Burton, JL (1982). Reduced levels of prostaglandin precursors in the blood of atopic patients: Defective delta-6-desaturase function as a biochemical basis for atopy. *Prostaglandins Leukotrienes Med*, 9(6):615-28.

Manns, A, Blattner, WA (1991). The epidemiology of HTLV-1. II: etiologic role in human disease. *Transfusion*, 31:67-75.

Matherson, S, Courpotin, C, Simon, F, et al. (1990). Vertical transmission of HIV-2 (letter). *Lancet*, 335:1103-04.

Mathiesen, B, Skuse, D, Wolke, D, et al. (1989). Oral-motor dysfunction and failure to thrive among inner-city infants. *Develop Med Child Neurol*, 31:293.

Matsumura, T, Kuroume, T, Oguri, M, et al. (1975). Egg sensitivity and eczematous manifestations in breast-fed newborns with particular reference to intrauterine sensitization. *Ann Allergy*, 35:221-29.

Matthew, DJ, Taylor, B, Norman, AP, et al. (1977). Prevention of eczema. *Lancet*, 1:321-24.

May, CD, Fomon, SJ, Remigio, L (1982). Immunologic consequences of feeding infants with cow milk and soy products. *Acta Paediatr Scand*, 71:43.

McDonald, PJ, Goldblum, RM, Van Sickle, GJ, et al (1984). Food protein-induced enterocolitis: altered antibody response to ingested antigen. *Pediatr Res*, 18:751-55.

McDonald, RE, Avery, D (1983). *Dentistry for the Child and Adolescent*, 4th ed. (pp. 169-71). St. Louis: Mosby.

McEvoy, G (1992). *American Hospital Formulary Service Drug Information* (p. 1720). Bethesda, MD: American Society of Hospital Pharmacists.

McMillan, JA, Landaw, SA, Oski, FA (1976). Iron sufficiency in breast-fed infants and the availability of iron from human milk. *Pediatrics*, 58:686-91.

McNeilly, AS (1993). Lactational amenorrhea [review]. *Endocrinology and Metabolism Clinics of North America*, 22(1):59-73.

McNeilly, AS, Glasier, AF, Howie, PW, Houston, MJ, Cook, A, Boyle, H (1983). Fertility after childbirth: pregnancy associated with breastfeeding. *Clin Endocrinol*, 18:167-74.

McNeilly, AS, Tay, CC, Glasier, A (1994). Physiological mechanisms underlying lactational amenorrhea [review]. *Ann NY Acad Sci*, 709:145-55.

Meier, PP, Engstrom, JL, Crichton, CL, Clark, DR, Williams, MM, Mangurten, HH (1994). A new scale for in-home test-weighing for mothers of preterm and high-risk infants. *J Hum Lact*, 10(3):163-68.

Meigel, W, Dettke, T, Meige, EM, Lenze, V (1987). Additional oral treatment of atopic dermatitis with unsaturated fatty acids. *Z Hautkr*, 62(1):100-103.

Mennella, JA, Beauchamp, GK (1991). The transfer of alcohol to human milk: effects of flavor and the infant's behavior. *N Engl J Med*, 325(14):981-85.

Menon, SD, Qin, S, Guy, GR, Tan, YH (1993). Differential induction of nuclear NF-kappa B by protein phosphatase inhibitors in primary and transformed human cells. Requirement for both oxidation and phosphorylation in nuclear translocation. *J Biol Chem*, 268(35):5-12.

Merrett, TG, Burr, ML, Butland, BK, et al. (1988). Infant feeding and allergy: 12-month prospective study of 500 babies born into allergic families. *Ann Allergy*, 61:13-20.

Mestyan, J, Soltesz, G, Schultz, K, Horvath, M (1975). Hyperaminoacidemia due to the accumulation of gluconeogenic amino acid precursors in hypoglycemia small-for-gestational age infants. *J Pediatr*, 87(3):409-14.

Michaelsen, KF, Skafte, L, Badsberg, JH, Jorgensen, M (1990). Variation in macronutrients in human bank milk: influencing factors and implications for human milk banking. *J Pediatr Gastroenterol Nutr*, 11:229-39.

Minami, J (1990). Helping mothers with chronic illness. *Leaven*, 26:52-53.

Mofenson, LM, Wolinsky, SM. (1994). Vertical transmission of HIV. Part C. Current insights regarding vertical transmission. In: Pizzo, PA, Wilfert, CM (Eds.), *Pediatric AIDS: The Challenge of HIV Infection in Infants, Children and Adolescents*, 2nd ed. (pp. 179-203). Baltimore: Williams & Wilkins.

Mohrbacher, N (1994). Breastfeeding and silicone breast implants: Are there risks? *Medela Rental Roundup*, 11(3):8-9.

Moore,WJ, Corbett, ME (1971). The distribution of dental caries in ancient British populations. I. Anglo-Saxon period. *Caries Res*, 5:151-68.

Moore, WJ, Corbett, ME (1973). The distribution of dental caries in ancient British populations. II. Iron Age, Romano-British and medieval periods. *Caries Res*, 7:139-53.

Morgan, G, Wilkins, HA, Pepin, J, et al. (1990). AIDS following mother-to-child transmission of HIV-2. *AIDS*, 4:879-82.

Morse, PF, Horrobin, DF, Manku, MS, Stewart, JCM, Allen, R, Littlewood, S, Wright, S, Burton, J, Gould, DJ, Holt, PJ, Janse, CT, Mattila, L, Meigel, W, Dettke, T, Wexler, D, Guenther, L, Bordoni, A, Patrizi, A (1989). Meta-analysis of placebo-controlled studies of the efficacy of Epogam in the treatment of atopic eczema: relationship between plasma essential fatty acid changes and clinical response. *Br J Dermatol*, 121:75-90.

Moutos, D (1996). Diarrhea. *Building Blocks for Life*, 20:3.

Moyer, MP, Huot, RI, Ramirez, A, et al. (1990). Infection of human gastrointestinal cells by HIV-1. *AIDS Res Hum Retroviruses*, 6:1409-15.

Myher, JJ, Kuksis, A, Steiner, G (1984). Milk fat structure of a patient with type I hyperlipidemia. *Lipids*, 19:673-82.

National Diabetes Data Group (1979). Classification and diagnosis of diabetes mellitus and other categories of glucose intolerance. *Diabetes*, 28:1039-59.

National Institute of Dental Research (NIDR), National Caries Program (1979–1980). Summary of Findings. In: *The Prevalence of Dental Caries in United States Children*. NIH Publication No. 82-2245:5-8. Washington, DC: National Institutes of Health.

Nau, H, Kuhnz, W, Egger, HJ, Rating, D, Helge, H (1982). Anticonvulsants during pregnancy and lactation: Transplacental, maternal and neonatal pharmacokinetics. *Clin Pharmacokinet*, 7:508.

Neifert, MR, Seacat, JM (1987). Lactation insufficiency: a rational approach. *Birth*, 14:182-88.

Neifert, MR (1990). The influence of breast surgery, breast appearance, and pregnancy-induced breast changes on lactation sufficiency as measured by infant weight gain. *Birth*, 17:31-38.

Neifert, MR, McDonough, S, Neville, M (1981). Failure of lactogenesis associated with placental retention. *Am J Obstet Gynecol*, 140:477-78.

Neifert, MR, Seacat, JM (1986). Medical management of successful breast-feeding. *Pediatric Clinics of North America*, 33(4):743-62.

Neifert, MR, Seacat, J (1987). Lactation insufficiency: a rational approach. *Birth*, 14:182-90.

Neifert, MR, Seacat, JM, Jobe, WE (1985). Lactation failure due to insufficient glandular development of the breast. *Pediatrics*, 76(5):823-28.

Nelson, LM, Franklin, GM, Jones, MC, et al. (1988). Risk of multiple sclerosis exacerbation during pregnancy and breastfeeding. *JAMA*, 259:3441.

Neubauer, SH (1990). Lactation in insulin-dependent diabetes. *Prog Food Nutr Sci*, 14(4):333-70.

Newburg, DS, Viscidi, RP, Ruff, A, et al. (1992). A human milk factor inhibits binding of human immunodeficiency virus to the CD4 receptor. *Pediatr Res*, 31:22-28.

Newman, TB, Maisels, MJ (1992). Evaluation and treatment of jaundice in the term newborn: a kinder, gentler approach. *Pediatrics*, 89:809-18.

Nice, FJ (1990). Breastfeeding and medications. *J Prac Nurs*, 40:119-25.

Nicholls, EB (1914). Teeth of Aboriginal children in Cape Barren Island. *Dent Record*, XXXIV:560-62.

Nikkila, EA (1983). Familial lipoprotein lipase deficiency and related disorders of chylomicron metabolism. In: Stanbury, J, Wynagaarden, JB, Fredrickson, DS, Goldstein, JL, Brown, MS (Eds.), *The Metabolic Basis of Inherited Disease*, 5th ed. (pp. 622-642). New York: McGraw-Hill.

Nowak, A, Bishara, S, Lancial, L, Heckert, A (1986). Changes in nutritive and non-nutritive sucking habits: birth to two years. *J Dent Res* (Abs), 65:1525.

Nowak, A, Crall, J (1988). Prevention of dental disease. In: Pinkham, JR (Ed.), *Pediatric Dentistry, Infancy through Adolescence* (p. 160). Philadelphia: Saunders.

Nursing Mothers' Association of Australia (1982). *Where There's a Will There's Usually a Way—Breastfeeding When the Mother Has a Disability*. Victoria, Australia: Hawthorn.

Oehler, J (1981). *Family-Centered Neonatal Nursing Care*. Philadelphia: Lippincott.

Ohto, H, Terazawa, S, Sasaki, N, et al. (1994). Transmission of hepatitis C virus from mothers to infants: the Vertical Transmission of Hepatitis C Virus Collaborative Group. *N Engl J Med*, 17(11):744-50.

Orloff, SL, Wallingford, JC, McDougal, JS (1993). Inactivation of human immunodeficiency virus type 1 in human milk and of pasteurization. *J Hum Lact*, 9:13-17.

Osborn, LM (1986). Management of neonatal jaundice. *Nurse Pract*, 11:41-52.

Oski, FA, Landaw, SA (1980). Inhibition of iron absorption from human milk by baby food. *Am J Dis Child*, 134:459-60.

Oxtoby, MJ (1988). Human immunodeficiency virus and other viruses in human milk: placing the issues in broader perspective. *Pediatr Infect Dis J*, 7:825-35.

Oxtoby, MJ (1994). Vertically acquired HIV infection in the United States. In: Pizzo, PA, Wilfert, CM (Eds.), *Pediatric AIDS: The Challenge of HIV-1 Infection in Infants, Children and Adolescents*, 2nd ed. (pp. 3-20). Baltimore: Williams & Wilkins.

Paccagnini, S, Principi, N, Massironi, E, et al. (1995). Perinatal transmission and manifestation of hepatitis C virus infection in a high-risk population. *Pediatr Infect Dis J*, 14(3):195-99.

Patton, S (1994). Detection of large fragments of the human milk MUCIN-1 in feces of breastfed infant. *J Pediatr Gastroenterol Nutr*, 18(2):225-30.

Pedersen, PO (1938). Investigations into dental conditions of about 3000 ancient and modern Greenlanders. *Dent Record*, 58:191-98.

Pereira, GR, Baker, L, Egler, J, et al. (1990). Serum myoinositol concentrations in premature infants fed human milk, formula for infants, and parenteral nutrition. *Am J Clin Nutr*, 51:589-93.

Perez, A, Labbok, MH, Queenan, JT (1992). Clinical study of the lactational amenorrhea method for family planning. *Lancet*, 339:968-70.

Peterson, KE, Washington, J, Rathburn, JM (1984). Team management of failure to thrive. *J Am Diet Assoc*, 84:810.

Pisacane, A, De Viziab, B, Valiante, A (1995). Iron status in breast-fed infants. *J Pediatr*, 127(3):429-31.

Pisacane, A, Graziano, L, Mazzarella, G, et al. (1992). Breastfeeding and urinary tract infection. *J Pediatr*, 120:87-89.

Pisacane, A, Impagliazzo, N, Russo, M, Valiani, R, Mandarini, A, Florio, C, Vivo, P (1994). Breastfeeding and multiple sclerosis. *Br Med J*, 308:1403-06.

Pizarro, F, Yip, R, Dallman, PR, et al. (1991). Iron status with different infant feeding regimens: relevance to screening and prevention of iron deficiency. *J Pediatr*, 118:687-92.

Polywka, S, Feucht, H, Zollner, B, Laufs, R (1997). Hepatitis C virus infection in pregnancy and the risk of mother-to-child transmission. *Eur J Clin Micro Inf Dis*, 16(2):121-24.

Porro, E, Antognoni, G, Midulla, F, et al. (1988). Breastfeeding and bronchiolitis. In: Pershewitz, R (Ed.), *Ambulatory Pediatric Association Program Book* (p. 4). Philadelphia: Lippincott Medical.

Powell, GF, Low, JF, Speers, MA (1987). Behavior as a diagnostic aid in failure-to-thrive. *J Dev Behav Pediatr*, 8-18.

Powell, GK (1978). Milk- and soy-induced enterocolitis of infancy: clinical features and standardization of challenge. *J Pediatr*, 93:553-60.

Priest, A (1994). Breastfeeding troubles "can backfire" on babies. *Vancouver Sun* (July 28).

The Providence Journal-Bulletin (1994a). Breast-feeding and uproar over "insufficient milk syndrome." Conspiracy debate on breast-feeding article (September 14), C:6.

The Providence Journal-Bulletin (1994b). Breast-feeding and uproar over "insufficient milk syndrome." R.I. experts say education eliminates risks (September 14), C:3.

Pukander, J, Luotonen, J, Timonen, M, Karma, P (1985). Risk factors affecting the occurrence of acute otitis media among 2–3-year-old urban children. *Acta Otolaryngol*, 100:260-65.

Quinn, PT, Lofberg, JV (1978). Maternal herpetic breast infection: another hazard of neonatal herpes simplex. *Med J Aust*, 2:411.

Rains, CP, Bryson, HM, Fitton, A (1995). Cabergoline. A review of its pharmacological properties and therapeutic potential in the treatment of hyperprolactinaemia and inhibition of lactation. *Drugs*, 49(2):255-79.

Rathburn, JM, Peterson, KE (1987). Nutrition in failure to thrive. In: Grand, RJ, Sutphen, JL, Dietz, WH (Eds.), *Pediatric Nutrition*, Boston: Butterworth.

Rayburn, WF (1996). Clinical commentary: the bromocriptine (parlodel) controversy and recommendations for lactation suppression. *Am J Perinatol*, 13:69-71.

Riordan, J, Auerbach, K (1993). *Breastfeeding and Human Lactation*. Boston: Jones and Bartlett.

Ripa, LW (1988). Nursing caries: a comprehensive review. *Ped Dent*, 10:268-82.

Roberts, GJ, Rugg-Gunn, AJ, Wright, WG (1983). The effect of human milk on plaque pH and enamel dissolution compared with cow's milk, lactose and sucrose. *J Dent Res*, 62:426.

Roddey, OF, Jr, Martin, ES, Swetenburg, RL (1981). Critical weight loss and malnutiriton in breastfed infants: four case reports. *Am J Dis Child*, 135:597-99.

Rogan, WJ (1989). Cancer from PCBs in breastmilk? A risk benefit analysis. [Abstract No. 612.] *Pediatr Res*, 25:105A.

Rogan, WJ, Gladen, BC, McKinney, JD, Carreras, N, Hardy, P, Thullen, J, Tingelstad, J, Tully, M (1986). Polychlorinated biphenyls (PCBs) and dichlorodiphenyl dichloroethene (DDE) in human milk: effects on growth, morbidity, and duration of lactation. *Am J Public Health*, 77:1294-97.

Rogan, WJ, Gladen, BC, McKinney, JD, Carreras, N, Hardy, P, Thullen, J, Tingelstad, J, Tully, M (1987). Polychlorinated biphenyls (PCBs) and dichlorodiphenyl dichloroethene (DDE) in human milk: effects of maternal factors and previous lactation. *Am J Public Health*, 76:172.

Rogers, AH (1981). The source of infection in the intrafamilial transfer of *Streptococcus mutans*. *Caries Res*, 15:26 31.

Rowland, TW, Zori, RT, Lafleur, WR, Reiter, EO (1982). Malnutrition and hypernatremic dehydration in breastfed infants. *JAMA*, 247(7):1016-17.

Rudolph, AJ (1985). Failure to thrive in the perinatal period. *Acta Paediatr Scand*, 319:55.

Ruff, AJ (1994). Breastmilk, breastfeeding, and transmission of viruses to the neonate. *Sem Perinatol*, 18(6):510-16.

Ruff, AJ, Halsey, NA, Coberly, J, et al. (1992). Breastfeeding and maternal–infant transmission of human immunodeficiency virus type I. *J Pediatr*, 121:325-29.

Rugg-Gunn, AJ, Roberts, GJ, Wright, WG (1985). Effect of human milk on plaque pH in situ and enamel dissolution in vitro compared with bovine milk, lactose, and sucrose. *Caries Res*, 19:327-34.

Rule, JT (1982). Recognition of dental caries. *Pediatr Clin North Am*, 29:439-56.

Saarinen, UM, Kajosaari, M, Backman, A, et al. (1979). Prolonged breast-feeding as prophylaxis for atopic disease. *Lancet*, 1:163-66.

Saarinen, UM, Siimes, MA (1979). Iron absorption from breast milk, cow's milk, and iron-supplemented formula: an opportunistic use of changes in total body iron determined by hemoglobin, ferritin and body weight in 132 infants. *Pediatr Res*, 13:143-47.

Salonen, JT, Nyyssonen, K, Korpela, H, Tuomilehto, J, et al. (1992). High stored iron levels are associated with excess risk of myocardial infarction in Eastern Finnish men. *Circulation*, 86:803-11.

Sampson, WEA (1932). Dental examination of the inhabitants of the island of Tristan da Cunha. *Br Dent J*, LII: 397-401.

Saylor, J, Bahna, S (1991). Anaphylaxis to casein hydrolysate formula. *J Pediatr*, 118:71-73.

Schultz, K, Mestyan, J, Soltesz, G, Horvath, M (1976). The metabolic effects of glucagon infusion in normoglycaemic and hypoglycaemic small-for-gestational-age infants. I. Changes in blood gluscose, blood lactate and plasma free fatty acids. *Acta Paediatr Acad Scientiarum Hungaricae*, 17(3):237-44.

Schneider, AP (1986). Breastmilk jaundice in the newborn: a real entity. *JAMA*, 255:3270-74.

Schwartz, RH, Amonette, MS (1991). Cow milk protein hydrolysate infant formulas not always "hypoallergenic." *J Pediatr*, 118:839-40.

Scialli, AR (1991). Breast milk. In: Scialli, AR (Ed.), *A Clinical Guide to Reproductive and Developmental Toxicology*. Boca Raton: CRC Press.

Seibold, JR (1993). Scleroderma. In: Kelley, WN, Harris, ED, Jr., Ruddy, S, Sledge, CB (Eds.), *Textbook of Rheumatology*, 4th ed. (p. 1114). Philadelphia: Saunders.

Seligman, PA, Schleicher, RB, Allen, RH (1979). Isolation and characterization of the transferrin receptor from human placenta. *J Biol Chem*, 254:9943.

Sergent, JS, Fuchs, H, Johnson, JS (1993). Polyarticular arthritis. In: Kelly, WN, Harris, ED, Jr, Ruddy, S, Sledge, CB (Eds.), *Textbook of Rheumatology*, 4th ed. (pp. 381-84). Philadelphia: Saunders.

Shelton, PG, Berkowitz, RJ, Forrester, DJ (1977). Nursing bottle caries. *Pediatrics*, 59:777.

Sherwen, LN, Scoloveno, MA, Weingarten, CT (1991). *Nursing Care of the Childbearing Family* (p. 1211). Norwolk, CT: Appleton & Lange.

Showers, J, Mandelkorn, R, Coury, DL, McCleery, J (1986). Non-organic failure to thrive: Identification and intervention. *J Pediatr Nurs*, 1:240.

Sigurs, N, Hattevig, G, Kjellman, B (1992). Maternal avoidance of eggs, cow's milk, and fish during lactation: effect on allergic manifestations, skin-prick tests and specific IgE antibodies in children at age 4 years. *Pediatrics*, 89:735-39.

Silprasert, A, Dejsarai, W, Keawvichit, R, et al. (1986). Effect of storage on the creamatocrit and total energy content of human milk. *Hum Nutr: Clin Nutr*, 40C:31.

Singer, L (1986). Long-term hospitalization of failure-to-thrive infants: developmental outcome at three years. *Child Abuse Negl*, 10:479.

Sioufi, A, Hillion, D, Lumbroso, P, Wainer, R, Olivier-Martin, M, Schoeller, JP, Colussi, D, Leroux, F, Mangoni, P (1984). Oxprenolol placental transfer plasma concentrations in newborn and passage into breast milk. *Br J Clin Pharmacol*, 18:453.

Skikne, B, Flowers, C, Cook, J (1990). Serum transferrin receptor: a quantitative measure of tissue iron deficiency. *Am Soc Hemat*, 75:1870-76.

Smith, L, Bickerton, J, Pilcher, G, et al. (1985). Creamatocrit, carbon content, and energy value of pooled banked human milk: implications for feeding preterm infants. *Early Hum Dev*, 11:75.

Solomon, G, Espinoza, L, Silverman, S (1994). Breast implants and connective-tissue disease. *N. Engl J Med*, 331:1231.

Sousa, PLR (1975). Metoclopramide and breast-feeding. *Br Med J*, 1:512.

Sowers, MF, Corton, G, Shaprio, B, et al. (1993). Changes in bone density with lactation. *JAMA*, 269:3130-35.

Sowers, M, Randolph, J, Shapiro, B, Jannausch, M (1995). A prospective study of bone density and pregnancy after an extended period of lactation with bone loss. *Obst Gynecol*, 85(2):285-89.

Spika, JS, Shaffer, N, Hargrett-Bean, N, Collin, S, MacDonald, KL, Blake, PA (1989). Risk factors for infant botulism in the United States. *Am J Dis Child*, 143:828-32.

Steele, S (1986). Nonorganic failure to thrive: A pediatric social illness. *Iss Comp Pediatr Nursing*, 9:47.

Steiner, G, Myher, JJ, Kuksis, A (1985). Milk and plasma lipid composition in a lactating patient with type I hyperlipoproteinemia. *Am J Clin Nutr*, 41:121-28.

Stephan, RM (1940). Changes in the hydrogen iron concentration on tooth surfaces and in carious lesions. *JADA*, 27:718-23.

Stephenson, LS (1995). Possible new developments in community control of iron deficiency anemia. *Nutr Rev*, 53(2):23-30.

Stocker, R, McDonagh, AF, Glazer, AN, Ames, BN (1990). Antioxidant activities of bile pigments: biliverdin and bilirubin. *Methods Enzymol*, 186:301-309.

Stocker, R, Yamamoto, Y, McDonagh, AF, et al. (1987). Bilirubin is an antioxidant of possible physiological importance. *Science*, 235:1043-46.

Sullivan-Boyai, JZ, Fife, KH, Jacobs, RF, et al. (1983). Disseminated neonatal herpes simplex virus type 1 from a maternal breast lesion. *Pediatrics*, 71:455.

Takahashi, K, Takezaki, T, Oki, T, et al. (1991). Inhibitory effect of maternal antibody on mother-to-child transmission of human T-lymphotrophic virus type I. *Int J Cancer*, 49:673-77.

Takala, AK, Eskola, J, Palmgren, J, Ronnberg, PR, Kela, E, Rekola, P, Makela, PH (1989). Risk factors of invasive *Haemophilus influenzae* type B disease among children in Finland. *J Pediatr*, 115:694-701.

Taylor, B, Norman, AP, Orgel, HA, et al. (1973). Transient IgA deficiency and pathogenesis of infantile atopy. *Lancet*, ii:111-13.

Thiry, L, Sprecher-Goldberger, S, Jonckheer, T, et al. (1985). Isolation of AIDS virus from cell-free breast milk of three healthy virus carriers (letter). *Lancet*, 2:891.

Thureen, PJ, Hay, WW (1993). Conditions requiring special nutritional management. In: *Nutritional Needs of the Preterm Infant* (pp. 243-65). Baltimore: Williams & Wilkins.

Torney, H (1995). Prolonged, on-demand breastfeeding and dental caries—An investigation (ABS). LLLI Annual Meeting, Chicago.

Torrence, C (1985). Neonatal seizures: Part I. A developmental and clinical understanding. *Neonatal Network*, 4(1):9-16.

Traisman, AS, Traisman, H (1958). Thumb and finger sucking: a study of 2,650 infants and children. *J Pediatr*, 52:566-77.

U.S. Department of Health, Education, and Welfare (1979). *Evaluatory Surveys of Long-Term Fluoridation Show Improved Dental Health*, Publication No. 84-22647. Atlanta: USPHS.

U.S. Food and Drug Administration (FDA) (1994). Study of children breastfed by women with breast implants. *FDA Talk Paper*, 94:6.

Uraizee, F, Gross, SJ (1989). Improved feeding tolerance and reduced incidence of sepsis in sick, very low birthweight (VLBW) infants fed maternal milk. *Pediatr Res*, 25:298A.

van Asperen, PP, Kemp, AS, Mellis, CM (1983). Immediate food hypersensitivity reactions on the first known exposure to the food. *Arch Dis Child*, 58:253-56.

van Asperen, PP, Kemp, AS, Mellis, CM (1984). A prospective study of the clinical manifestations of atopic disease in infancy. *Acta Paediatr Scand*, 73:80-85.

van Beusekom, CM, Zeegers, TA, Martini, IA, Velvis, HJ, Visser, GH, Van Doormaal, JJ, Muskiet, FA (1993). Milk of patients with tightly controlled insulin-dependent diabetes mellitus has normal macronutrient and fatty acid composition. *Am J Clin Nutr*, 57(6):938-43.

Van de Perre, P, Lepage, P, Homsy, J, et al. (1992). Mother-to-infant transmission of human immunodeficiency virus by breast milk: Presumed innocent or presumed guilty? *Clin Infect Dis*, 15:502-7.

Van de Perre, P, Simonon, A, Hitimana, DG, et al. (1993). Infective and anti-infective properties of breastmilk from HIV-1 infected women. *Lancet*, 341:914-18.

van der Heijden, PF, Kremer, JA, Brownell, J, Rolland, R (1991). Lactation inhibition by the dopamine agonist CV 205-502. *Br J Obstetr Gynecol*, 98(3):270-76.

Van Dyke, RB, Heneine, W, Perrin, M, et al. (1994). Vertical transmission of HTLV-II in the presence and absence of breast feeding. *AIDS Res Hum Retroviruses*, 10:483.

Van Esterik, P, Latham, MC (1981). Response to Gussler and Briesemeister's reply. *Med Anthropol*, 5:253-54.

Victoria, CG, Smith, PG, Vaughan, JP, Nobre, LC, Lombardi, C, Teixeira, AM, Fuchs, SC, Moreira, LB, Gigante, LP, Barros, FC (1989). Infant feeding and deaths to diarrhea: a case-control study. *Am J Epidemiol*, 129(5): 1032-41.

Vorherr, H (1974). *The Breast: Morphology, Physiology, and Lactation*. New York: Academic.

Wada, HD, Hass, PE, Sussman, HH (1979). Transferrin receptor in human placental brush border membranes. *J Biol Chem*, 254:12629-35.

Walter, T, Dallman, PR, Pizarro, F, Belozo, L, et al. (1993). Effectiveness of iron fortified infant cereal in prevention of iron deficiency anemia. *Pediatrics*, 91:976-82.

Walter, T, Kovalskys, J, Stekel, A (1983). Effect of mild iron deficiency on infant mental development scores. *J Pediatr*, 102:519-22.

Warner, JO (1980). Food allergy in fully breast-fed infants. *Clin Allergy*, 10:133-36.

Webb, TE, Oski, FA (1973). Iron deficiency anemia and scholastic achievement in young adolescents. *J Pediatr*, 82(5):827-30.

Webster, J (1996). A comparative review of the tolerability profiles of dopamine agonists in the treatment of hyperprolactinaemia and inhibition of lactation. *Drug Safety*, 14(4):228-38.

Welliver, RC, Wong, DT, Sun, M, McCarty, N (1986). Parainfluenza virus bronchiolitis. *Am J Dis Child*, 140:34-40.

Whittle, BJR, Esplugues, JV (1989). PAF. In: Barnes, PJ, Page, CP, Henson, PM (Eds.), *Platelet-Activating Factor and Human Disease* (pp. 198-219). Oxford, England: Blackwell Scientific Publishers.

Wiktor, SZ, Pate, EJ, Murphy, EL, et al. (1993). Mother-to-child transmission of human T-cells lymphotrophic virus type I (HTLV-I) in Jamaica: association with antibodies to envelope glycoprotein (gp46) epitopes. *J Acquir Immune Defic Syndr*, 6:1162-67.

Wilkerson, NN (1988). A comprehensive look at hyperbilirubinemia. *MCN*, 13:360-64.

Wilson, JT (1983). Determinants and consequences of drug excretion in breast milk. *Drug Metabolism Rev*, 14(4):619-52.

Wilson, NW, Hamburger, RN (1988). Allergy to cow's milk in the first year of life and its prevention. *Ann Allergy*, 61(5):323-37.

Winnikoff, B, Semeraro, P, Zimmerman, M (1987). *Contraception During Lactation*. New York: Population Council Publishers.

Woodruff, CW, Latham, BA, McDavid, S (1977). Iron nutrition in the breast-fed infant. *J Pediatr*, 90:36-38.

Woolridge, M (1995). Paper presented at the International Lactation Consultant Association annual meeting and conference, Scottsdale, AZ.

Wong, YK, Wood, BS (1971). Breast-milk jaundice and oral contraceptives. *Br Med J*, 4(784):403-4.

World Health Organization (WHO) (1992). Consensus statement from the consultation on HIV transmission and breastfeeding. *J Hum Lact*, 8:173-4.

Wright, A, Luffingham, GH, North, D (1989). Breastfeeding and lower respiratory tract illness in the first year of life. *Br Med J*, 299:946-49.

Wright, S, Bolton, C (1989). Breast milk fatty acids in mothers of children with atopic eczema. *Br J Nutr*, 62(3):693-97.

Yeager, AS, Palumbo, PE, Malachowski, N, et al. (1983). Sequelae of maternally derived cytomegalovirus infections in premature infants. *J Pediatr*, 102:918.

Youdim, MBH, Ben-Shachar, D (1987). Minimal brain damage induced by early iron deficiency: modified dopaminergic neurotransmission. *Isr J Med Sci*, 23:19-25.

Zeigler, RS, Heller, S, Mellon, M, et al. (1986). Effectiveness of dietary manipulation in the prevention of food allergy in infants. *J Allergy Clin Immunol*, 78:224-38.

Zeigler, RS, Heller, S, Mellon, MH, et al. (1989). Effect of combined maternal and infant food-allergen avoidance on development of atopy in early infancy: a randomized study. *J Allergy Clin Immunol*, 84:72-89.

ADDITIONAL READINGS

Adlard, BPF, Lathe, GH (1970). Breast milk jaundice: Effect on 3 alpha, 20 beta-pregnanediol on bilirubin conjugation by human liver. *Arch Dis Child*, 45:186-89.

Alhford, CE (1994). Criteria for exchange transfusion in jaundiced newborns. *Pediatrics*, 93:488-94.

American Academy of Pediatrics, Committee on Fetus and Newborn (1993). Routine evaluation of blood pressure, hematocrit, and glucose in newborns. *Pediatrics*, 92(3):474-76.

Arias, IM, Gutsteen, S, Biempical, L (1967). Prolonged neonatal unconjugated hyperbilirubinemia associated with breastfeeding and steroid pregnane-3 alpha, 20 B-dial in maternal milk that inhibits glucuronide formation in vitro. *J Clin Invest*, 43:2037.

Bauchner, H, Leventhal, JM, Shapiro, ED (1986). Studies of breastfeeding and infections. How good is the evidence? *JAMA*, 256:887-97.

Berlin, CM, Jr (1992). Drugs and human milk. *Breastfeeding Abstracts*, 11(3):1-3.

Berlin, CM, Jr (1994). Silicone breast implants and breastfeeding. *Pediatrics*, 94:547-49.

Black, RF (1996). Transmission of HIV-1 in the breastfeeding process. *J Am Diet Assoc*, 96:267-74.

Businco, L, Loppi, M, Morse, NL, Nisini, R, Wright, S (1993). Breastmilk from mothers of children with newly developed atopic eczema has low levels of long chain polyunsaturated fatty acids. *J Allergy Clin Immunol*, 91:1134-39.

Casey, PH, Wortham, B, Nelson, JY (1984). Management of children with failure-to-thrive in a rural ambulatory setting. *Clin Pediatr*, 23:325.

Centers for Disease Control and Prevention, USPHS Working Group (1993). Guidelines for counseling persons infected with human T-lymphotrophic virus type I (HTLV-I) and type II (HTLV-II). *Ann Intern Med*, 118:448-54.

Corbett, JV, Yaros, PS (1994). Metoclopramide (Reglan). *MCN*, 19:296.

Dennery, PA, Rhine, WD, Stevenson, DK (1995). Neonatal jaundice—What now? *Clin Pediatr*, 34:103-7.

Duncan, B, Schiffman, RB, Corrigan, JJ, Schaefer, C (1985). Iron and the exclusively breast-fed infant from birth to 6 months. *J Pediatr Gastroenterol Nutr*, 4:421-25.

Ferris, A, Jensen, R (1984). Lipids in human milk: A review. I. Sampling determination and content. *J Pediatr Gastroenter Nutr*, 3:108.

Gartner, LM (1994). On the question of the relationship between breastfeeding and jaundice in the first 5 days of life. *Semin Perinatol,* 18(6):502-9.

Gaskin, KJ, Waters, DL (1994). Nutritional management of infants with cystic fibrosis. *J Pediatr Child Health,* 30(1):1-2.

Gruskay, FL (1982). Comparison of breast, cow, and soy feedings in the prevention of onset of allergic disease. *Clin Pediatr,* 21:486.

Guzman, V, Toscano, G, Canales, ES, Zarate, A (1979). Improvement of defective lactation by using oral metoclopramide. *Acta Obstet Gynecol Scand,* 58:53-55.

Habbick, BF, Gerrard, JW (1984). Failure to thrive in the contented breast-fed baby. *Can Med Assoc J,* 131(7):765-68.

Hackett, AF, Rugg-Gunn, AJ, Murray, JJ, Roberts, GJ (1984). Can breast feeding cause dental caries? *Hum Nutr: App Nutr,* 38A:23-28.

Haddock, RL, Cousens, SN, Guzman, CC (1991). Infant diet and salmonellosis. *Am J Public Health,* 81(8):997-1000.

Hall, DM, Kay, G (1977). Effect of thyrotrophin-releasing factor on lactation [letter]. *Br Med J,* 1(6063):777.

Hallman, M, Bry, K, Hopper, K, et al. (1992). Inositol supplementation in premature infants with respiratory distress syndrome. *N Engl J Med,* 326:1233-39.

Hide, DW, Guyer, BM (1981). Clinical manifestations of allergy related to breast and cows' milk feeding. *Arch Dis Child,* 56:172.

Johnstone, DE, Dutton, AM (1966). Dietary prophylaxis of allergic disease in children. *N Engl J Med,* 274:715.

Kaufman, HS, Frick, OL (1976). The development of allergy in infants of allergic parents: a prospective study concerning the role of heredity. *Ann Allergy,* 37:410.

Kaufman, HS, Frick, OL (1981). Prevention of asthma. *Clin Allergy,* 11:549.

Kauppila, A, et al. (1983). Metoclopramide and breast feeding: transfer into milk and the newborn. *Eur J Clin Pharm,* 25:819-23.

Kent, GN, Price, RI, Gutteridge, DH, Allen, JR, Blakeman, SL, Bhagat, CI, St. John, A, Barnes, MP, Smith, M, Evans, DV (1991). Acute effects of an oral calcium load in pregnancy and lactation: findings on renal calcium conservation and biochemical indices of bone turnover. *Mineral and Electrolyte Metabolism,* 17(1):1-7.

Kent, GN, Price, RI, Gutteridge, DH, et al. (1991). The efficiency of intestinal calcium absorption is increased in late pregnancy but not in established lactation. *Calcif Tissue Int,* 48:293-95.

Lewis, PJ, Devenish, C, Kahn, C (1980). Controlled trial of metoclopromide in the initiation of breast feeding. *Br J Clin Pharmacol,* 13:731.

Maisels, MJ (1994). Neonatal jaundice. In: Avery, JB, Fletcher, A, MacDonald, MG (Eds.), *Pathophysiology and Management of the Newborn* (pp. 630-725). Philadelphia: Lippincott.

Michel, SH, Mueller, DH (1994). Impact of lactation on women with cystic fibrosis and their infants—A review of five cases. *J Am Diet Assoc,* 94(2):159-65.

Moore, WJ, Midwinter, RE, Morris, AF, et al. (1985). Infant feeding and subsequent risk of atopic eczema. *Arch Dis Child,* 60:722.

Newman, TB, Maisels, MJ (1990). Does hyperbilirubinemia damage the brain of healthy full-term infants? *Clin Perinatol,* 71:660-63.

Neubauer, SH, Ferris, AM, Chase, CG, Fanelli, J, Thompson, CA, Lammi-Keefe, CJ, Clark, RM, Jensen, RG, Bendel, RB, Green, KW (1993). Delayed lactogenesis in women with insulin-dependent diabetes mellitus. *Am J Clin Nutr,* 58(1):54-60.

Oski, F (1992). Hyperbilirubinemia in the term infant: an unjaundiced approach. *Contemporary Pediatrics,* 9:148-54.

Peter, G (1994). Summary of major changes in the 1994 Red Book: American Academy of Pediatrics. Report of the Committee on Infectious Disease. *Pediatrics,* 93(6, Part 1):1000-2.

Poulsen, AG, Kvinesdal, BB, Aaby, P, et al. (1992). Lack of evidence of vertical transmission of the human immunodeficiency virus type 2 in a sample of the general population in Bissau. *J Acquir Immune Defic Syndr,* 5:25-30.

Ruff, AJ, Coberly, J, Halsey, NA, et al. (1994). Prevalence of HIV DNA and p24 antigen in breast milk and correlation with maternal factors. *J Acquir Immune Defic Synd,* 7:68-73.

Saarinen, UM (1978). Need for iron supplementation in infants on prolonged breast feeding. *J Pediatr,* 93:177-80.

Saarinen, UM, Siimes, MA (1977). Iron absorption from infant milk formula and the optimal level of iron supplementation. *Acta Paediatr Scand,* 66:719-22.

Saarinen, UM, Siimes, MA (1978). Developmental changes in red blood cell counts and indices of infants after exclusion of iron deficiency by laboratory criteria and continuous iron supplementation. *J Pediatr,* 92:412-16.

Saarinen, UM, Siimes, MA, Dallman, PR (1977). Iron absorption in infants: high bioavailability of breast milk iron as indicated by the extrinsic tag method of iron absorption and by the concentration of serum ferritin. *J Pediatr,* 91(1):36-39.

Siimes, MA, Vuori, E, Kuitunen, P (1979). Breast milk iron—A declining concentration during the course of lactation. *Acta Paediatr Scand,* 68:29-31.

Specker, BL, Vieira, NE, O'Brien, KO, Ho, ML, Heubi, JE, Abrams, SA, Yergey, AL (1994). Calcium kinetics in lactating women with low and high calcium intakes. *Am J Clin Nutr,* 59:593-609.

Thappa, S, Short, R, Potts, M (1988). Breastfeeding, birth spacing, and their effect on child survival. *Nature,* 355:679-82.

Watchki, J, Oski, F (1983). Bilirubin 20 mg/dL = vigintiphobia. *Pediatrics,* 71:4.

Welch, MJ, Phelps, DL, Osher, AB (1981). Breast-feeding by a mother with cystic fibrosis. *Pediatrics,* 67:664-66.

CHAPTER 3

Special Lactation Circumstances

SECTION A

Breastfeeding Infants with Special Needs

Jan B. Simpson, RN, BSN, IBCLC
Rebecca F. Black, MS, RD/LD, IBCLC
Bryn Hamilton, RD/LD, IBCLC

LEARNING OBJECTIVES

At the completion of this section, the learner will be able to do the following:

1. Discuss suggestions for the successful initiation and continuation of breast-feeding of the infant who is born prematurely.
2. Discuss tongue and jaw movements that are disorganized and/or dysfunctional and how these variations and movements impact feeding.
3. Discuss suggestions for the successful initiation and continuation of breastfeeding of the neurologically impaired infant.
4. Discuss suggestions for the successful initiation and continuation of breastfeeding of the infant with Down syndrome.
5. Identify classifications of cleft lip and/or cleft palate.
6. Discuss suggestions for the successful initiation and/or continuation of breastfeeding of the infant with cleft lip and/or cleft palate.

OUTLINE

I. Introduction

II. The Premature Infant

    A. Problems of prematurity
        1. Breathing problems
        2. Patent ductus arteriosus

3. Necrotizing enterocolitis
4. Interventricular hemorrhage
B. Advantages of breastmilk for the preterm infant
C. Nutritional management for the preterm infant
    1. Fluid management
    2. Enteral nutrition
    3. Human milk fortifiers
    4. Feeding methods
    5. Total parenteral nutrition
D. Introducing breastfeeding to premature infants
E. Management suggestions for breastfeeding premature infants
F. Breastfeeding multiple preterm infants
G. Equipment and personnel to assist with breastfeeding assessment of the preterm infant
H. Breastmilk expression
I. Kangaroo care
J. Resources

III. Functional Variations of the Palate, Tongue, and Jaw

A. Structural abnormalities
B. Oral–motor dysfunction versus disorganization

IV. The Neurologically Impaired Infant

A. The hypotonic infant
B. The hypertonic infant
C. Introducing breastfeeding to neurologically impaired infants
D. Resources

V. The Infant with Down Syndrome

A. Breastfeeding benefits
B. Introducing breastfeeding to infants with Down syndrome
C. Resources

VI. The Infant with Cleft Lip and/or Cleft Palate

A. Embryology of facial clefting
B. Epidemiology of facial clefting
    1. Racial influence
    2. Sex ratio influence
    3. Parental age influence
    4. Genetic influences
    5. Environmental influences
C. Clefting of the lip
D. Clefting of the palate
E. Advantages of breastmilk for infants with cleft lip and/or palate
F. Problems encountered when feeding infants with cleft palate

PRE-TEST

For questions 1 to 13, choose the best answer.

1. A mother who has given birth to a 30-week gestational-age infant produces breastmilk that

   A. is exactly the same as a mother who delivers a full-term infant.

   B. has higher concentrations of protein, lipids, sodium, potassium, and chloride than the breastmilk produced by the mother of a full-term infant.

   C. is tailor-made for her infant and meets the nutritional needs required by her infant to grow and thrive.

   D. has a higher concentration of protein, sodium, potassium, chloride, calcium, and phosphorus.

2. Human milk fortifiers are

   A. added to breastmilk because some premature infants may require extra amounts of certain nutrients for optimal growth.

   B. prescribed by physicians for all infants who are breastfeeding as a supplemental feed.

   C. considered the same as any type formula preparation.

   D. none of the above.

3. Alternative methods of feeding for the premature infant who is unable to breastfeed right away include

   A. intravenous feeds.

   B. gavage feeds.

   C. intraoral feeds

   D. Both A and B.

   E. A, B, and C.

4. Breastfeeding is more stressful on the infant than bottle feeding.

   A. Yes

   B. No

   C. Most of the time.

   D. They're both extremely stressful.

5. A mother delivers a 29-week gestational-age infant who is not able to be put to the breast for feedings right away. You discuss which of the following with her?

   A. She should not plan on breastfeeding because her infant is premature.

   B. She should not plan on breastfeeding because her breastmilk is inadequate for the premature infant.

    C. She should pump a minimum of five times a day with a total duration exceeding 100 minutes.

    D. Encourage pumping every two to three hours when awake, and once during the night if she awakens.

    E. Both A and B.

6. When a health-care worker handles breastmilk,

    A. no precautions are required because it is a sterile fluid.

    B. she or he shouldn't wear gloves because it might offend the mother.

    C. she or he should wear gloves because OSHA guidelines consider breastmilk a bodily fluid.

    D. she or he should inquire about the mother's past before deciding whether wearing gloves is necessary.

7. _____ describes kangaroo care.

    A. Skin-to-skin contact with the premature infant

    B. The mother of a preterm infant holds her infant underneath her clothing placed in a prone position between her breasts, allowing for self-regulatory breastfeeding

    C. Infants who show decreased periodic breathing and apnea

    D. All of the above.

8. The hypotonic infant

    A. exhibits extremely weak oral and facial muscle tone.

    B. is a sleepy infant.

    C. is an infant with a low hemoglobin.

    D. is not interested in breastfeeding.

9. The hypertonic infant

    A. cries constantly.

    B. exhibits exorbitant body arching, often lying in an extended position.

    C. overreacts to various forms of stimulation with muscle spasticity causing jerkinglike movements.

    D. All of the above.

    E. Only B and C.

10. The infant with Down syndrome

    A. has 46 chromosomes in each cell instead of 47.

    B. can be successfully and completely breastfed.

    C. is in need of extra stimulation through frequent touching, which breastfeeding skin-to-skin can help provide.

    D. All of the above.

    E. Only B and C.

11. The infant with Down syndrome may be hypotonic as with many neurologically impaired infants. This may cause

    A. a weak suck.

    B. tiring easily.

    C. difficulty remaining on the breast.

    D. Only A and C.

    E. All of the above.

12. Facial clefting
    A. involves the lip; the palate will always be involved also.
    B. can never occur as a cleft palate only.
    C. may involve only the lip, or extend into the hard and soft palate.
    D. is always related to an environmental influence such as maternal disease or alcohol abuse.

13. The _____ is often considered the best position to use when breastfeeding the infant with a bilateral cleft palate defect.
    A. straddle position
    B. cradle hold position
    C. Australian cleft hold
    D. All of the above.

14. Nutritional concerns about using unsupplemented preterm human milk for low and very low-birth-weight infants are that
    A. the fats are undigestible.
    B. the energy, protein, sodium, calcium, and phosphorus levels do not meet the needs of these infants.
    C. the sodium and protein levels exceed the needs of these infants.
    D. the iron content is too low.

15. The most common cause of rickets in preterm infants on total parenteral nutrition is
    A. vitamin D deficiency.
    B. hypocalcemia.
    C. hypophosphatemia.
    D. hyperphosphatemia.

For questions 16 to 20, choose the best answer from the following key:

A. True   B. False

16. When able to tolerate it, the premature infant should be offered a pacifier to suck when receiving gavage feeds.

17. Guidelines set by OSHA do not consider breastmilk a bodily fluid.

18. Infection problems are the only problems associated with kangaroo care of the premature infant.

19. The hypotonic infant should be offered increased lower jaw and chin support while nursing, especially if a nonrhythmic suck is noted.

20. Breastfeeding the hypertonic infant is much more effective if the infant is in a flexed position, chin downward and spine rounded, rather than an extended position.

Introduction

Optimally, a woman is able to put her infant to breast immediately following birth, but for some mothers this is not an option and the breastfeeding relationship is delayed. For some the delay lasts only minutes; for others, it may be hours, days, or weeks. Many mothers experience little to no difficulty when putting their infants to the breasts to feed, but some mothers confront difficulties, which may require them to seek the assistance of a lactation consultant (LC) for successful management and continuation of the breastfeeding relationship. Whether the obstacle is caused by the mother's or the infant's health, the age of the new mother, lifestyle, returning to work or school, lack of support, or any other special circumstance, she can be assisted to a successful and rewarding relationship by support, encouragement, and counseling techniques that include current breastfeeding information.

The Premature Infant

When a baby arrives before the expected due date, not only do parents feel unprepared for what is happening, but often they are in a state of disbelief because of what is happening to them. Many feelings and emotions accompany this event, and much support and encouragement is required. *Preterm infant* is an all-inclusive term used to describe a wide range of infants born at less than 37-weeks gestational age. When discussing the nutritional suitability of preterm human milk, broad categorizations cannot be made. The needs of the infant born at 34 to 36 weeks gestation are far different from the micropreemie of 24 to 26 weeks gestation. Therefore, even though the milk of the mother may be higher in many nutrients, the infant needs more of some nutrients in order to approximate interuterine growth.

PROBLEMS OF PREMATURITY

Several medical problems are associated with and are fairly predictable after the birth of a premature infant. The severity of the conditions varies depending on the gestational age of the baby. Infants born between 24 and 30 weeks usually weigh more than 1,500 g, which is considered very low birth weight (VLBW). Infants born between 31 and 36 weeks generally weigh more than 2,500 g, which is considered low birth weight (LBW). Logically, the smaller the infant, the more critical the problems associated with prematurity can be.

Breathing Problems

Respiratory Distress Syndrome (RDS) is a common disorder that occurs with prematurity. The lungs of a fetus are the last organ to develop. RDS occurs when the lungs are immature and lack surfactant. *Surfactant* is a substance produced by the lungs that prevents the alveoli from collapsing when a breath is taken. An infant with RDS usually requires some type of mechanical ventilation.

Apnea and bradycardia are other breathing problems associated with prematurity. *Apnea* is the absence of breathing (> 20 seconds) and *bradycardia* is a decreased or low heart rate (< 100 beats per minute). Excessive episodes of apnea and/or bradycardia can be treated with gentle stimulation of the baby. If these spells persist, a central nervous system (CNS) stimulant is initiated (theophylline or caffeine). Apnea and bradycardia usually resolve at about 35 to 36 weeks postconceptive age.

Patent Ductus Arteriosus

Patent ductus arteriosus (PDA) occurs when the ductus arteriosus fails to close. This occurs in approximately two-thirds of all infants less than 1,970 g. The ductus is important in fetal circulation as it shunts blood away from the lungs. The ductus usually closes in five to seven days (allowing blood to circulate through the lungs) in term infants and at 20 days in preterm infants. If the ductus fails to close, blood continues to shunt away from the lungs, which in turn decreases the oxygenated blood flowing to the stomach, intestines, kidneys, and other organs. Without adequate oxygenation, these organs can suffer serious asphyxia. Some PDAs can be closed by fluid restriction, others require medication (indomethacin), and severe PDAs may need to be surgically repaired.

Necrotizing Enterocolitis

Necrotizing enterocolitis (NEC) is primarily a disease of low-birth-weight infants, but it can also occur in term infants (5%). The cause of NEC is thought to be injury to the intestinal mucosa resulting from an eschemic insult. The result is reduced mesenteric blood flow, especially to the small intestine. Clinical signs of NEC can include abdominal distention, gastric residuals, bloody stools, apnea and/or bradycardia, temperature instability, and decreased activity. Treatment of NEC includes nothing by mouth (NPO) status for 10 to 14 days, antibiotic therapy, and surgery (if intestinal perforation occurs). Total parenteral nutrition (TPN) is the sole source of nutrition while NPO. Feeding should be restarted very slowly and advanced cautiously.

Interventricular Hemorrhage

Interventricular hemorrhage (IVH) occurs in 40% of infants weighing less than 1,500 g. Blood vessels surrounding the ventricles are very fragile and sometimes rupture, resulting in a bleed in the brain. IVHs are labeled according to severity—grade I, II, III, IV. Infants with a grade I or II IVH can lead relatively normal lives. Infants with a grade III or IV IVH can have neurological impairment, including motor or cognitive impairment, language delay, fine-motor disability, and cerebral palsy.

ADVANTAGES OF BREASTMILK FOR THE PRETERM INFANT

There are multiple advantages to feeding the premature infant breastmilk over the formula counterparts. Human milk provides more than just nutrients. It provides a number of bioactive components that influence neonatal development (Hamosh, 1992).

Many assume that breastfeeding is much more stressful on the infant than bottle feeding is; however, studies show the opposite is true. Due to this assumption, an infant may not be allowed to breastfeed until he or she can consume a complete bottle feeding without signs of distress. Several small studies report that bottle feeding was significantly more stressful for the infant than breastfeeding (Meier, 1988, Meier & Anderson, 1987). Infants in these studies demonstrated better coordination of sucking, swallowing, and breathing while breastfeeding. Transcutaneous (tc) PO_2 during bottle feeding declined. During breastfeeding, tc PO_2 values remained at baseline. Skin temperatures of the infants increased more during breastfeeding. The mean duration of breastfeeding was greater than the duration of bottle feedings.

A mother's breastmilk contains anti-infective components that may help protect her vulnerable premature infant from illnesses such as NEC, diarrhea, and other infections (Ashraf et al., 1991; Barlow et al., 1974; Countryman, 1984; Cunningham, 1977). Many of these components are proteins that stay intact because of the high degree of glycosylation in milk proteins, the antiprotease system in human milk, and the immature digestive system of the infant. The presence of proteins that are intact results in immune and nonimmune protection, growth factors, and digestive enzymes.

Ashraf and associates (1991) reported a lower rate of neonatal sepsis in a partially breastfed group, suggesting that even partial breastfeeding can help protect the vulnerable infant from neonatal sepsis. Lucas and Cole (1990) found that for exclusively formula-fed preterm infants, NEC was six to ten times more common than for those fed breastmilk alone and three times more common for those fed formula plus breastmilk.

Breastmilk has very long-chain polyunsaturated fatty acids that are not currently available in formulas or fat emulsions for TPN and that have been shown to be important in retinal function (Uauy et al., 1990) and in brain development (Innis, 1992). These fatty acids are also precursors for prostaglandins, leukotrienes, and cytokines. They are provided to the fetus in the last trimester of pregnancy and thus the premature infant will not have reaped the benefits of deposition of these fatty acids unless they are provided after birth.

The very long-chain fatty acids (VLCFA) are considered conditionally essential because the premature infant lacks the ability to synthesize these fatty acids from the precursors linoleic and linolenic acid. In addition, the premature infant greatly benefits from the specific milk digestive lipase present in human milk (often called bile salt–stimulated lipase). Because pancreatic lipase and bile salts needed for the digestion and solubilization of fat during digestion are deficient in premature infants, milk digestive lipase becomes very important. As much as 95% of the fat in human milk is reported to be absorbed (Armand et al., 1993) in contrast to the lower absorption rates (83% to 85%) for premature infants fed formulas with specially modified fat blends to optimize digestion (Hamosh et al., 1989; Hamosh et al., 1991).

The fat globules of preterm milk are smaller than those in term milk (Simonin et al., 1984); this results in a greater total concentration of globule membrane components such as phospholipids and cholesterol (Bitman et al., 1983; Bitman et al., 1984). Epidermal growth factor has been shown to be absorbed from the gastrointestinal tract in human preterm infants and could be involved in tissue growth and maturation (Gale et al., 1989). Finally, human milk contains medium-chain fatty acids that can be absorbed directly from the stomach (Hamosh et al., 1989) to provide a readily accessible energy source. See Module 3, *The Science of Breastfeeding*, Chapter 2, for a discussion of very long-chain polyunsaturated fatty acids and enzymes in human milk.

The role of nutrition in early life on long-term neurodevelopment has been studied in preterm infants and breastmilk feedings have been associated with higher developmental scores at 18 months (Morley et al., 1988). Subsequent follow-up of this cohort of preterm infants at 7½ to 8 years has found that children who had consumed mother's milk in the early weeks of life had a significantly higher intelligence quotient (IQ) as measured by the Weschler Intelligence Scale for Children (WISC). For the 300 children assessed, an 8.3-point advantage (over half a standard deviation) remained even after adjustment for differences in mother's education and social class ($p < 0.0001$) between groups (Lucas et al., 1992).

NUTRITIONAL MANAGEMENT FOR THE PRETERM INFANT

The goal of nutrition support in premature, low-birth-weight infants is to simulate interuterine growth. Achieving interuterine growth levels is very difficult because nutrients delivered to the infant via the placenta are many times greater than the nutrients that can be delivered via enteral feeding or TPN.

Fluid Management

Fluid requirements of premature infants vary depending on gestational age, current medical condition, and postconceptive age. Generally, the smaller the infant, the greater the fluid requirements. The very tiny micropreemie has increased insensible water losses because his or her skin is so thin and there is a larger surface area in proportion to body mass. A heavier infant has more developed skin and less insensible fluid losses.

Fluid balance should be monitored closely especially if the infant is under *phototherapy*—a radiant heat warmer—or has increased gastrointestinal (ostomy output) or renal losses, because all these factors can increase fluid needs. Patent ductus arteriosus, severe respiratory distress syndrome (RDS), bronchopulmonary dysplasia (BPD), and renal failure are indications for fluid restriction. General guidelines to follow for fluid management are shown in Table 3A–1.

Table 3A–1 Fluid Management Guidelines

Day of Life	Fluids
1	80–100 mL/kg/d
2	80–100 mL/kg/d
3	100–120 mL/kg/d
4	130–150 mL/kg/d

Enteral Nutrition

Energy expenditure in premature infants is shown in Table 3A–2 (Tsang et al., 1993). Preventing protein catabolism by providing 50 kcal/kg for basal metabolic needs is the first nutritional goal. Advancement of the kcal/kg intake should be made as quickly as tolerated, always observing for signs of feeding intolerance such as vomiting, abdominal distension, gastric residuals, and bloody stools.

Adequate growth is present when weight gain is 10 g to 40 g per day or 1% to 2% of body weight and head circumference and length increase by 0.5 cm to 1.0 cm per week. If adequate growth does not occur with 120 kcal/kg, modular components can be added to increase the caloric density of the feeding. If the infant is formula fed, a modular carbohydrate source or fat source can be added.

The liquid form of one modular carbohydrate source (Polycose) has 2 kcal/mL and the powder form has 8 kcal/tsp (1 tsp = 2 g). A fat source commonly used is Microlipid, which contains 4.5 kcal/mL. Neonatal nutritionists report that Microlipid mixes well with preterm formulas and stays in suspension well. Adding modular units of carbohydrate or fat to breastmilk is not recommended because doing so leads to an excessively high energy-to-protein ratio. Instead, protein modular components or human milk fortifiers are usually used.

The nutritional needs of preterm infants are greater than the nutritional needs of term infants. Special preterm infant formulas have been developed to meet the in-

Table 3A–2 Premature Infants' Energy Expenditure

Condition	Amount Needed
• Basal metabolic needs	50 kcal/kg
• Activity	15 kcal/kg
• Cold stress	10 kcal/kg
• Specific dynamic action	8 kcal/kg
• Fecal loss	12 kcal/kg
• Growth allowance	25 kcal/kg

creased nutritional needs of preterm infants whose mothers choose not to breast-feed. Unfortunately, these formulas cannot provide the immunologic factors or long-chain fatty acids needed by the preterm infant. Current preterm formulas are higher in protein (2.7 g/100 kcal), energy (24 kcal/oz), sodium (43 mg/100 kcal), calcium (180 mg/100 kcal), phosphorus (90 mg/100 kcal), copper (250 µg/100 kcal), zinc (1,500 µg/100 kcal), and selected micronutrients than term formulas. As with term formula, multivitamin supplementation is not recommended if the infant is consuming adequate amounts of formula.

Most Western neonatal units recommend iron supplementation for premature infants beginning at two weeks of age until one year of age. The requirement is 4 mg to 6 mg/kg per day of elemental iron. Term infants require 1 mg/kg per day if provided by formula but less if breastfed because of the higher bioavailability of iron in human milk.

Calcium and vitamin D supplements are not recommended when adequate amounts are provided in proprietary preterm formulas, but are of concern for the infant receiving breastmilk. Rickets is a concern in preterm infants because of decreased bone mineralization. The majority of calcium transported to the infant via the placenta occurs during the third trimester. The most common cause of rickets in premature infants is hypophosphatemia, not hypocalcemia or vitamin D deficiency. Hypophosphatemia usually occurs in infants on TPN.

Studies have shown that the milk produced by the mother of a preterm infant has higher concentrations of protein, nonprotein nitrogen, lipids, sodium, chloride, potassium, magnesium, iron, copper, zinc, and IgA than the breastmilk produced by the mother of a full-term infant (ADA, 1986; Atinmo & Omololu, 1982; Atkinson et al., 1978; Gross et al., 1980, 1981; Lemons et al., 1982; Schanler & Oh, 1980). Calcium, phosphorus, and energy levels are similar in the milk of women delivering preterm and term infants.

Premature infants who weigh less than 2,000 g require extra amounts of certain nutrients (especially calcium, phosphorus, sodium, protein, and energy) for optimal growth; the physician may recommend adding a human milk fortifier to the breastmilk. Human milk fortifiers have been made available to increase the calcium, phosphorus, energy, and other nutrients' content in human milk so that preterm infants whose mothers desire to express breastmilk or breastfeed can reap the immense immunologic and developmental benefits of human milk. When added to a mother's preterm milk, human milk fortifier reduces the time needed to grow from 1,500 g to 1,800 g by 25% and achieves significantly better alkaline phosphatase levels. If unsupplemented, preterm breastmilk is fed to a low or very low-birth-weight infant, osteopenia and rickets are likely to occur.

A recent study by Bishop and associates (1996) is calling into question whether bone disease resulting from decreased bone mineralization, common among preterm infants, is fully understood. In this study, 54 children born preterm, who received preterm infant formula or banked pasteurized donor human milk as a supplement to their mother's milk during their early weeks, were tested at five years of age for bone mineral content. The study reported that the greater the intake of human milk, the higher the later bone mineral content. Two mechanisms to explain their results were postulated by Bishop and associates (1996):

1. One or more of the growth hormones present in donor milk survives pasteurization and is active in producing the higher bone mineralization.

2. Early mineral depletion somehow programs preterm infants to conserve bone mineral and to limit growth until a time when mineral intakes are normal and increased growth can occur.

Obviously, this study raises more questions than it answers, and the subject needs further exploration.

In most cases, unfortified, preterm human milk fails to meet the estimated nutrient needs for protein, energy, sodium, calcium, phosphorus, magnesium, iron, copper, zinc, and vitamins B_{12}, B_6, C, D, E, K, and folic acid. The reader is referred to *Nutritional Needs of the Preterm Infant—Scientific Basis and Practical Guidelines* edited by Tsang, Lucas, Uauy, and Zlotkin (1993) and *Neonatal Nutrition and Metabolism* edited by W. W. Hay (1991) for in-depth discusssions of the preterm infant's nutritional needs.

One area that the LC should be familiar with is protein. Lucas and Hudson (1984) suggest that the high protein content of preterm milk is due to the small volume produced when mothers of preterm infants express their milk. To support this, the author cites data which shows that when mothers are able to express larger quantities of milk, the protein content of their preterm milk is similar to term milk. This concept is supported by evidence that by the 14th day the nitrogen content of the breastmilk of women delivering prematurely is similar to mothers who deliver at term (Micheli & Schutz, 1993; Raiha, 1991). By day 14, milk volume has increased to mature levels.

The European Society of Paediatric Gastroenterology and Nutrition (ESPGAN) recommends a protein intake of 2.9 g/kg to 4.0 g/kg per day of protein. To achieve such high intakes, 185 mL/kg to 200 mL/kg per day of a mother's fresh milk must be consumed by the moderately low-birth-weight infant. This is an achievable goal; however, care must be taken to use fresh milk (heat and freezer treatment decrease the nutritionally available protein) and to support the mother so that she can continue to express this quantity of milk. To approach this amount of bioavailable protein through human bank milk, an amount of 250 mL/kg per day must be provided—a high intake not commonly used in Western neonatal units.

Another area that cannot be overlooked is energy intake. The energy cost of growth depends on protein metabolism. High protein intake without adequate energy is not optimal. The energy level should be optimal in proportion to protein intake in order to increase fat deposition. According to Putet (1993), for growing very low-birth-weight infants, 120 kcal/kg per day is recommended to achieve the following:

- A weight gain of 18 g/kg to 20 g/kg per day
- A protein retention of 2 g/kg per day
- A fat retention of 20% to 25% of weight gain

These are optimal values—energy at levels greater than 80 kcal/kg per day can result in growth in the transitional period, with further increases achieving adequate growth implemented as quickly as tolerated by the infant. Again, to achieve these energy levels with human milk, and within the volume preterm infants (very low and low-birth-weight) are capable of consuming, requires fortification.

Human milk from milk banks is not recommended for very low-birth-weight infants, according to reports of failure to thrive and delayed psychomotor development (Lucas et al., 1990; Micheli & Schutz, 1993). However, supplementation from milk banks can increase the suitability of human milk for these preterm infants despite temperature treatments necessary to process and maintain banked human milk, and provides many of the components unique to human milk. Although it fell out of favor in many neonatal units during the 1980s, a resurgence of interest in how banked human milk can be fortified and used is occurring as more and more is being realized about the nonnutritional properties of human milk and their benefit to preterm infants.

Human Milk Fortifiers

Use of a mother's fresh milk is especially important if the infant is very immature and very low birth weight (< 1,000 g) but is able to take enteral feeds. This is a critical period for survival and the protective factors of breastmilk should not be underestimated. Soon thereafter the metabolic needs for growth and development have to be matched and fortification of a mother's milk is necessary. Table 3A–3 shows the nutritional composition of commercial human milk fortifiers; it shows the nutrient content for the amount of fortifier that would be added to 25 mL of preterm milk in the last column. By adding the nutrient amounts listed for one of the four fortifiers to values for the preterm milk, the nutrient content of 25 mL of fortified preterm milk can be obtained.

It is standard practice in Western neonatal intensive care units (NICU) to keep a premature infant on preterm formula or supplemented breastmilk until a weight of 2,000 g has been achieved. At this point, the infant can be changed to unsupplemented breastmilk or term formula. The following are four ways to supplement breastmilk for the preterm infant (Robertson & Bhatia, 1993):

1. 1:1 breastmilk with a premature infant formula (24 kcal/oz.) in the liquid form, which will provide 22 kcal/oz.
2. 1:1 breastmilk with a liquid human milk fortifier, which is almost identical to premature formula, which will provide 22 kcal/oz.
3. One packet of powdered human milk fortifier mixed with 25 mL of breastmilk, which will provide 24 kcal/oz.
4. For those who do not want to mix breastmilk with any other supplement or fortifier due to concerns over the stability of immunologic factors in human milk, alternating feedings of breastmilk and premature infant formula may be an option.

Although the fortification of human breastmilk may meet the requirements for the supplementation of calcium, phosphorus, and other minerals, the methods by which it can be delivered to the preterm infant may result in incomplete delivery of nutrients. A study conducted by Bhatia and Rassin (1988) showed that there were significant losses of energy, calcium, and phosphorus (especially large for calcium and phosphorus), with greater losses developing when powder fortification was used.

Evidence also shows that the length of time it takes for usual syringe-pump feedings possibly contributes to the loss of nutrients by precipitation or adherence to the wall of the delivery system if an efficient agitation method is not used. Use of liquid fortifiers did not show as much of a pronounced loss. Little to no change was noted in concentrations of the various nutrients that were given with simu-

Table 3A–3 Nutritional Composition of Commercial Human Milk Fortifiers

Nutrient	Enfamil HMF (g)	Similac Natural Care (mL)	Eoprotein (g)	FM 85 (g)	Preterm Human Milk (mL)
Volume or weight	0.96	4.34	0.96	0.96	25
kcalories (kcal)	3.5	3.5	3.5	3.5	16.75
Protein g	0.18	0.095	0.19	0.18	0.402
Fat g	0.025	0.19	0.01		0.89
Carbohydrate	0.68	0.37	0.66	0.71	1.84
Vitamins					
Vitamin A, IU	237.5	23.8	31.15		12.06
Vitamin D, IU	52.5	5.25			2.01
Vitamin K, μg	1.1	0.42	0.06		0.50
Vitamin E, IU	1.15	0.14	0.06		0.10
Thiamine, μg	37.75	8.75			2.18
Riboflavin, μg	52.5	21.7			6.87
Vitamin B_6, μg	28.5	8.75			1.51
Vitamin B_{12}, μg	0.05	0.08			0.01
Niacin, μg	750	175			0.05
Folic acid, μg	6.25	1.3			0.84
Pantothenic acid, μg	182.5	6.5			0.05
Biotin, μg	0.68	1.3			0.13
Vitamin C, mg	2.9	1.3	4.73		1.12
Minerals					
Calcium, mg	22.5	7.35	11.73	9.77	6.37
Phosphorus, mg	11.25	3.68	8.05	6.65	3.69
Zinc, μg	177.5	52.5	4.73		93.8
Manganese, μg	1.18	0.42	0.95		0.09
Copper, μg	15.5	8.75	0.95		9.55
Sodium, mg	1.75	1.51	6.37	5.25	7.37
Potassium, mg	3.9	4.52	0.74	2.21	12.4
Chloride, mg	4.43	2.84	4.73	3.75	14.91
Magnesium, mg	0.25	0.42	0.67	0.39	0.84
Iron, mg		0.013	0.005		0.023
Selenium, μg		0.06			NA
Iodine, μg		0.21	0.14		4.52
Taurine, mg		0.23	0.56		
Inositol, mg		0.19			
Choline, mg	0.35				

Source: Information compiled from Gross (1983); Moran et al. (1983); Atkinson et al. (1987); Tsang (1985); Ford (1983); Atkinson et al. (1980); Mendelson et al. (1982); Ehrenkranz (1984); Atkinson et al. (1989); Tsang et al. (1993).

lated bolus feedings. Bhatia and Rassin suggest that human milk fortifiers be carefully monitored while being fed to prevent large amounts of residue from being left in the syringes. They also suggest that all infants receiving such feedings be closely monitored to ensure an adequate nutritional status (Bhatia & Rassin, 1988). This study prompted manufacturers to reformulate the powder fortifiers so this problem has now been minimized.

Feeding Methods

Some premature infants are able to be put to the breast for feedings soon after birth, while others may require more time depending on gestational age, maturity, and physical condition. For infants who will not be able to tolerate full enteral feedings quickly after birth, TPN is provided via a central catheter. Gestational age is often used as a general guideline for what to expect regarding feeding method, and the weight of the infant is useful in determining how much to feed and how quickly once enteral feedings are begun. For healthy infants born at 34 to 36 weeks gestation, breastmilk may be fed as usual after birth. For infants born between 32 and 34 weeks gestation, small amounts of milk feedings may be tolerated with additional nutrients added to the expressed breastmilk if the infant is under 2,000 g. Gavage (tube feeding through mouth or nose into stomach) feeding is often used for this infant age group initially. If the infant is less than 30 weeks gestation, he or she may be unable to tolerate enteral feedings until he or she is a few weeks older.

For those who are unable to breastfeed at first, various means, such as intravenous (IV), TPN, or gavage feeds may be required to nourish the infant until breastfeeding is possible. Depending on hospital policies, protocols, or the infant's physician, bottle feeding may be required before the infant is allowed to be put to the breast although the justification for this practice is weak.

Once an appropriate feeding method has been chosen, the feeding route should be established. Most feeding decisions are based on the weight of the infant, not the gestational age. Every NICU has its own feeding protocol and no one practice is necessarily better than the other if it works to promote growth and maintain the nutritional needs of the infant. However, some protocols are more protective of the breastfeeding relationship than others. It should be noted that feeding schedules are guidelines and as with any patient, the nutrition plan and goals should be tailored to the individual infant.

Most infants less than 1,250 g tolerate continuous feeding better than intermittent or bolus feeds. Orogastric or nasogastric tube positions can be used, but orogastric is preferred due to the commonly held belief that infants are obligate nose breathers. If an infant does not tolerate continuous gastric feeds because of slow gastric emptying or gastric distention due to ventilatory support, continuous transpyloric feedings should be inititated. Once an infant weighs more than 1,250 g, bolus feeds can be started. Bolus feedings must be gastric, not transpyloric, because of the volume being infused. Table 3A–4 shows suggested feeding guidelines for infants of different birthweights (MCG, 1994).

Table 3A–4   Infant Feeding Guidelines

Body Weight	Volume
< 750 g	0.5 mL/hr, increase by 0.5 mL/24 hr
750–1,000 g	1.0 mL/hr, increase by 1.0 mL/24 hr
1,001–2,500 g	3.0 mL/hr, increase by 1.0 mL/24 hr
1,251–1,500 g	5.0–8.0 mL every 3 hr, increase by 1.0–2.0 mL/24 hr
1,501–1,800 g	5.0–10.0 mL every 3 hr, increase by 3.0 mL/24 hr
1,801–2,000 g	8.0–10.0 mL every 3 hr, increase by 5.0–8.0 mL/24 hr
> 2,000 g	10.0–30.0 mL every 3 hr, increase by 5.0–10.0 mL/24 hr

Total Parenteral Nutrition

Premature infants probably receive more TPN than any other pediatric population. Preterm infants should be started on TPN if they have been NPO for more than 2 to 3 days or their nutritional needs cannot be adequately met through the enteral route (see Table 3A–5). Infants in the NICU are almost always given dextrose water (D_5 if < 1,000 g or D_{10} if > 1,000 g) on admission. A decision is then made whether to feed the infant enterally or begin TPN.

Most hospitals have a standard TPN form which usually has standard electrolyte additives. The percent of dextrose, amino acids, and fat can be specified and specific electrolytes can be increased or decreased according to daily laboratory values (see Table 3A–6). Calorie needs for an infant on TPN are lower, approximately 80 kcal/kg to 90 kcal/kg, than the calorie needs for an infant on enteral feedings because digestion, absorption, and so on, are not required (Tsang et al., 1993). Glucose, up to 12.5%, can be given via a peripheral line and dextrose, up to 30%, can be given through a central line.

Several pediatric amino acid solutions, which should be used as the protein source, are available. Infants weighing less than 1,000 g can start at 1.0 g/kg per day of protein and infants more than 1,000 g can tolerate 1.5 g/kg per day. Both should be increased by 0.5 g/kg per day to a maximum of 3.0 g/kg per day (Robertson & Bhatia, 1993). Protein tolerance can be measured by monitoring blood urea nitrogen (BUN).

Several lipid sources are also available for use in TPN solutions. All of them are appropriate for use in pediatric populations. A 20% solution should be used as opposed to a 10% solution because larger amounts of lipids can be given with a smaller increase in triglycerides, phospholipids, and cholesterol (Robertson & Bhatia, 1993; Tsang et al., 1993). Infants weighing less than 1,500 g should be started at 0.5 g/kg per day and infants weighing more than 1,500 g can start at 1.0 g/kg per day. Both should be increased by 0.5 g/kg per day to a maximum of 3.0 g/kg per day. Lipids are better tolerated when given over an 18- to 24-hour period with the minimum being 15 hours. Infants can only tolerate an infusion rate of 0.15 g/kg to 0.25 g/kg per hour of lipids. Triglyceride levels are used to monitor lipid tolerance. If infant serum levels are more than 200 mg/dL, the lipid infusion rate should be checked and decreased if above 0.15 g/kg to 0.25 g/kg per day.

In addition to standard electrolytes, a standard multivitamin and trace mineral package is added to the TPN. Protein, lipids, electrolytes, vitamins, minerals, and trace

Table 3A–5   Typical TPN Order for a Low-Birth-Weight Infant

Weight 1.32 kg
130 cc/kg/d
12.5% dextrose
2.5 g/kg/d protein
2.0 g/kg/d lipid
standard electrolyte
standard multivitamin and mineral

Calculations for the above TPN order are as follows:

CHO = 12.5% dextrose = .125 g × 130 cc/kg × 1.32 kg × 3.4 kcal/g = 72.9 kcal from carbohydrate

PRO = 2.5 g/kg × 1.32 kg × 4.0 kcal/g = 13.2 kcal from protein

FAT = 2.0 g/kg × 1.32 kg × 5 cc/g = 13.2 cc × 2 kcal/cc = 26.4 kcal from fat

72.9 + 13.2 + 26.4 = 112.5 kcal ÷ 1.32 (hypothetical weight) = 85.2 kcal/kg

Table 3A–6 Recommended daily parenteral requirements for neonate, infant, and pediatric patients[a]

Nutrient	Preterm neonate	Neonate	Infant	Children	Adolescents
Energy	120–140 non-protein kcal/kg	90–120 non-protein kcal/kg	90–120 non-protein kcal/kg —< 6 mo 80–100 non-protein kcal/kg —6–12 mo	75–90 non-protein kcal/kg —1–7 yr 60–75 non-protein kcal/kg —7–12 yr	30–60 non-protein kcal/kg
Protein	2.5–3.0 g/kg	2.5–3.0 g/kg	2.0–2.5 g/kg	1.5–2.0 g/kg	0.8–2.0 g/kg
Fat	< 32 weeks provide up to 3 g/kg	SGA infants provide up to 3 g/kg AGA up to 4 g/kg	Up to 4 g/kg	Up to 4 g/kg	Individualized—do not exceed 2.5 g/kg
Carbohydrate	70–85% of non-protein calories	70–85% of non-protein calories	70–85% of non-protein calories	70–85% of non-protein calories	Individualized—do not exceed 7 g/kg/day
L-cysteine HCL	40 mg/g protein	40 mg/g protein	40 mg/g protein	—	—
Sodium	Individualized	2–5 mEq/kg	2–6 mEq/kg	2–6 mEq/kg	Individualized
Chloride	Individualized	1–5 mEq/kg	2–5 mEq/kg	2–5 mEq/kg	Individualized
Potassium	Individualized	1–4 mEq/kg	2–3 mEq/kg	2–3 mEq/kg	Individualized
Calcium	Individualized	3–4 mEq/kg	1–2.5 mEq/kg	1–2.5 mEq/kg	10–20 mEq
Phosphorus	Individualized	1–2 mmol/kg	0.5–1 mmol/kg	0.5–1 mmol/kg	10–40 mmol
Magnesium	Individualized	0.3–0.5 mEq/kg	0.3–0.5 mEq/kg	0.3–0.5 mEq/kg	10–30 mEq
Zinc	400 µg/kg	300 µg/kg	100µg/kg	100 µg/kg—< 5 yr 2–5 mg—> 5 yr	2–5 mg
Copper	20 µg/kg	20 µg/kg	20 µg/kg	20 µg/kg—< 5 yr 200–500 µg—> 5 yr	200–500 µg
Manganese	1 µg/kg	1 µg/kg	1 µg/kg	2–10 mg—< 5 yr	50–150 µg
Chromium	0.2 µg/kg	0.2 µg/kg	0.2 µg/kg	0.14–0.2 µg/kg—< 5 yr 5–15 µg—> 5 yr	5–15 µg
Selenium	2–3 µg/kg	2–3 µg/kg	2–3 µg/kg	2–3 µg/kg—5 yr[b] 30–40 µg—> 5 yr	30–40 µg
Iodine	1 µg/kg[c]	1 µg/kg[c]	1 µg/kg[c]	1 µg/kg—< 5 yr	—
Pediatric multiple vitamin formulation[d]	Weight < 2.5 kg provide 2 mL/kg	Weight < 2.5 kg provide 2 mL/kg Weight > 2.5 kg provide 5 mL	Weight > 2.5 kg provide 5 mL	Individualized	Individualized

[a]Single pediatric multitrace products do not meet the recommended intakes of trace elements. Individualized trace element products are required to meet the recommended intakes of trace elements.

[b]Do not exceed 40 µg.

[c]Percutaneous absorption from protein-bound iodine may be adequate.

[d]Note: 5 mL contains A, 2300 IU; D, 400 IU; E, 7 IU; K, 200 µg; C, 80 mg; B_1, 1.2 mg; B_2, 1.4 mg; B_3, 17 µg; B_5, 1 g; B_6, 1 mg; B_{12}, 1 µg; Biotin, 20 µg; Folic acid, 140 µg.

Source: Adapted from National Advisory Group on Standards and Practice Guidelines for Parenteral Nutrition (1998). Safe practices for parenteral nutrition formulations. *JPEN*, 22:49-66.

Table 3A–7   Suggested Monitoring Schedule During TPN

Variable Monitored	Suggested Frequency	
	Initial Period*	Later Period†
Serum electrolytes	3–4 times/wk	2–3 times/wk
Serum urea nitrogen	3 times/wk	2 times/wk
Serum calcium, magnesium, phosphorus	3 times/wk	2 times/wk
Serum glucose	††	††
Serum acid-base status	3–4 times/wk	2–3 times/wk
Serum ammonia	2 times/wk	Weekly
Serum protein (electrophoresis or albumin/ globulin, prealbumin/transferrin)	Weekly	Weekly
Liver function studies	Weekly	Weekly
Hemoglobin	2 times/wk	2 times/wk
Urine glucose	Daily	Daily
Clinical observations (activity, temperature, etc.)	Daily	Daily
Blood cell count and differential count	As indicated	As indicated
Cultures	As indicated	As indicated
Serum triglyceride	As indicated	As indicated

*Initial period is the period before full glucose, protein, and lipid intake is achieved, or any period of metabolic instability.

†Later period is the period during which patient is in a metabolic steady state.

††Blood glucose should be monitored closely during a period of glucosuria and for 2 to 3 days after cessation of parenteral nutrition to determine the degree of hypoglycemia or hyperglycemia. Frequent Dextrostix determination constitutes adequate screening. After a month or more on total parenteral nutrition, measurements can be decreased to once a week or longer.

Source: Barness, LA (Ed.) (1993). *Pediatric Nutrition Handbook,* p. 157. Elk Grove Village, IL: AAP. Reprinted with permission of American Academy of Pediatrics.

elements are all given on a per kilogram basis (i.e., 2.0 g/kg per day protein, 3 mEq Na kg per day). All ingredients in TPN can be added on the first day of parenteral nutrition. Protein should not exceed 3.5 g/kg per day and lipids should not exceed 5 g/kg per day. An ideal caloric distribution for TPN is protein 7% to 12%, carbohydrate 35% to 55%, and fat 35% to 55% (Robertson & Bhatia, 1993; Tsang et al., 1993).

One of the biggest concerns about TPN is the amount of calcium and phosphorus that can be given. It is difficult to add the recommended amounts without causing a precipitation of the TPN mixture. This can lead to osteopenia and rickets, especially if the infant is on TPN for a long period of time. Another complication of long-term TPN is cholestatic jaundice. It is not clear which TPN component contributes to this condition, but amino acids are believed to play an important role. Possible complications of TPN can be monitored (see Table 3A–7) with serial laboratory measurements (ALT, AST, GGT, bile acids, albumin, cholesterol, triglycerides, bilirubin) (Greene et al., 1988).

INTRODUCING BREASTFEEDING TO PREMATURE INFANTS

There continues to be controversy surrounding when the preterm infant can be put to the breast for feeds. Much of the confusion is from the prevalence of research on bottle-fed infants, and from the lack of published information regarding the expected breastfeeding behavior of preterm infants of different gestational ages.

Research on bottle feeding has reported that at 28 weeks mouthing movements are noticeable in the preterm infant and by 32 weeks a burst–pause pattern of sucking emerges, with a regular rhythm of sucking, swallowing, and breathing developed by 34 weeks. By 37 weeks, the rhythm and rate of sucking is similar to that of a full-term infant (Hack et al., 1985). Also in bottle-feeding populations, immature, transitional, and mature suck–swallow patterns have been identified (McGowan et al., 1991; Medcoff-Cooper, 1991; Medcoff-Cooper et al., 1993; Palmer, 1993).

Several clinical tools have been developed for assessing healthy, term breastfed infants and are described in Module 2, *The Process of Breastfeeding*, Chapter 1. Tools to assess breastfeeding behavior of preterm infants have not been available until the recent work of Nyqvist and associates (1996), who developed a preterm infant-breastfeeding behavior scale (PIBBS) in collaboration with mothers, and they tested it for interobserver agreement between observers and between observers and mothers. This tool scores the following:

- Behavior related to rooting
- How much of the breast was inside baby's mouth
- Latching and fixing to the breast
- Sucking
- The longest sucking burst
- Swallowing
- What the infant looked like during feedings
- The milk-ejection reflex

The PIBBS tool was compared across three groups according to gestational age: (1) full-term infants, (2) infants who had reached 34- to 36-weeks gestational age, and (3) infants born at less than 33 weeks. Significant differences among the three groups were found in the percentage of infants who scored the highest on all items analyzed. The PIBBS has promise for clinical use, not only as a useful assessment tool for determining the appropriateness of the breastfeeding behavior observed for an individual infant, but also as an educational tool for mothers to learn how to watch for maturational signs in their breastfeeding infant. Results from using this tool should give mothers, LCs, and health-care workers a realistic picture of what behavior to expect for an infant of a particular gestational age.

The mother of the premature infant should initiate the discussion of her desire to breastfeed with the infant's physician and nursery staff. When able to tolerate it, the infant should be offered a pacifier to suck when receiving gavage feeds. This encourages the development and strengthening of the muscles used for sucking, and also helps the infant associate the feeling of fullness with the action of sucking (Walker & Driscoll, 1989). Several studies report that sucking on a pacifier improved weight gain, reduced hospital stay, and enhanced the maturation of the sucking reflex (Bernbaum et al., 1983; Field et al., 1982; Measal & Anderson, 1979). Ernst and associates (1989), however, were not able to show an improved growth outcome related to nonnutritive sucking. In some NICUs, infants are allowed to suck at the breast after pumping by the mother rather than using a pacifier for nonnutritive sucking. Narayanan and associates (1991) reported on the duration of breastfeeding in two groups of preterm infants:

1. One group of 16 low-birth-weight infants (mean weight 1,559 g–228 g SD) was allowed brief periods of nonnutritive sucking (sucking after the mother pumps her milk) prior to full tube feeds.

2. A control group of 16 low-birth-weight infants (mean weight 1,605 g–198 g SD), who were not allowed the nonnutritive sucking, and were allowed to breastfeed only after it was determined the infants could tolerate adequate volumes from trial feeds.

The intervention group had a significantly higher mean duration of exclusive breastfeeding (3.7 months vs. 1.9 months; $p < 0.001$) and a significantly higher mean duration of total lactation (5.1 months vs. 3.3 months; $p < 0.05$). The positive outcomes of early sucking on the breast demonstrated in this study are encouraging and challenge the widely held concept that low-birth-weight infants cannot go to breast at all until they are able to take full feeds.

Gavage feeding while skin-to-skin next to mother's breasts is an optimal situation when able to be tolerated by the infant. Among the many known benefits of this type of kangaroo care (see pages 240–41 for a description) is that it provides a warm and secure place for the infant as she or he is being introduced to the breast (Anderson, 1990). As soon as the infant is able, the process of introducing the breast should begin. For some infants, the transition to all nipple feeds occurs quickly but the mother may not be available for all feedings. The staff can employ other methods, including finger feeding, cup feeding, or feeding with a peridontal syringe, for the feedings missed by the mother. This is especially important if the infant shows signs of nipple confusion (difficulty switching back to the breast for feeds after bottle feedings). For other infants, fatigue sets in early and only a small portion of the desired intake is provided to the infant, with the remaining amount gavage-fed. For some infants, the time from the introduction of the breast to full breastfeeding may be as long as a month.

Some of the obstacles premature infants must overcome as they transition from gavage feedings to breastfeedings include respiratory compromise, lack of coordination of swallowing muscles, weakness, and, often, a mother's low milk supply (Stine, 1990). Also, traveling to the hospital can be difficult for many mothers because of the expense, distance, and other family responsibilities. Other problems experienced by the premature infant learning to breastfeed include an inability to maintain latch, dysfunctional suck, or a mother with flat or large nipples. The use of a silicone nipple shield has been reported to be helpful in facilitating the process of successful breastfeeding for these latter situations (Clum & Primomo, 1996).

The introduction of breastfeeding to the premature infant is a slow process that will require much patience and support. The early breastfeeding sessions may be difficult, and encouragement needs to be given for even the smallest of accomplishments. In the beginning, the majority of the infant's nourishment may continue to be received via the gavage tube, bottle, or a lactation supplementation aid depending on his or her condition and strength, and until enough milk to meet his or her nourishment and growth requirements can be adequately removed by sucking the breasts.

The LC should encourage the mother to pump following a breastfeeding session with her infant if it has lasted less than 10 minutes, if the baby continues to have a very weak suck, or if the breasts are still full. Not only will this help stimulate the mother's breasts to maintain a milk supply, but it will also obtain the hind milk that is higher in fat and is essential for the infant's weight gain. This will enable the infant to be supplemented with the mother's hind milk until he or she is strong enough to obtain it through breastfeeding.

MANAGEMENT SUGGESTIONS FOR BREASTFEEDING PREMATURE INFANTS

An infant born prematurely may not feed effectively when she or he is able to begin breastfeeding and will need to be worked with in a slow and patient manner. The mother will require continued support, encouragement, and instruction as she endeavors to enter a new phase of her breastfeeding relationship and motherhood. Breastfeeding suggestions for this special group of mothers include the following:

1. The mother should wash her hands with soapy water. She should prepare her breast by gently cleansing the nipple and areola areas with sterile gauzes moistened with sterile water (Meier & Mangurten, 1993). This practice is not necessary for the healthy full-term infant and in many NICUs may not be considered necessary.

2. The mother should make herself as comfortable as possible.

3. Prior to putting the infant to breast, suggest techniques that will help encourage the milk to eject, and elongate the nipple for easier latching-on. Techniques such as warm compresses, breast massage, nipple rolling, or pumping have worked well for many mothers.

4. The infant should be breastfed at frequent intervals. The feeding sessions may not last long if the infant tires easily, and frequent feedings will allow him or her to get more milk.

5. Feedings will vary in length as the premature infant grows and becomes stronger. The mother should refrain from setting time limitations for breastfeeding sessions.

6. When positioning the premature infant at the breast, it is important to bring him or her to breast level and maintain good support throughout the feeding. Position the infant in flexion; the cross-cradle or modified clutch hold is recommended. (See Appendix: Specialty Positions at the end of this section.) The mother needs to support her breast by encircling it with the "same side" hand and support the infant's head with her other hand. This type of positioning allows her good control and visibility while breastfeeding. Some infants who have low muscle tone will be able to breastfeed better if their buttocks and head are at the same level while supported. This can be done easily by putting pillows on the mother's lap to bring the infant to breast level (Danner & Cerutti, 1990a).

7. The mother should express a small amount of breastmilk onto the nipple or infant's lips to entice the infant and encourage licking and latching-on. Some mothers have found using a dropper to dribble earlier expressed milk on the nipple helpful while the infant is at the breast if he or she is having a difficult time becoming interested (Danner & Cerutti, 1990a). Eliciting the milk-ejection reflex prior to offering the breast is another option. Pump the breasts one to two minutes prior to breastfeeding or use a single pump on one breast while nursing on the other (Bocar, 1993).

8. The "dancer hand position," where the hand forms a U shape, is an optional hand position to use while the infant is weak. The techniques used with this position help support the infant's weak mandibular control

because he or she may tire easily, and will also assist in keeping the breast from falling out of the baby's mouth while nursing.

9. Assess the infant to see that she or he is latched on and sucking properly by gently pulling downward on his or her lower lip while nursing. The infant's tongue should be troughed and extended over the lower gum-ridge, and the upper and lower lips flanged. If the tongue is noted to be elsewhere, such as to the side or on top of the nipple, suction should be broken and the infant removed for repositioning. If a lip is curled under, this can be corrected easily by gently uncurling the lip while nursing.

10. Because the premature infant is usually weak and has low muscle tone, he or she may often get choked. If this is noted, try positioning the infant so that the back of his or her throat is at a higher level than the mother's nipple. This will cause the flow of the mother's milk to work against gravity, slowing the force at which it is flowing into the infant's mouth.

11. For some mothers, the use of a nipple shield can be very helpful in transitioning the infant to the breast. Guidelines for the use of nipple shields are provided in Module 2, *The Process of Breastfeeding*, Chapter 2.

12. Encourage the family to join a local support group. Introduce them to other families who have been through this experience and have had a successful breastfeeding relationship.

A growing trend in NICUs supportive of breastfeeding is the concept of a transition stay for the mother. The infant who is ready to be discharged is moved to a pediatric floor with a bed for the mother, and the mother and infant room together as they transition from gavage and/or nipple feeds to full breastfeeds. This allows the mother to watch her infant for signs of feeding cues and to receive specialized support from LCs and nurses or nutrition specialists. The need for alternative feeding devices such as supplemental nursing systems can be assessed and a care plan for discharge to home can be developed. Once the infant shows a satisfactory weight gain on breastmilk, the mother and infant can go home. Table 3A–8 summarizes how health-care providers can increase breastfeeding in the preterm population (Spangler, 1994).

BREASTFEEDING MULTIPLE PRETERM INFANTS

Only a few reports of the successful breastfeeding management of multiples can be found in the literature (Mead et al., 1992; Saint et al., 1986). Yet, with more liberal use of fertility drugs, multiple births are increasing. Saint and associates (1986) reported on the management of eight mothers who breastfed twins and one mother who breastfed triplets. Test-weighing was used to determine milk yield. Feeding frequency and milk yield were recorded for the mothers at periodic intervals during the 12 months after delivery.

In the case report by Mead and associates (1992), a mother's successful experience breastfeeding quadruplets (delivered at 34 weeks gestation and weighing between 1,820 g and 2,240 g) was shared. Two of the four were able to go to breast within a couple of days of birth while the other two infants required ventilator

Table 3A–8 How to Increase Breastfeeding Rates Among Preterm Infants

A. Mobilize a support team (depending on your facility, resources will vary—NICU nurse, postpartum nurse, neonatologist, social worker, nutritionist, physical therapist, occupational therapist, family, friends, clergy, or (even better) *another mother who has breastfed a preterm infant*

B. The support team will provide the following:
   1. Information on anatomy of the breast, physiology of lactation, management of lactation
   2. Information on expression, collection, and storage of breastmilk—parent becomes an active participant in the care of the infant when milk of mother is provided

C. Establish and maintain a milk supply—*Requirements:* Food, fluid, rest, routine stimulation, and support
   1. Milk expression should begin within 12 to 24 hours after delivery if possible
   2. Provide an environment conducive to breastfeeding
   3. Establish a routine
   4. Establish realistic expectations
   5. Pump a minimum of 100 minutes a day (5 sessions × 20 minutes—every 2 to 4 hours during the day and 4 to 6 hours at night)
      Pump choice considerations: time and money
   6. Anticipate problems (low milk supply, inadequate milk-ejection reflex, nipple pain, mastitis)

D. Maintain adequate nutrition for the infant without compromising transition to the breast
   1. Parenteral
   2. Enteral (gavage, cup, medicine dropper, peridontal syringe, syringe and/or feeding tube, bottle)

E. Assess readiness to breastfeed
   1. PCA (postconceptual age)—not research-based
   2. Ability to bottle feed without distress—not research-based
   3. Weight—not research-based
   4. Ability to coordinate suck–swallow–breathe
      a. Finger feed with peridontal syringe
      b. Breastfeed with eye dropper
      c. Positioning critical (head flexion, c-shape, chest-to-chest, clutch or football hold, dancer's hand position)

F. Facilitate early transition to the breast
   Why:
   1. Limit the need for long-term expression, collection and storage
   2. Decrease the possibility of contamination and alteration of milk composition caused by freezing and/or heating
   3. Prevent the development of a sucking mechanism specific to artificial nipples
   How:
   1. Hunger cues
   2. 24-hour intake
   3. Alternate massage
   4. Frequency and duration (watch your baby, not the clock)
   5. Transition stay
   6. Home follow-up

Source: Spangler, Amy (1994). Lecture Outline—Can I Breastfeed When I Have a Preterm/Low Birth-weight Infant? Reprinted with permission.

support, which delayed breastfeeding for a few more days. Interventions that helped this mother included the following:

- Information received prenatally
- Use of test-weighing as an estimate of milk intake during breastfeeding
- Frequent feedings and/or pumpings with an electric pump and double collection kit
- Self-regulatory feeds
- Early introduction of feeds in the hospital
- Technical assistance from experienced clinicians
- Supportive family and health-care staff

This mother was able to minimize her use of supplemental formula and managed to maintain a rigorous feeding schedule (12–34 times daily during the first 28 days after hospital discharge). The neonates gained weight well, averaging 30 g to 54 g. These two case reports are encouraging to lactation professionals who encounter doubting physicians and fearful mothers, and offer insight into the appropriate management of breastfeeding multiple preterm infants.

EQUIPMENT AND PERSONNEL TO ASSIST WITH BREASTFEEDING ASSESSMENT OF THE PRETERM INFANT

One of the latest developments in the lactation profession is the acceptance of test-weighing for premature infants and infants with medical problems. Test-weighing is a process that involves weighing the baby immediately before and after breastfeeding and subtracting the pre- from the post-feed weight. An assumption is made that the weight change in grams is equivalent to the milk intake in milliliters.

Meier and associates (1994) studied 30 preterm and/or high-risk infants within five days of hospital discharge during a single breastfeeding session by weighing the infants on two scales. One was a previously tested scale from Olympic Medical (Seattle) called the Smart Model 20 (Meier et al., 1990) and one was a new scale marketed by Medela for home use—the BabyWeigh™ scale. Estimates of intake by the mother and investigator were also recorded and compared to measured intakes from the two scales. The BabyWeigh™ scale provided an accurate estimate of intake when compared to the Smart Model 20; however, the investigator and maternal estimates of intake were not sufficiently accurate.

The Whitney strain gage is a new instrument used in research for measuring nutritive sucking in preterm infants. Sucking events that can be measured with the gage include number of sucking bursts, number of sucks per burst, duration of bursts, and pauses between bursts. This instrument was found to be valid for measuring sucking events (deMonterice et al., 1992) and is adaptable to breastfeeding infants. This device will be beneficial to research conducted on breastfeeding preterm infants.

Many health-care professionals are involved in the care of the preterm infant with the neonatologist retaining the ultimate responsibility for overseeing the management. It is not uncommon for NICUs to routinely employ occupational, physical, and speech therapists; dietitians; lactation consultants; and neonatal nurses. Clinical rounds are an important time for group sharing of information and decision making regarding feeding regimens. The LC must participate in rounds on a regular basis to support, protect, and promote breastfeeding.

One concept that is gaining popularity is the feeding team. The professionals participating on the feeding team vary depending on the particular needs of an infant and the choice of substance fed to the infant. The feeding team meets regularly each week to discuss each discipline's care plan for an individual infant and to ensure that plans are compatible and support one another. By sharing expertise among disciplines, the professionals learn more about how to be effective within their own realm of care, the infant receives better care, and the parents are not confronted with oftentimes conflicting information. This concept can be especially helpful to the LC who may not have the depth of experience in dealing with the oral–motor assessements needed for assisting the more complex preterm infant.

BREASTMILK EXPRESSION

If the premature infant is unable to breastfeed soon after birth, the mother should be instructed on breastmilk expression. Use of an electric breast pump is an easy and efficient way to establish and maintain lactation if a long-term separation prevents nursing. Encourage the mother to pump every 2 to 3 hours when awake, and once during the night if she awakens. If the infant is ill and will be unable to nurse for a period of time, pumping the breasts a minimum of 5 times a day for 20 minutes per session, with a total duration exceeding 100 minutes, should be adequate stimulation for maintaining lactation and milk supply (Hopkinson et al., 1988). Bilateral pumping of the breasts is optimal because it requires less time and produces higher prolactin levels (Neifert & Seacat, 1985). Module 2, *The Process of Breastfeeding*, Chapter 3, discusses breastmilk expression in more detail.

For the mother who notices a decline in her milk production after pumping for several weeks, an increase in her pumping to as many as 12 sessions per day may be needed. Medications that can increase the maternal milk supply are discussed in Chapter 2 of this module.

A prospective, placebo-controlled, double-blind trial of the successful use of human growth hormone (hGH) for mothers of premature infants with inadequate lactation has been recently published (Gunn et al., 1996). In this study, 10 mothers received hGH, 0.2 IU/kg per day subcutaneously to a maximum of 16 IU per day for 7 days, and 10 mothers received the same volume of placebo. Outcome measures evaluated included maternal milk production (milk expression plus amount consumed by the infant as measured by test-weighing), plasma concentrations of insulin-like growth factor-1 (IGF-1), insulin-growth factor binding protein-3 (IGFBP-3), and growth hormone (GH). Milk production increased in all the treated mothers by 31%, from 139 mL ± 49 mL per day to 175 mL ± 46 mL per day, but decreased in 4 of the 9 placebo mothers. Plasma concentrations of IGF-1 and IGFBP-3 increased in the hGH-treated mothers but not the placebo-treated mothers. GH did not increase in either group. No adverse effects were seen in the mothers or the infants. Growth hormone has been reported to be important to galactopoiesis in other species but the exact mechanism of action has not been worked out. Presently, the use of hGH is experimental and expensive.

Guidelines set by OSHA as well as infection control policies of individual institutions direct the implementation of certain protocols related to working with lactating mothers. Breastmilk is a body fluid and those health-care providers who come into contact with or handle the expressed milk may be required to wear gloves. Expressed breastmilk represents an investment of the mother, both physically and emotionally. Careless handling or storage of this "liquid gold" may be demoralizing and discouraging. Most NICUs have a designated storage area for expressed breastmilk. Every effort should be made to use fresh, expressed breastmilk for every preterm infant.

KANGAROO CARE

Kangaroo care, or skin-to-skin contact, is a method of preterm infant care being used in South America, Scandinavia, Europe, and in some facilities in the United States. The concept has been attributed to Dr. Edgar Rey and Dr. Hector Martinez of the Maternal Child Institute in Bogota, Colombia. When using kangaroo care, the mother of the preterm infant holds her infant underneath her clothing, placed in a prone position between her breasts, allowing for self-regulatory breastfeeding. Kangaroo care provides the stable, premature infant with warmth and comfort through skin-to-skin contact.

Kangaroo care can begin early for the stable infant weighing as little as 700 g to 1,000 g. Infants have been shown to maintain stable temperatures, respirations, and heart rate and improve weight gain while being cared for in this manner for up to three hours (Ludington-Hoe et al., 1991; Whitelaw, 1986; Whitelaw et al., 1988). In most of the studies, no crying occurred during kangaroo care and sleep was increased. Lactation is enhanced and supported as well through this method of care (Schmidt & Wittreich, 1986; Tuomikoski-Koiranen, 1988). Kangaroo care can be initiated before the infant is ready to breastfeed or while the infant is on the ventilator.

There are four levels of kangaroo care—late K, intermediate K, early K, and very early K (Anderson, 1991):

1. The late K phase begins after the preterm infant has stable respiration and is on room air, having completed the intensive care phase.
2. Intermediate K usually occurs seven days postbirth, after the early intensive care phase; often the infants are on oxygen and periods of apnea and bradycardia are seen. This group also may be on ventilator support.
3. Early K care can be provided to infants who are easily stabilized.
4. Very early K care begins during the first minute postbirth.

Infants who receive kangaroo care have been reported to come out of incubators sooner, go home sooner (Affonso et al., 1989), and have parents who are very happy to participate in their care.

One interesting finding of the studies to date has been the thermal synchrony mothers showed with their infants, with increases and decreases in the maternal temperature documented to maintain their infant in a thermoneutral range (Ludington-Hoe et al., 1990). Kangaroo care can be delivered by fathers and grandparents as well.

The benefits and advantages of kangaroo care are many and no infection problems have been documented (Acolet et al., 1989; Affonso et al., 1989; de Leeuw, 1988;

Ludington-Hoe, 1990). Design limitations, such as lack of control groups, and small sample sizes, confine the widespread applicability of these studies but have provided enough promising information to warrant further larger-scale investigations.

One larger prospective, randomized trial has been reported from Ecuador (high altitude) by Sloan and associates (1994), who described an intervention using kangaroo care, with 128 infants assigned to kangaroo care and 147 to standard incubator care. The infants were less than 2,000 g and satisfied out-of-risk criteria of food tolerance and weight stabilization.

The infants were followed for six months and the kangaroo-care group had a significantly lower rate than the control group of lower respiratory-tract disorders, aspiration, pneumonia, apnea, septicemia, and general infections (7, 5%, vs. 27, 18%; $p < 0.002$) and had fewer readmissions; thus, the cost was lower for the kangaroo-care group. This study reported no significant differences between groups in less severe morbidity, in growth, or in breastfeeding (the proportion of breastfeeding was high in both groups). A summary of the benefits of kangaroo care is shown in Table 3A–9.

Table 3A–9   Summary of the Benefits of Kangaroo Care

- Adequate oxygenation
- Adequate temperatures
- Decreased periodic breathing and apnea
- Energy conservation
- Fathers receive equal responsiveness from infants when also involved in kangaroo care
- Increased warmth
- Mothers are more inclined to breastfeed
- Mothers breastfeed longer
- Moved to open-air cribs sooner
- Optimal behavioral states (alert inactivity)
- Parents have an increased level of confidence in monitoring the infant's health
- Slightly elevated heart rate

RESOURCES

The following organizations may be helpful to the family with a low-birth-weight infant:

Intensive Caring Unlimited
910 Bent Lane
Philadelphia, PA 19118
   (Newsletter subscription)

International Lactation Consultant Association
200 North Michigan Avenue
Chicago, IL 60601
Phone: (312) 541-1710

Lactation Associates
254 Conant Road
Weston, MA 02193-2756
Phone: (617) 893-3553
Fax: (617) 893-8608
   (Pamphlets)

La Leche League International
1400 North Meacham Road
P.O. Box 4079
Schaumburg, IL 60168-4079
Phone: (847) 519-7730 (for orders) / (800) 525-3243
Fax: (847) 519-0035

Parents of Premature and High Risk Infants International, Inc.
c/o The National Self-Help Clearinghouse
33 West 42nd Street
New York, NY 10036
Phone (212) 840-1259
   (Support group referral)

Functional Variations of the Palate, Tongue, and Jaw

STRUCTURAL ABNORMALITIES

The central nervous system regulates the normal buccal, lingual, and pharyngeal movements necessary for sucking and swallowing. Thus, intact brainstem pathways and the effective transmission of impulses through cranial nerves to a healthy mouth, tongue, and pharynx musculature are necessary for sucking and swallowing. When the regulatory centers or pathways for impulse transmission are injured or dysfunctional, abnormalities in sucking and swallowing may occur. Structural abnormalities of the face, mouth, or pharynx and neurologic dysfunction are most often independent of one another. Neurologic dysfunction includes a diminished or absent suck reflex, a weak suck, an uncoordinated suck, and a combination of suck disorders (McBride & Danner, 1987).

For many years, lactation consultants at The Lactation Institute have used a mouth model to illustrate different palatal variations such as concave, bubble, and high-arched palates. They contend that variations in infant palatal stucture (VIPS) can contribute to breastfeeding problems. To further study this theory, Snyder (1995) studied retrospectively the charts of 200 infants assessed at the Institute and Breastfeeding Clinic and found that palatal variations were found in 50% of the babies assessed and in the group with VIPS, 74% sucked incorrectly compared to 26% in the reference group. More testing of the definition tool for VIPS is needed, as are intervention strategies for VIPS. The reader is referred to occupational and speech therapy texts for more information.

ORAL–MOTOR DYSFUNCTION VERSUS DISORGANIZATION

Feeding problems are often seen by LCs who work with growing premature infants transitioning to full breastfeeding after a period of TPN and/or nasogastric feeding. Also, infants recovering from perinatal and neonatal complications often have some feeding problems. How quickly the transition to nipple feeds can be made depends on developmental maturity and any neurologic damage present. Ideally, a team of professionals, including the LC, speech pathologist, occupational and physical therapist, physician, nurse, and nutritionist monitor and evaluate the infant as feeding progresses. Oral–motor performance is best measured or evaluated using a neonatal oral–motor assessment scale (NOMAS) such as the one copyrighted by Palmer in 1990. This scale differentiates tongue and jaw movements, identifies normal and deviant oral–motor patterns (dysfunctional vs. disorganized), and allows one to quantify oral–motor skills.

Palmer (1990) describes the tongue and jaw movements on the NOMAS as follows: In normal tongue movements, a cupped tongue configuration is maintained during sucking, there are rhythmical movements to the tongue, the movements occur at the rate of one per second, liquid is efficiently sucked into the oropharynx for swallowing, and extension–elevation–retraction movement occurs in an anterior–posterior direction.

Disorganized tongue movements include the following: arrhythmical movements; excessive protrusion beyond the labial border during the extension phase of sucking without interrupting sucking rhythm; and the inability to sustain the suck pattern for two minutes due to habituation, poor respiration or fatigue, and an incoordination of the suck and swallow and respiration, which results in nasal flaring, head turning, and extraneous movement.

In dysfunctional tongue movements, the tongue may be retracted, humped, and pulled back into the oropharynx; there may be assymmetry and lateral tongue deviation; the tongue may be flaccid and flattened with an absent tongue groove; there may be an excessive protrusion beyond the labial border before or after nipple insertion; and there may be an absence of movement a certain percent of the time.

In normal jaw movements, there is a consistent degree of jaw depression; there are rhythmical excursions; jaw movement occurs at the rate of approximately one per second during nutritive sucking and two per second during nonnutritive sucking; spontaneous jaw excursions occur on tactile presentation of the nipple up to 30 minutes prior to a feed; and there is sufficient closure on the nipple during the expression phase to express fluid from the nipple.

Disorganized jaw movements include the following: arrhythmical jaw movements; an inconsistent degree of jaw depression; difficulty initiating movements such as an inability to latch on; small, tremorlike start-up movements noted and no response to the initial cue of the nipple until jiggled; and the persistence of an immature suck pattern beyond the appropriate age.

Dysfunctional jaw movements may be identified by minimal jaw excursions and clenching; excessively wide excursions that interrupt the intra-oral seal on the nipple; asymmetry and lateral jaw deviation; a lack of the rate change in jaw movements between nutritive and nonnutritive sucking; or an absence of jaw movement a certain percentage of the time.

In a pilot study of the NOMAS (Braun & Palmer, 1985), oral–motor performance tended to be disorganized or dysfunctional for infants with intraventricular hemorrhage (IVH) and asphyxia neonatorum. Oral–motor dysfunction correlated with generalized hypotonia on neurologic examination and was found in infants of 40 weeks corrected age. Disorganization was seen at earlier corrected ages (35 and 37 weeks) and raised the question of whether oral–motor function deteriorates with loss of normal movement so that by term age dysfunction is noted.

The Neurologically Impaired Infant

As with all infants, breastfeeding can offer the neurologically impaired infant many benefits. Not only is the mother–infant bonding enhanced, but the infant receives protection from infections while working on the development and improved coordination of muscles, and is using the nervous system while breastfeeding.

An infant who has been classified as being neurologically impaired has a nervous system that does not function normally. This could be caused by physical problems or immaturity. Neurologically impaired infants can generally be classified in one of two categories: infants who are hypotonic (have low muscle tone) and exhibit a weak suck, and those that are hypertonic (have overactive muscle tone) and exhibit an uncoordinated suck (Danner & Cerutti, 1990b).

THE HYPOTONIC INFANT

The hypotonic infant may exhibit extremely weak oral and facial muscle tone. Symptoms that may be associated with this include a weak suckle-and-swallow reflex, nonrhythmic sucking, and gulping and choking while breastfeeding. His or her tongue may remain in the back of the mouth, not coming forward to form a trough around the nipple and areola, which will result in ineffective breastfeeding patterns.

Before putting the hypotonic infant to the breast, the following suggestions may help:

- Gently tap or stroke the infant's cheeks, lips, and tongue in a rhythmic pattern (Mohrbacher & Stock, 1991).
- Stroke the infant's tongue, causing an increased awareness, possibly helping him or her to use it more effectively when breastfeeding (Mohrbacher & Stock, 1991).
- Offer the infant increased lower jaw and chin support while breastfeeding, especially if a nonrhythmic suckling is noted. Many times this nonrhythmic suckle causes the infant to have difficulty keeping the mother's breast in his or her mouth, and often more air than usual is swallowed. This infant may need to be burped at more frequent intervals.

THE HYPERTONIC INFANT

The hypertonic infant may exhibit exorbitant body arching often lying in an extended position, overreacting to various forms of stimulation with muscle spasticity causing jerking-like movements, and/or eliciting excessive rooting and biting movements. This hyperreflexive characteristic of biting while swallowing is referred to as a tonic bite reflex. Hypertonic infants may also exhibit a nonrhythmic suckle, which is characteristic of hypotonic infants as well. When putting hypertonic infants to the breast, they may be helped by the following suggestions:

1. Breastfeeding is much more effective if the infant is in a flexed position, chin downward and spine rounded, rather than an extended position. The mother may find that wrapping the baby securely in a blanket helps maintain this position while feeding (Mohrbacher & Stock, 1991).

2. The mother should try to sit somewhat still during nursing sessions and avoid additional outside stimulation.

3. The mother should talk to the infant in a soft, calm voice, which can be very soothing to the infant.

4. An infant who is eliciting the tonic bite reflex by biting down with the jaws while swallowing, thrusting the tongue forward, or sometimes gagging if the tip of his or her tongue is touched, may breastfeed more effectively if his or her face is washed with cold water then warm water several times before being put to the breast (Mohrbacher & Stock, 1991).

5. Offer the infant increased lower jaw and chin support while nursing, especially if a nonrhythmic suckling is noted. Many times this nonrhythmic suckling causes the infant to have difficulty keeping the mother's breast in his or her mouth, often swallowing more air than usual. This infant may need to be burped at more frequent intervals (Mohrbacher & Stock, 1991).

INTRODUCING BREASTFEEDING TO NEUROLOGICALLY IMPAIRED INFANTS

If the infant with a neurologic impairment is not ready for oral feedings, it is optimal that the mother and infant have the chance for skin-to-skin contact at the breast as soon as it is possible and that the infant have the opportunity to comfort nurse if desired. The mother should maintain her milk supply by pumping until the infant is able to begin breastfeeding (McBride & Danner, 1987).

Neurologically impaired infants may be unable to nurse effectively in the beginning and will need to be worked with in a slow and patient manner. The mother will require continued support, encouragement, and instruction as she endeavors to enter a new phase of motherhood. Breastfeeding suggestions include the following:

1. The mother should wash her hands with soap and water.

2. The mother should make herself as comfortable as possible. The environment should be kept calm and quiet, reducing any external stimulation.

3. Prior to putting the infant to breast, suggest techniques that will help encourage the milk-ejection reflex and assist in elongating the nipple for easier latching by the infant. Techniques such as warm compresses, breast massage, nipple rolling, or pumping have worked well for many mothers.

4. When positioning the neurologically impaired infant at the breast, it is important to bring him or her to breast level and maintain good support throughout the feeding. Some babies who have low muscle tone will be able to breastfeed better if their buttocks and head are at the same level

while supported. This can easily be done by putting pillows on the mother's lap to bring the infant up to breast level (Danner & Cerutti, 1990b). See the Appendix, Specialty Positions, that follows this section for positioning ideas.

5. The mother may support her breast using the C-hold or palmar grasp (thumb on top of the breast and four fingers below). While cupping the breast in this manner, tickle the infant's lips with the nipple, eliciting the rooting reflex. As the infant opens his or her mouth, gently press down on the chin while centering the nipple and areola in the mouth. While the infant is nursing, the mother can support the lower mandible by putting her index finger under his or her chin, or if this is not enough support, she may use the dancer hand position, where the hand forms a U shape. While the infant is weak, these techniques will help support the mandible because he or she may tire easily, and will also assist in keeping the breast from falling out of the infant's mouth while nursing (Danner & Cerutti, 1990b).

6. Assess to see that the infant is latched on properly by gently pulling downward on her or his lower lip while nursing. The infant's tongue should be troughed and extended over the lower gum ridge, with upper and lower lips flanged. If the tongue is noted to be elsewhere, such as to the side or on top of the nipple, suction should be broken and the infant removed for repositioning. If a lip is curled under, this may be corrected easily by gently uncurling with a finger (Danner & Cerutti, 1990b).

7. The neurologically impaired infant with low muscle tone often may gulp milk and choke easily because his or her airway is not being well protected while swallowing. If this is noted, try positioning the infant so that the back of his or her throat is at a higher level than the mother's nipple. This will cause the flow of the mother's milk to work against gravity, slowing the force at which the milk is flowing into the infant's mouth.

8. Encourage the mother and father to join a local support group. Introduce them to other families who have been through this type of experience and have accomplished a successful breastfeeding relationship.

RESOURCES

The following organizations may be helpful to the family with an infant who is neurologically impaired.

International Lactation Consultant Association
200 North Michigan Ave.
Chicago, IL 60601
Phone: (312) 541-1710

La Leche League International
1400 North Meacham Rd.
P.O. Box 4079
Schaumburg, IL 60168-4079
Phone: (847) 519-7730 (for orders) / (800) 525-3243
Fax: (847) 519-0035

The Infant with Down Syndrome

Down syndrome (Trisomy of Chromosome 21) occurs in approximately one in 600 to 800 live births; there are 47 chromosomes in each cell instead of 46 (Timko et al, 1986). Characteristics of the infant may include a sloping forehead; a flat nose or absent bridge of the nose; ears that are set low; a large protruding tongue, which is sometimes not evident at birth; a dwarfed physique; epicanthal folds; and broad hands (Good, 1991). Incomplete cardiac development frequently accompanies Down syndrome and surgery may be required.

BREASTFEEDING BENEFITS

Many infants with Down syndrome are successfully and completely breastfed. Breastfeeding the Down syndrome infant has many benefits, one of which being the antibodies and other white blood cells she or he receives from breastmilk to help fight off infections. Down syndrome infants have an increased susceptibility to respiratory-tract and ear infections. Breastfed infants are known to have fewer incidences of these infections than those fed formula. See Module 1, *The Support of Breastfeeding,* Chapter 2, for a review of the benefits of human milk feeding.

Another benefit is the stimulation of oral and facial muscles that are used when breastfeeding. Enhanced development and coordination of these muscles assists in improving the infant's muscle control. Breastfeeding also helps give the infant increased jaw stability and specific muscle action of the infant's tongue, which may later contribute to building language-related skills (Timko et al., 1986).

Infants with Down syndrome are in need of extra stimulation through frequent touching. Skin-to-skin contact with the mother helps provide direct sensory stimulation to the infant's body and face, and helps interest them in breastfeeding.

INTRODUCING BREASTFEEDING TO INFANTS WITH DOWN SYNDROME

Some infants with Down syndrome have other physical problems, which may interrupt the beginning of breastfeeding. Cardiac or respiratory problems may require them to remain hospitalized in an intensive care nursery for a period of time. While being cared for in the hospital setting, they may be nourished by a nasogastric tube. The mother should be encouraged and instructed on expressing her breastmilk to be given to her infant until the infant is able to breastfeed for nourishment. She should also be encouraged to pump following a nursing session with her infant if it has lasted less than 10 minutes, if the infant continues to have a weak suck, or if the mother's breasts remain full. When the infant is being fed by a nasogastric tube, it is desirable to offer the breast or a pacifier for nonnutritive sucking because the sensory input for both infant and mother is beneficial. The mother should discuss her options with the physician.

Infants with Down syndrome may be hypotonic as with many neurologically impaired infants. This may cause ineffective suckling and breastfeeding as a result of a weak suckle, tiring easily, and difficulty remaining on the breast (Timko et al., 1986). A flattened tongue also may cause some difficulty for the Down syndrome infant until muscle tone begins to improve. Feeding at the breast may take longer, but will improve with time, as will the infant. Being unable to form a trough around the areola and nipple with the tongue causes the breastmilk to go to the sides of the infant's mouth rather than being swallowed immediately. Less of the milk will be swallowed each time this occurs. Feedings will go better as the infant's muscle tone improves.

Infants with Down syndrome may be unable to nurse effectively in the beginning and will need to be worked with in a slow and patient manner. The mother will require continued support, encouragement, and instruction as she endeavors to enter a new phase of motherhood. Breastfeeding suggestions include the following:

1. The mother should wash her hands with soap and water.

2. The mother should make herself as comfortable as possible. The environment should be kept calm and quiet, reducing any external stimulation.

3. Prior to putting the infant to breast, suggest techniques that will help encourage the milk ejection reflex and assist in elongating the nipple for easier latching by the infant. Techniques such as warm compresses, breast massage, nipple rolling, or pumping have worked well for many mothers.

4. The infant should be breastfed at frequent intervals of at least every two to three hours. The nursing sessions may not last long if the infant tires easily, and frequent feedings will allow him or her to get more milk. Infants with Down syndrome may learn best with frequent short feeding sessions (Timko et al., 1986).

5. The mother should express a small amount of breastmilk onto the nipple or infant's lips to entice the infant and encourage licking and latching on. Some mothers have found that using a dropper to dribble earlier expressed milk on the nipple helpful while the infant is at the breast if he or she is having a difficult time becoming interested (Danner & Cerutti, 1990c).

6. When positioning the infant with Down syndrome at the breast, it is important to bring him or her to breast level and maintain good support throughout the feeding. Some babies who have low muscle tone will be able to breastfeed better if their buttocks and head are at the same level while being supported. Pay special attention to supporting the head because infants with Down syndrome tend to have floppy heads. For efficient feeding, the head must not become too drastically flexed. Placing pillows on the mother's lap will bring the infant up to breast level (Danner & Cerutti, 1990c). See the Appendix, Specialty Positions, for ideas for positioning the infant with low muscle tone at the breast.

7. The mother can support her breast using the C-hold (thumb on top of the breast and four fingers below). While cupping the breast in this manner, tickle the infant's lips with the nipple, eliciting the rooting reflex. As the infant opens his or her mouth, gently press down on the chin while centering the nipple and areola in the mouth. While the infant is nursing, the mother can support the lower jaw by putting her index finger under his or her chin, or if this is not enough support, she may use the dancer

hand position, where the hand forms a U shape. While the infant is weak, these techniques will help support the mandible because he or she may tire easily, and will also assist in keeping the breast from falling out of the infant's mouth while nursing (Danner & Cerutti, 1990c).

8. Assess to see that the infant is latched on properly by gently pulling downward on his or her lower lip while nursing. The infant should be using the gums to compress the milk sinuses located beneath the areola and then, using his or her tongue, to stroke the milk out of the nipple. Infants who are hypotonic may compress the areola with the gums two or three times before stroking the nipple to get milk. A rhythm develops as the infant breastfeeds, each infant finding a rhythmic pattern that is right for him or her. At the beginning of the feeding, a more rapid suckle will be noted (nonnutritive). As the feeding progresses and the infant has picked up a rhythmic pattern for breathing, suckling, and swallowing, a slower gum movement will be noted (nutritive suckle) (Danner & Cerutti, 1990c).

9. The infant with Down syndrome who is hypotonic often may gulp milk and may choke easily because his or her airway is not being well protected when swallowing. If this is noted, try positioning the infant so that the back of the throat is at a higher level than the mother's nipple. This will cause the flow of the mother's milk to work against gravity, slowing the force at which the milk is flowing into the infant's mouth. This infant may need to be frequently burped because of the increased amount of air swallowed (Mohrbacher & Stock, 1991).

10. The Down syndrome infant who has a large tongue that protrudes may experience difficulty latching on to the mother's breast, as a result of pushing the breast out of the mouth with her or his tongue. Exercises and suck training may help this (Mohrbacher & Stock, 1991).

11. If the infant is unable to be put to the breast, or if the infant is being put to the breast but is not breastfeeding effectively, the mother should be instructed on breastmilk expression.

12. Encourage the mother and father to join a local support group. Introduce them to other families who have been through this type of experience and have accomplished a successful breastfeeding relationship.

RESOURCES

The following organizations may be helpful to the family of the infant with Down syndrome.

International Lactation Consultant Association
200 North Michigan Ave.
Chicago, IL 60601
Phone: (312) 541-1710

La Leche League International
1400 North Meacham Rd.
P. O. Box 4079
Schaumburg, IL 60168-4079
Phone: (847) 519-7730 (for orders) / (800) 525-3243
Fax: (847) 519-0035

March of Dimes Defects Foundation
1275 Mamaroneck Ave.
White Plains, NY 10605
Phone: (914) 428-7100
e-mail: Resourcecenter@modimes.org

National Association for Down Syndrome
P.O. Box 4542
Oak Brook, IL 60522-4542
Phone: (708) 325-9112

National Down Syndrome Congress
1605 Chantilly Dr., Suite 250
Atlanta, GA 30324
Phone: (404) 633-1555 / (800) 232-6372
e-mail: ndsc@charitiesusa.com

National Down Syndrome Society (NDSS)
666 Broadway
New York, NY 10012
Phone: (212) 460-9330 / (800) 211-4602
http://www.ndss.org

State Departments of Human Resources
and Mental Health Services
   (Community health center referrals)
U.S. Department of Health and Human Services
Washington, DC 20201

The Infant with Cleft Lip and/or Cleft Palate

Cleft lip with or without cleft palate is a common congenital malformation seen in approximately 1:700 live births occurring in the United States (Slavkin, 1992; Warkany, 1971). Clefting of the lip or palate is a congenital defect that has varying degrees of severity. Although clefting is an anomaly that tends to be genetically determined, some cases of clefting are of unknown causes or result from in utero environmental influences, including maternal diseases, alcohol, chemotherapy, radiation, anticonvulsant medications, and maternal folate deficiency (Ferguson, 1991; Heinonen et al., 1977; Slavkin, 1979; Warkany, 1971; Wilson, 1963).

EMBRYOLOGY OF FACIAL CLEFTING

Although often associated, clefting of the lip and clefting of the palate are distinct malformations and originate at different times during the developmental process. Facial clefting may involve only the lip, or extend into the hard and soft palate. The clefting may be unilateral or bilateral (see Figure 3A–1). A blend of failure in normal fusion and deficient development may influence the soft tissue and bony components of the upper lip, alveolar ridge, and hard and soft palates (see Figure 3A–2). The general classifications of facial clefting are CL (cleft lip only), CL/P (cleft lip and palate), and CP (cleft palate only).

During the second and third months of development, the face of the fetus endures rapid and considerable changes (Hayward, 1984). Malformation occurs during embryonic development between the fourth and tenth weeks of the gestational period (Bixler, 1981; Ferguson, 1991; Slavkin, 1979; Warkany, 1971). Ultrasound techniques can provide the professional with a noninvasive diagnostic tool for identifying facial clefting by 16 to 20 weeks gestation (Marsh & Vannifer, 1988; Slavkin, 1992).

EPIDEMIOLOGY OF FACIAL CLEFTING

Facial clefting appears to be influenced by race, sex, parental age, genetics, and environmental factors.

Racial Influence

Clefting tends to occur more frequently in the Oriental population, with a report of approximately 2.1 per 1,000 for cleft lip and palate, and a cleft palate incidence of 0.00055. The Caucasian population has an incidence rate of cleft lip and palate of approximately 1 per 1,000 population. The African American population in the United States has a less frequent risk for cleft lip and palate, with an estimated incidence of 0.41 per 1,000 (Bennett, 1988).

Figure 3A–1

Changes in embryology of the face.

Source: Hayward, JR (1984). Cleft lip and cleft palate. In: Kruger, GO. *Textbook of Oral and Maxillofacial Surgery*, 6th ed., p. 457. St. Louis: Mosby. Adapted from Avery, JK (1957). In: Bunting, RW. *Oral Hygiene*, 3rd ed., Philadelphia: Lea & Febiger. Reprinted with permission of Gustav Kruger and publishers.

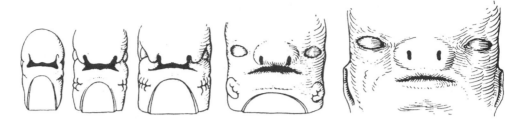

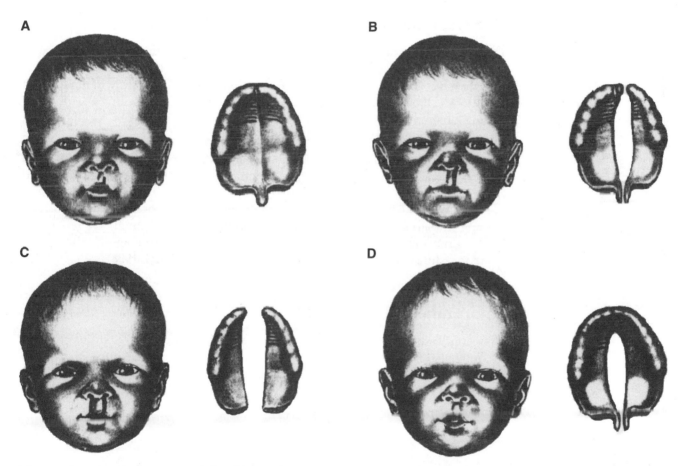

Figure 3A–2   Variations in clefts of lip and palate: **A**—Notch in vermilion border at birth; **B**—Unilateral cleft lip and palate; **C**—Bilateral cleft lip and cleft palate; **D**—Cleft palate.

Source: Whaley, LF, Wong, D (1991). *Nursing Care of Infants and Children*, p. 491, 4th ed. St. Louis: Mosby. Used with permission.

Sex Ratio Influence

Males have a higher incidence of cleft lip and/or cleft palate, while also having defects of a more serious nature. Females tend to be more affected with cleft palate alone (Bennett, 1988).

Parental Age Influence

Some evidence has shown a possible correlation between increasing parental age and an increased risk of producing a child with cleft lip and cleft palate. The father's age may be more of a significant factor than that of the mother (Bennett, 1988).

Genetic Influences

There is a significant increase of cleft lip and/or cleft palate among relatives, but it is very possible for isolated cases to occur (Bennett, 1988). If parents without facial clefting have a child with a cleft, the chance that a following child will have a cleft is 2% to 4%. If one of the parents has facial clefting, the risks become 4% to 5% for having a baby with clefting. If both of the parents of the child have facial clefting, the risk becomes even more significant (Slavkin, 1992).

When a child presents having cleft lip and/or cleft palate, other defects can often be associated. The occurrence of related anomalies in all cleft cases is 29%, isolated cleft palate having the highest (Bennett, 1988). Some of the associated anomalies include central nervous system malformations, cardiac abnormalities, club foot, hearing impairment, and impaired speech development (Bennett, 1988; Slavkin, 1992). Almost all children who have cleft palates will require speech therapy to overcome difficulties at some stage in their lives (King & Wei, 1988).

Environmental Influences

Shaw and associates (1995) reported that if a mother used multivitamins containing folic acid from one month before to two months after conception, an overall reduction in the risk of orofacial clefts of 25% to 50% occurred.

CLEFTING OF THE LIP

Clefting of the lip (cheiloschisis) occurs when portions of the upper lip do not fuse together in utero. Cleft lip with or without cleft palate is produced between the period of four to ten weeks gestation (Slavkin, 1992). This malformation of the lip, with or without involvement of the palate, may be unilateral (one-sided) or bilateral (two-sided). While there are various clefting classifications by different authors, Veau (1931) suggested what is probably one of the most frequently used classifications of variations of clefting of the lip and palate. Veau's classification of clefting of the lip is shown in Table 3A–10 (Garner & Davis, 1983).

Table 3A–10   Veau's Cleft Lip Classifications

Class	Description
I	A unilateral notch of the vermilion border (where the pink area of the lips meets the surrounding skin) that does not extend into or involve the lip
II	A unilateral notch of the vermilion border that does extend into the lip
III	A unilateral clefting of the vermilion border and lip that extends into the floor of the nasal cavity
IV	Any bilateral clefting of the lip, whether it be incomplete notching or complete clefting

Table 3A–11   Veau's Cleft Palate Classifications

Class	Description
I	Clefting of the soft palate only
II	Clefting of the hard and soft palates, but not extending to or involving the alveolar ridge
III	Clefting of the hard and soft palates, and alveolar ridge, on one side of the premaxilla; usually associated with clefting of the lip
IV	Clefting of the hard and soft palates, and alveolar ridge, affecting the premaxilla bilaterally; usually associated with clefting of the lip

CLEFTING OF THE PALATE

Clefting of the palate (palatoschisis) occurs from failure of the medial nasal, lateral nasal, and maxillary processes on either left, right, or both sides of the forming skull and face to fuse together midline (Slavkin, 1992). Cleft lip, with or without cleft palate, is produced between four and ten weeks gestation. The process of palatal fusion should occur during the seventh or eighth week of embryonic development. Secondary fusion of the palate takes place during the ninth week (Slavkin, 1992). This malformation of the palate may be unilateral (one-sided) or bilateral (two-sided). Veau's classification of clefting of the palate is shown in Table 3A–11 (Veau, 1931; Garner & Davis, 1983).

ADVANTAGES OF BREASTMILK FOR INFANTS WITH CLEFT LIP AND/OR PALATE

In addition to the numerous known benefits of human milk, the following are six of the multiple advantages to feeding the infant with cleft lip and/or palate breastmilk instead of formula.

1. Breastfeeding helps offer additional protection from various types of infections. Infants with clefting of the lip and/or palate tend to be more susceptible to otitis media than the average infant because of the eustachian tubes filling with fluid when the infant swallows (Danner & Cerutti, 1990d). Protection from infections may be especially significant for the infant who is confronting surgery.

2. Breastmilk is a natural bodily fluid, unlike formula, so it is not irritating to mucous membranes as formula would be (Mohrbacher & Stock, 1991). Choking is a common problem when there is clefting of the hard or soft palate. Milk may leak into the nose through the opening in the palate, or may be aspirated into the lungs.

3. The muscles used during breastfeeding help promote improved oral and facial muscular development. Breastfeeding requires more specific movements of the tongue, muscles of mastication and jaws, and encourages normal formation of the infant's face through increased muscle strength. The orificial muscle involvement may assist in the promotion of a more accurate speech development later on (Danner & Cerutti, 1990d).

4. The breast is pliable and will allow molding into the defect of the lip or alveolar ridge. This pliability assists the infant in obtaining a better seal on the breast for feeding. It also allows the infant more control over the flow of milk he or she is receiving (Mohrbacher & Stock, 1991).

5. By using the various nursing positions, breastfeeding can be adapted to fit each individual infant's feeding needs, whether it be the suckling sequence or location of the cleft. The direction of the flow of the breastmilk can be altered to adapt to the rate at which it flows by using a position that puts the infant above or below the breast (Danner & Clay, 1986).

6. Breastfeeding allows for nonnutritive suckling (comfort nursing) by the infant with cleft lip and/or palate, which is beneficial for both mother and child. Infants with clefts often find it trying to manage pacifiers, so nonnutritive suckling at the end of a nursing becomes even more important for the infant who is not only suckling for nourishment, but for comfort and pleasure (Mohrbacher & Stock, 1991).

PROBLEMS ENCOUNTERED WHEN FEEDING INFANTS WITH CLEFT PALATE

Two major problems encountered when feeding an infant with a cleft palate are nasal regurgitation and aspiration. In nasal regurgitation, liquids come out of the nose. These fluids may irritate the nasal cavity and can lead to ear infections because fluids can back up in the eustachian tube. To prevent this from happening, position the infant's head up when feeding so fluids are allowed to run down the throat, not up into the nose. Expect some nasal regurgitation; it is not completely preventable. Burp the infant frequently to help minimize spitting up. Aspiration is breathing liquids into the lungs, and digestive fluids are very irritating. Aspiration results in choking and can lead to colds, upper-respiratory infection, pneumonia, and possible allergies. Without a palate to protect the nasal cavity, liquid runs up into the nasal cavity; as it runs back, the infant aspirates the liquid.

INTRODUCING BREASTFEEDING TO INFANTS WITH CLEFT LIP AND/OR PALATE

To many new parents, the thought of breastfeeding their infant with facial clefting may seem impossible. The parents should be offered increased emotional support and encouragement, as well as techniques and instruction on how to breastfeed. Breastfeeding suggestions include the following:

1. The mother should wash her hands with soap and water.

2. Encourage the mother to begin breastfeeding her infant as soon as possible after birth. These early breastfeedings will help the infant to adapt and learn to cope with the defect. Also, the breasts are softer and more pliable during the first couple of days, which helps make it easier for the mother and infant to experiment with various nursing positions and find the one that works best for them (Mohrbacher & Stock, 1991).

3. The mother should make herself as comfortable as possible, indulging in whatever she finds comfortable and relaxing.

4. Prior to putting the infant to breast, suggest techniques that will encourage the milk-ejection reflex and elongate the nipple for an easier latch-on. Techniques such as warm, moist compresses; breast massage; nipple rolling; or pumping have worked well for many mothers. Suggest to the lactating mother that she might rhythmically squeeze her breast during a feeding, which might help the infant to receive multiple milk ejections.

5. The infant should be breastfed at goal intervals of at least every two to three hours. The nursing sessions may not last long if the infant tires easily, and frequent feedings allow him or her to obtain more breastmilk.

6. The breastfeeding mother should strive for at least 10 minutes of active breastfeeding on each breast, and build on that.

7. The mother should express a small amount of breastmilk onto the nipple to entice the infant and encourage licking and latching on. Some mothers have found that using a dropper to dribble earlier expressed milk on the nipple helpful while the infant is at the breast if she or he is having a difficult time becoming interested.

8. When positioning the infant with cleft lip and/or palate at the breast, it is important to bring him or her to breast level and maintain good support throughout the feeding. Some infants who have low muscle tone will be able to breastfeed better if their buttocks and head are at the same level while supported. This can be done easily by putting pillows on the mother's lap to bring the infant to breast level. Experimentation by the mother is highly encouraged to see which angle or position works best for her and her infant (Danner & Cerutti, 1990d). See the Appendix, Specialty Positions, for ideas on positioning for facial clefting.

   When the hard and/or soft palates are involved in the clefting, breastfeeding is more difficult. The infant has to gulp the breastmilk between breaths to prevent regurgitation through the nostrils because there is a direct space into the nasal cavity. This is impossible unless the breastmilk flows easily and rapidly into the back of the infant's oral cavity where it can be swallowed quickly.

   Encourage the mother to try different breastfeeding positions in the first few days while her breasts are soft and pliable. The clutch (football) position and straddle position (the infant sits upright on the mother's lap straddling her abdomen) may work well if the infant is having an especially difficult time latching on to the breast, and are often considered best if the infant has a bilateral palate defect. In these positions, gravity works with you in positioning the nipple and areola in the infant's mouth. These positions may also reduce the incidence of choking or milk leaking into and out of the infant's nose.

The infant may tend to prefer one breast over the other because the positioning at the preferred breast allows him or her to angle the mother's nipple to one side of the cleft. To encourage bilateral nursing, slide the infant over to the second breast (i.e., if the infant prefers nursing this way, have the mother slide him or her across her lap to the other breast without turning the orientation of the infant's head to the breast).

9. The mother may support her breast using the C-hold or palmar grasp (thumb on top of the breast and four fingers below and back from the areola). While cupping the breast in this manner, the mother can also slightly compress her breast between her fingers to firm the tissue. This will assist the infant in keeping the breast in his or her mouth during a feeding. As the infant opens the mouth, gently press down on the chin while centering the nipple and areola in his or her mouth. The index finger can then slide under the infant's chin to provide additional support.

If this is not enough support, the mother may choose to use the dancer hand position, where the hand forms a U shape. This position will help support the infant's jaw because he or she may tire easily, and will also assist in keeping the breast from falling out of the infant's mouth during breastfeeding (Danner & Cerutti, 1990d).

10. Encourage the family to join a local support group. Introduce them to other families who have been through this experience and have had a successful breastfeeding relationship.

THE PALATAL OBTURATOR

An obturator is an orthodontic appliance that is sometimes used to prevent the cleft in the hard palate from closing improperly and changing the correct facial contour. It serves as an artificial or temporary roof to the mouth and can assist the infant in sucking at the breast until surgical repair can be done (Danner & Cerutti, 1990d). Whether the palatal obturator is used depends on the medical team treating the infant. If the infant's doctor uses the palatal obturator in the treatment plan, it should be requested that a smooth plate be made so it will be less of an irritant to the breastfeeding mother's nipples.

SURGICAL REPAIR OF CLEFT LIP

When repair of the cleft lip takes place is individualized and depends on the surgical team performing the procedure. Some cleft teams use the "three tens law" to determine the appropriate time for surgical repair of the lip. This rule states that the child should have the following (Bennett, 1988; King & Wei, 1988):

- Hematocrit of 10 grams
- Weight of 10 pounds
- Age of 10 weeks
- White blood cell count of no more than 10,000

Elective surgery is generally considered safe after the three tens law has been accomplished. Surgical teams have begun cleft lip repairs within the first three months of the infant's life with success (Mohrbacher & Stock, 1991).

After surgical correction of the cleft lip, the breastfeeding relationship may be delayed for only a few hours or up to few days, depending on the surgeon. Some surgeons allow mothers to put their infants to breast immediately on discharge from the recovery room (Weatherly-White et al., 1987). These same infants are unable to tolerate the bottle so soon following surgery, so if artificial feeding must resume, spoon or cup feedings are initiated.

SURGICAL REPAIR OF CLEFT PALATE

When repair of the cleft palate takes place depends on the discretion of the surgical team involved. Surgical repair of the cleft palate may occur within the first year of life, but sometimes does not occur until in the second or third year of life. This allows time for increased maturation of the oral and facial features. Following surgical correction of the palate, the toddler may find it uncomfortable to nurse immediately, but may take great comfort in holding the mother's nipple in his or her mouth (Mohrbacher & Stock, 1991). If the child is unable to breastfeed, methods of expressing the breastmilk should be discussed with the mother to assist her in maintaining her milk supply, and allowing the infant to be supplemented with her breastmilk until able to actively breastfeed.

RESOURCES

The following organizations may be helpful to the parents of an infant with facial clefting:

Cleft Palate Foundation
1218 Grandview Ave.
Pittsburgh, PA 15211
Office: (412) 681-9620
Cleftline: (800) 242-5338
e-mail: cleftline@aol.com
http://www.cleft.com

International Lactation Consultant Association
200 North Michigan Ave.
Chicago, IL 60601
Phone: (312) 541-1710

La Leche League International
1400 North Meacham Rd.
P.O. Box 4079
Schaumburg, IL 60168-4079
Phone: (847) 519-7730 (for orders) / (800) 525-3243
Fax: (847) 519-0035

Appendix: Specialty Positions

Type Position	Baby's Position	Mother's Position	Indications for Use
Horizontal Prone	Baby lies horizontally across mother's chest, his or her body perpendicular to hers	Mother lies on her back with her head slightly elevated	Baby having problems coping with fast milk flow, baby having trouble extending tongue, baby having trouble staying on the breast, mother with a persistent plugged duct
Vertical Prone	Baby lies parallel to mother, feet resting on the same-side leg as the breast he or she is latched onto	Mother lies on her back with her head slightly elevated	Baby having problems coping with fast milk flow, baby having trouble extending tongue, baby having trouble staying on the breast, mother with a persistent plugged duct
Lateral Prone	Baby lies parallel to mother but slightly off to the side, most of weight is on side of his or her body nearest mother's arm and he or she is cradled by her arm	Mother lies on her back with her head slightly elevated	The mother of twins can use this position with a baby at each arm. Baby having problems coping with fast milk flow, baby having trouble extending tongue, baby having trouble staying on the breast, mother with a persistent plugged duct
Diagonal Prone	Baby's body is on angle to mother's, feet against mother's opposite side	Mother lies on her back with her head slightly elevated	Baby having problems coping with fast milk flow, baby having trouble extending tongue, baby having trouble staying on the breast, mother with a persistent plugged duct
Over-the-Shoulder Prone	Baby lies on a pillow, approaches breast over the mother's shoulder	Mother lies on her back with her head slightly elevated	Works best with older baby who has some head control. Baby having problems coping with fast milk flow, baby having trouble extending tongue, baby having trouble staying on the breast, mother with a persistent plugged duct
Upside Down Side Lying	Baby lies on his or her side upside down in relation to her, feet point toward mother's head	Mother lies on her side	Mother with sore nipples, baby with poor suck, mother with persistent plugged ducts
Hands and Knees	Baby lies flat on back elevated by pillows to breast height	Mother raises herself on her hands and knees above baby	Mother of twins, persistent plugged ducts

Type Position	Baby's Position	Mother's Position	Indications for Use
Straddle Position	Baby sits in mother's lap, faces mother with legs straddling mother's abdomen	Mother is sitting with baby in lap, facing her and straddling legs around mother's abdomen. Mother uses pillow to bring small baby to breast level and tips head back as baby latches to position better	Baby having problems coping with fast milk flow, baby with a cleft palate
Combination Cradle and Clutch Hold	One baby in cradle hold, other baby in clutch hold with head on sibling's abdomen	Mother is sitting upright with pillows under mother's elbows and babies	Breastfeeding two babies simultaneously
Criss Cross	Two babies' bodies in cradle hold, criss-crossed in mother's lap	Mother is sitting upright with pillows under mother's elbows and babies	Breastfeeding two babies simultaneously
Parallel	Babies' bodies extend in same directions, one baby in cradle hold, head in crook of mother's arm and body across mother's lap, other baby's body extends in same direction as sibling off mother's lap, with head supported by mother's hand and arm	Mother is sitting upright with pillows under mother's elbows and on her lap	Breastfeeding two babies simultaneously
Double Clutch Hold	Both babies in clutch hold, lying on firm pillows at mother's sides	Mother is sitting upright with feet propped on footstool, chair, books, low horizontal structure such as table, base of hospital tray table	Breastfeeding two babies simultaneously

Appendix: Specialty Positions *Continued*

Type Position	Baby's Position	Mother's Position	Indications for Use
Babies at Side	Babies lie at mother's sides, partly on their sides facing each other with feet in mother's lap	Mother is sitting upright	Breastfeeding two babies simultaneously
V-Position	Babies' heads are at mother's breasts, forming V with knees touching in her lap	Mother is lying nearly flat on back with two pillows under head and upper body	Breastfeeding two babies simultaneously, safe and comfortable for night position
Slide-Over	Baby begins nursing on preferred breast and mother slides baby over to less preferred breast without changing baby's body position	Mother nurses first on preferred breast; after milk-ejection reflex, mother slides baby over to less preferred breast without changing baby's orientation to mother's body and finishes feeding at less preferred breast	Persuading baby who is refusing one breast to nurse on the less preferred breast
Cross-Cradle, Modified Clutch, or Transitional Hold	Baby is supported in mother's lap on a pillow or cushion in horizontal or semi-upright position, baby's mouth at level of nipple or slightly lower, baby's body on his or her side facing her extends along length of mother's forearm, baby's neck and head supported by mother's hand	Mother holds baby using the arm opposite the breast to be used for feeding, right arm when nursing left breast, mother's hand opposite the breast to be used for feeding supports baby's neck and head, baby's body extends along length of forearm, uses same-side hand to support breast	Babies having difficulty latching on, low-birthweight babies, babies with low muscle tone, babies with weak rooting reflex, babies with weak suck

Source: Compiled from information in Mohrbacher N, Stock J (1997). *The Breastfeeding Answer Book*. Schaumburg IL: La Leche League International, pp. 50-52, 321-323. Art by Donna Wilson used with permission.

POST-TEST

For questions 1 to 7, choose the best answer from the following key:
  A. The premature infant
  B. The hypertonic infant
  C. The hypotonic infant
  D. The cleft lip or cleft palate infant
  E. The Down syndrome infant

1. Symptoms associated with this include a weak suck-and-swallow reflex, non-rhythmic sucking, and gulping and choking while breastfeeding.

2. Characteristics may include a sloping forehead, flat nose, ears that are set low, a large protruding tongue, dwarfed physique, epicanthal folds, a simian crease, and varying degrees of mental retardation.

3. Symptoms associated with this include exorbitant body arching, often lying in an extended position, overreacting to various forms of stimulation with muscle spasticity causing jerkinglike movements, and/or excessive rooting and biting movements.

4. Cheiloschisis or palatoschisis

5. These infants may require extra amounts of certain nutrients for optimal growth, and a human milk fortifier may be required and added to the breastmilk by the physician.

6. When breastfeeding, this infant may have to gulp the breastmilk between breaths to prevent regurgitation through his or her nostrils because there is a space directly into the nasal cavity.

7. Incomplete cardiac and intestinal development is common in these children.

For questions 8 to 12, choose the best answer:

8. When positioning the infant with cleft lip or palate at the breast,
   A. bring him or her to breast level and maintain good support throughout the feeding.
   B. the straddle position may work well if the infant is having an especially difficult time latching on to the breast, and is considered best if the infant has a bilateral palate defect.
   C. the infant may prefer one breast over the other if positioning at the preferred breast allows her or him to angle the mother's nipple to one side of the cleft.
   D. All of the above.

9. The neurologically impaired infant
   A. has a nervous system that does not function normally.
   B. may be hypertonic.
   C. may be hypotonic.
   D. All of the above.

10. Before putting the hypotonic infant to breast, he or she may be helped by which of the following suggestions?
   A. The mother should try to sit still during a nursing session, and avoid additional outside stimulation.

B. Gently tap or stroke the infant's cheek, lips, and tongue in a rhythmic pattern.

C. Breastfeed the infant in an extended position at all times.

D. Never touch the infant's tongue with anything other than the breast prior to breastfeeding.

11. Benefits of breastfeeding the infant with Down syndrome include which of the following?

A. Stimulation of oral and facial muscles that are used when breastfeeding will assist in improving infant's muscle control.

B. Breastfeeding helps give the infant increased jaw stability.

C. Specific muscle action of the infant's tongue may later contribute to building of language-related skills.

D. All of the above.

12. Facial clefting

A. can involve only the palate.

B. affects the lip whenever the palate is affected.

C. never involves only the lip.

D. None of the above.

For questions 13 to 20, choose the best answer from the following key:

A. True   B. False

13. The breastmilk produced by a mother of a preterm infant is exactly the same as the milk produced by the mother of a full-term infant.

14. Bottle feeding is less stressful on an infant than breastfeeding.

15. The mother who is facing a long-term separation from her newborn infant as a result of her or his illness should be instructed to pump her breasts no more than five times a day.

16. Bilateral pumping of the breasts requires less time and produces higher prolactin levels.

17. Cleft lip with or without cleft palate is produced between the periods of four to ten weeks gestation.

18. An infant with clefting of the lip or palate tends to be more susceptible to otitis media than the average infant because the eustachian tubes fill with fluid when he or she swallows.

19. The palatal obturator can assist in the infant's ability to suckle at the breast by acting as an artificial or temporary roof to the mouth.

20. The infant who has Down syndrome and is hypotonic often may gulp milk and choke easily because the airway is not well protected when she or he is swallowing.

SECTION B

Breastfeeding in Special Situations

Jan B. Simpson, RN, BSN, IBCLC

LEARNING OBJECTIVES

At the completion of this section, the learner will be able to do the following:

1. Provide information and guidance to the mother who chooses to continue breastfeeding while pregnant.
2. Provide breastfeeding management suggestions for the mother who chooses to tandem nurse.
3. Provide breastfeeding management suggestions for the mother who is nursing multiples.
4. Offer guidance and information to the adolescent who is considering breastfeeding or who is breastfeeding.
5. Identify ways to help the lactating mother who will be separated from her infant for brief or extended lengths of time to have a successful breastfeeding relationship.
6. Advise the breastfeeding mother who is returning to work or school about methods for continuing a successful breastfeeding relationship.

OUTLINE

I. Breastfeeding While Pregnant

    A. Nipple soreness

    B. Fatigue

    C. Decreased milk supply

    D. Colostrum production

E. Nutrition

F. Weaning

II. Tandem Nursing

III. Breastfeeding Multiples

A. Managing multiples during breastfeeding

B. Supplementing multiples

C. Resources

IV. Adolescents and Breastfeeding

A. Psychosocial concerns

B. Counseling techniques

V. When Mother and Infant Are Separated

A. Short-term separation

B. Long-term separation

C. Returning to work or school

D. Care plan for mothers

PRE-TEST

For questions 1 to 10, choose the best answer.

1. A woman is pregnant and continues to breastfeed her other child. You should advise her as follows:

    A. She should be strongly encouraged to wean because her unborn child will be deprived of required nutrients.

    B. She should be encouraged and informed about changes she may or may not encounter.

    C. She will harm her older child if she breastfeeds while pregnant.

    D. Breastfeeding after conception is contraindicated.

2. Ms. Smith is 11 weeks pregnant and continues to breastfeed her two-year-old child. She is complaining of sore nipples, but no cracking, blistering, or bleeding is reported. You should

    A. work with Ms. Smith on the proper positioning of her child at the breast.

    B. encourage her by telling her these are due to her pregnancy and will disappear after the first trimester.

    C. tell her sore nipples are often reported in breastfeeding and pregnant mothers and are caused by hormonal changes that occur during pregnancy.

    D. Both B and C.

3. The mother who is pregnant and breastfeeding should consider weaning

   A. in all cases.
   B. if she has a history of difficult pregnancies such as those with uterine pain, bleeding, or weight loss while pregnant.
   C. never.
   D. if she has a history of giving birth to an infant of 37 weeks gestational age or less.

4. Tandem nursing is

   A. nursing two or more children of different ages during the same period of time.
   B. nursing triplets.
   C. unacceptable in our society and should not be encouraged.
   D. is extremely dangerous to the younger child.

5. Mothers who give birth to twins

   A. must supplement at least one of the infants.
   B. must breastfeed every hour in order for the milk supply to meet the demands and requirements of her infants.
   C. should only nurse them one at a time.
   D. can exclusively breastfeed both infants.

6. Select the statement that best describe the adolescent mother:

   A. It is physically impossible for the teen mother to adequately nourish her infant by breastfeeding him or her.
   B. The quality and quantity of breastmilk produced by a teen mother is inadequate to completely support the needs of her infant.
   C. It is physically possible for the teen mother to successfully breastfeed her infant.
   D. Both B and C.

7. According to Erikson, the adolescent is experiencing the psychosocial crisis of

   A. anatomy versus shame and doubt.
   B. identity versus role confusion.
   C. basic trust versus mistrust.
   D. initiative versus guilt.

8. Ms. Johnston is planning to return to work when her breastfed son is eight weeks old and plans to leave him at a day-care facility. She should discuss _____ with the day-care workers.

   A. not feeding the infant within one hour of the mother's return
   B. always feeling free to supplement the infant with any formula should he or she become hungry
   C. giving the supplemental formula required at the end of the day, just prior to the mother arriving
   D. None of the above.

9. When developing a plan of care for the lactating mother who is returning to work or school, it should include

   A. choices of milk expression.
   B. where she plans to store her expressed milk.
   C. how to transport her expressed milk.

    D. where she plans to express her milk while at work or school.

    E. All of the above.

10. For the mother who chooses to supplement her infant with bottles of her expressed milk when she is away at work, but whose infant repeatedly refuses to take the bottle,

    A. suggest warming the artificial teat under warm running tap water before offering it to the infant.

    B. suggest having someone other than the mother offer the bottle to the infant.

    C. suggest freezing the artificial teat before offering it to the infant because this will be soothing.

    D. Both A and B.

    E. Both B and C.

For questions 11 to 20, choose the best answer from the following key:

    A. True   **B. False**

11. A mother cannot breastfeed and work too.

12. Studies have shown that if breastfeeding continues during pregnancy, the unborn child will be deprived of required nutrients.

13. Sore nipples are often reported by breastfeeding women who are pregnant, and are caused by hormonal changes occurring as a result of the pregnancy.

14. The pregnant woman who is breastfeeding may notice a decreased milk supply during the last four to five months, which is caused by the hormones being produced to maintain the pregnancy.

15. If the pregnant mother continues to breastfeed her older child at the end of her pregnancy, there will not be colostrum available for the new infant after birth.

16. As the pregnancy nears term, there is a change in the composition of the breastmilk, and the production of colostrum for the new infant begins.

17. When counseling a pregnant teen regarding breastfeeding, her support systems, her perception of self-worth, her body image perception, her dietary habits, and her reaction to her pregnancy should be included in the discussion.

18. If the infant must remain hospitalized after birth, the mother should be encouraged to consider breastfeeding for her sake as well as for her infant's well-being.

19. The mother who will be separated from her infant may want to consider avoiding artificial teats, and supplement her infant with a cup, spoon, or dropper to avoid possible nipple confusion.

20. Breastfeeding after conception is contraindicated.

Breastfeeding While Pregnant

If a mother becomes pregnant while she is still nursing another child, she may face periods of confusion as to whether she should wean her child or continue the breastfeeding relationship. Studies have shown no evidence that proves breastfeeding during pregnancy will deprive the unborn child of any required nutrients if the mother is healthy. Therefore, breastfeeding after conception is not contraindicated.

Concerns that continued suckling stimulation may cause contractions or carry potential fetal risks or have adverse effects on the physical and emotional health of the mother are still found in some health-care professionals' texts (Lawrence, 1989; Moscone & Moore, 1993; Neifert, 1983). Any woman who decides that she will continue to breastfeed during her pregnancy should be encouraged and informed about changes she may or may not encounter. She should be advised of a possible change in the infant's or child's behavior while breastfeeding as well as a change in her milk supply and its appearance. This may or may not affect the nursing child's desire to nurse (Moscone & Moore, 1993).

NIPPLE SORENESS

Sore nipples are often reported and are caused by hormonal changes occurring in the woman because of the pregnancy (Huggins, 1990). Counseling methods to help prevent soreness, such as proper positioning, will not work in this case. The degree of severity and the duration of soreness is individualized. Some women may not experience it; however, a large number of mothers have reported sore nipples lasting throughout the pregnancy, which disappears after the birth of the new child (Mohrbacher & Stock, 1991).

FATIGUE

Fatigue is a natural symptom of pregnancy for many women, and may be increased if the woman is also breastfeeding, although this is not true in many cases. Adequate rest and a nutritious diet are essentials. Encourage the pregnant mother to nurse while lying down in order to get more rest if she is feeling fatigued.

DECREASED MILK SUPPLY

A decreased milk supply may be noticed in the last four to five months of pregnancy, caused by the hormones being produced to maintain the pregnancy. This may or may not cause the nursing child to lose interest in breastfeeding (Huggins, 1990; Mohrbacher & Stock, 1991).

COLOSTRUM PRODUCTION

As the pregnancy nears term, there is a change in the composition of the breast-milk, and the production of colostrum for the new infant begins. This change in flavor may or may not cause the nursing child to lose interest in breastfeeding (Lauwers & Woessner, 1990; Moscone & Moore, 1993). If the child continues to nurse, reassure the pregnant mother that colostrum will be available for the new infant (Mohrbacher & Stock, 1991).

NUTRITION

The mother who chooses to continue breastfeeding while pregnant should pay close attention to eating a nutritious diet that will provide nutrients for her, as well as her developing fetus and breastfeeding child. Nutrient needs of the mother who is breastfeeding while pregnant logically are increased. The recommended dietary allowance charts do not include a category for the pregnant woman who is lactating. It appears prudent that a multivitamin and mineral supplement, such as a prenatal supplement, should be encouraged and the need for additional iron, calcium, and so on, be assessed on an individualized basis.

It is known that malnourished women can produce quality breastmilk, although the quantity produced is less than their better nourished counterparts produce. See Module 3, *The Science of Breastfeeding*, Chapter 2, for more factors that influence milk composition and volume. Milk composition studies of poorly nourished women who are breastfeeding while pregnant have not been done.

WEANING

If the mother is experiencing a difficult pregnancy or has had other difficult pregnancies, weaning may need to be considered. A history of uterine pain, bleeding, or weight loss by the mother while pregnant also are reasons to consider weaning (Mohrbacher & Stock, 1991).

Tandem Nursing

Breastfeeding two or more children of different ages during the same period of time is referred to as *tandem nursing*. A mother may have continued her nursing relationship with one child while pregnant with another, and this relationship continues after the other child's birth; or the older child, previously weaned from the breast, may have renewed interest when seeing the new infant nursing.

During the first few days after birth, when the colostrum alone is present, the mother may need to pay special attention that the new infant receives the colostrum he or she needs. The mother may need to take measures to ensure that the infant has priority at the breast if the older child is still breastfeeding often (Mohrbacher & Stock, 1991). Because breastmilk is produced on a supply-and-demand basis, as the mature breastmilk comes in, there will be enough milk available to nurse both children; however, because the new infant has a physical need for the milk, it would be best for him or her to breastfeed first the majority of the time (Lauwers & Woessner, 1990).

Breastfeeding Multiples

The mother who gives birth to more than one baby at one time should be reassured that she can successfully breastfeed her infants. Because breastmilk is produced on a supply-and-demand basis, she can easily produce enough milk to nourish her infants. Lack of time, not milk production, seems to be the problem that mothers of multiples encounter.

Breastfeeding encourages the mother to spend an increased amount of time with each of the infants. This helps with the bonding process and is important in distinguishing the individuality of each of the infants. While breastfeeding simultaneously is recommended for saving time and increasing the mother's prolactin level, thus increasing her milk production, it is also recommended that the mother try to spend time alone breastfeeding each individual infant to promote bonding.

MANAGING MULTIPLES DURING BREASTFEEDING

Following the birth of her infants, the mother should obtain breastfeeding assistance from all available resources. Although it seems awkward at first, management of breastfeeding multiples may become routine in time. If breastfeeding is delayed because one or more of her infants remain in the high-risk nursery for special care, encourage the mother to express milk for them until they are able to breastfeed, while continuing to breastfeed any other infants. This will help provide the best possible nourishment for them while building her milk supply. (See the previous section on breastfeeding the premature infant for a description of a mother who successfully breastfed preterm quadruplets.)

If each of the infants is able to begin a breastfeeding relationship after birth, encourage the mother to have them room-in with her if possible, or have them brought out to her for feedings together instead of individually. One resource for mothers is the book *Mothering Multiples* by Karen K. Gromada.

A mother of multiples may find it more convenient, or time-saving at the least, to breastfeed her infants simultaneously. Breastfeeding this way also causes an increase in prolactin levels, which in turn increases the mother's milk production (Mohrbacher & Stock, 1991). She may need assistance with the positioning of the infants at the breast early in the relationship, but as the infants become more mature, breastfeeding simultaneously should become easier.

There are several positions the mother who is breastfeeding multiples may want to try when breastfeeding more than one child. (*See also* Appendix in Section A of this module.) Descriptions of four of the more common positions follow (Lauwers & Woessner, 1990; Mohrbacher & Stock, 1991):

1. *Combination Cradle and Clutch (Football) Hold*—The mother supports one of the infants in the cradle (Madonna) hold and the other in the clutch hold. Increased pillow support for the mother's comfort, as well as aid in supporting the infants, is extremely helpful. This position tends to be the

most discreet for nursing in public, and is most helpful if the infants are having a difficult time latching on properly.

2. *Double Cradle Hold (Criss-Cross)*—The mother supports both infants in the cradle (Madonna) hold while breastfeeding. The infants will cross over one another in the mother's lap. Pillow support for the mother's arms is important because this can be tiring for her arms.

3. *Double Clutch (Football) Hold*—The mother supports both infants in the football hold while breastfeeding. Pillow support under the infants, bringing them up to breast level, is important so the mother will not be positioning herself and putting undue strain on her back. This position is especially good for a mother who has had a cesarean section because it helps keep the infants off of her incision line.

4. *Parallel Hold*—While the mother is sitting up, one infant is in the cradle hold, and the other infant is lying in the same direction with his or her body extending off of the mother's lap. Pillows are helpful for support and comfort.

The mother of multiples will need to experiment with various nursing positions and breast-alternating methods to see which will work satisfactorily for her and her infants. She may choose to offer a different breast to each baby at each feeding, or she may choose to assign each baby a breast, and breastfeed him or her only on that breast. Another alternative is for the mother to choose a combination of two methods and breastfeed each infant exclusively on one breast, alternating the breast each day instead of each feeding.

SUPPLEMENTING MULTIPLES

Many mothers of twins have breastfed exclusively for six months, while others have chosen some form of supplementation for occasional or regular use. This may result from working outside the home or the increased time needed or emotional demands. Mothers of triplets, or more, may find an even bigger demand, and since there is no possible way a mother can breastfeed more than two infants at one time, she may be breastfeeding two while someone else is offering the other infant(s) a supplemental feed. The mother should take special note to see that each infant spends about the same amount of time at the breast.

Each mother is an individual and will have individual ways to nourish her infants. Providing increased emotional support and encouragement while allowing the mother to make her own informed decision regarding supplementation is important during this time. Regular supplementation may contribute to various breastfeeding difficulties, and it should not be assumed that a mother with multiples must supplement.

RESOURCES

The following organizations may be helpful to the parents of multiples:

Center for Study of Multiple Births
333 East Superior St., Suite 464
Chicago, IL 60611
Phone: (312) 266-9093

International Lactation Consultant Association
200 North Michigan Ave.
Chicago, IL 60601
Phone: (312) 541-1710

La Leche League International
1400 North Meacham Rd.
P.O. Box 4079
Schaumburg, IL 60168-4079
Phone: (847) 519-7730 (for orders) / (800) 525-3243
Fax: (847) 519-0035

National Mother of Twins Club
5402 Amerwood Ln.
Rockville, MD 20853
Phone: (301) 460-9108

Twinshock Training
Twin Services, Inc.
P.O. Box 10066
Berkeley, CA 94709
Phone: (510) 524-0863
Fax: (510) 524-0494

Adolescents and Breastfeeding

In the United States, teenage mothers are less likely to breastfeed than older women. Teenage mothers tend to have characteristics associated with lower likelihood of breastfeeding among all women (lower income, lower educational level, and an unmarried status). However, Peterson and DaVanzo (1992) report that the nearly 40% difference in numbers of mothers who breastfeed between teenage mothers aged 15 or less and mothers between 20 and 29 years of age remains unexplained by these factors. They believe developmental aspects of adolescence, such as greater egocentricity and concern over body image, play a role in explaining the lower breastfeeding incidence in teen mothers. Lizarraga and associates (1992) report that in a primarily Hispanic population of 64 primiparous, adolescent females, ages 14 to 18 years, breastfeeding was more likely to be initiated if the teen had been breastfed herself or had been exposed to other women who breastfed.

It is physically possible for the teen mother to successfully breastfeed her infant despite rumors to the contrary. There has been no proven difference in the quality of the milk produced, or the quantity produced by the teen mother. Young mothers experience the same successes as older mothers, as well as possibly experiencing the same obstacles (Lauwers & Woessner, 1990). The bigger differences seem to stem from the support system the adolescent has available and her level of maturity. When the older mother experiences breastfeeding difficulties, she may be more apt to work through them and overcome the problems, whereas the adolescent mother may tend to stop breastfeeding altogether because of the difficulties.

PSYCHOSOCIAL CONCERNS

According the works of E. H. Erikson, the adolescent is experiencing the psychosocial crisis of "identity vs. role confusion" (see Figure 3B–1). Her radius of significant relationships may consist of peers and leadership models, with psychosocial modalities of being, or not being, oneself, and sharing being oneself (Erikson, 1963). The following are a few concerns she may or may not be experiencing:

- She may be easily encouraged or discouraged about breastfeeding, because she is strongly influenced by peers and those in leadership roles.
- She may fear the restrictions breastfeeding will put on her lifestyle (i.e., diet, smoking, birth control pills, social activities, and so on).
- She may fear being teased by her peers or others if she breastfeeds.
- She may be concerned about how breastfeeding will affect her physical appearance.

COUNSELING TECHNIQUES

Adolescence is a normal phase of increased conflict characterized by fluctuation of ego strength. Because of the various emotions and concerns the adolescent mother experiences, it may be of great benefit to emphasize the multiple benefits of

	1	2	3	4	5	6	7	8
VIII. Maturity								Ego integrity vs. despair
VII. Adulthood							Generativity vs. stagnation	
VI. Young Adulthood						Intimacy vs. isolation		
V. Puberty and Adolescence					Identity vs. role confusion			
IV. Latency				Industry vs. inferiority				
III. Locomotor–genital			Initiative vs. guilt					
II. Muscular–Anal		Autonomy vs. shame, doubt						
I. Oral Sensory	Basic trust vs. mistrust							
	1 Birth–1 yr	**2** 2nd yr	**3** 3rd–5th yr	**4** 6th yr–onset of puberty	**5** Adolescence	**6** Early adulthood	**7** Young and middle adulthood	**8** Later adulthood

Figure 3B–1 The Span of Life—E. H. Erikson's eight stages of psychosocial development.
Source: Kaluger G, Kaluger MF (1979). *Human Development: The Span of Life,* 2nd ed., pp. 303-304. Reprinted with permission of Prentice Hall, Upper Saddle River, NJ.

breastfeeding to her. According to Mohrbacher and Stock (1991), the benefits to stress include the following:

- Breastfeeding will encourage a strong emotional bond with her infant.
- Breastfeeding allows her to do something for her infant that no one else can do.
- Breastfeeding will help her to get back in shape faster than she would if she does not breastfeed.
- Breastfeeding saves money.

When counseling the teen mother who is considering breastfeeding or is breastfeeding, her support systems, or lack of support systems, should be determined and discussed. Discussion of the teen mother's reaction to her pregnancy, to becoming a parent, and her perception of her self-worth and body image are also important issues to discuss. Become aware of her dietary habits and discuss the importance of a nutritious and well-balanced diet but realize the difficulties adolescence places on the teen's ability to select a nutritious diet. Also, remember that worrying about too many dietary rules is a barrier to breastfeeding for some population groups. Nutrition counseling from a dietitian who is also a lactation consultant may be helpful. It is good to refer a teen mother to a support group if one is available in her area.

When Mother and Infant Are Separated

After birth, more than likely there will be a time when the breastfeeding mother will be absent from her child. Whether the separation results from illness, returning to work or school, or just going out for the evening, emotional and physical adjustments to make this transition easier for both the lactating mother and breastfeeding infant will be required.

SHORT-TERM SEPARATION

The breastfeeding mother may sometimes need to be away from her infant for a brief period of time and a feeding may be missed. It may be because of an appointment that must be kept, outside interests or hobbies, or just needing to take a break. If the infant is not going to accompany the breastfeeding mother on the outing, arrangements must be made for child care and nourishment if regular feedings will be missed. A mother may express her breastmilk and store it in the refrigerator or freezer for use at the missed feeding time. If the infant is still very young, the mother may want to consider not using artificial teats by feeding with a cup, spoon, or dropper to avoid possible nipple confusion.

The mother's comfort level and health must also be considered during a separation. While the mother is away, her breasts may become full after this missed feeding and she will need to hand-express or pump her breasts to relieve the fullness, avoid potential problems, and increase her comfort.

LONG-TERM SEPARATION

Sometimes the breastfeeding mother and infant are separated for a long period of time. In many cases the separation cannot be avoided and must be dealt with in the best way possible. Whether the separation is planned or unplanned, increased encouragement and support will be necessary.

Sometimes the breastfeeding duo is separated because the mother or infant is ill. If the infant must remain hospitalized after birth, the mother should be instructed on breastmilk expression and storage, especially if the breastfeeding relationship is delayed and the infant is unable to be put to the breast. If the infant is hospitalized at any period during the breastfeeding relationship, the mother may inquire about staying with the infant to continue their feeding relationship. If the infant is going to have a surgical procedure done, the mother should inquire about the permitted time limits for breastfeeding prior to and following surgery. Since breastmilk is so easily and quickly digested, some physicians allow breastfed infants to nurse close to surgery time and soon afterward.

If the separation is caused by the illness and/or hospitalization of the mother, the situation is individualized and unique. Not only must the mother be treated as a patient with the illness she is presenting with, but she must be treated as a lactating mother. The fact that she is breastfeeding must be considered in her plan of care and during the recovery period.

In many situations, the breastfeeding relationship can continue without much interruption. The mother may inquire about a room in which she may be able to room-in with her breastfeeding infant, having another caregiver assist her. If this is not feasible, she may consider having someone bring the infant to her at feeding times or pumping her breasts so her infant can be fed while she is away. Many mothers have continued a successful and satisfying breastfeeding relationship while being hospitalized. If the mother chooses to do this, support must be given and options discussed.

For some mothers, the stress of hospitalization, illness, and separation may be too much and the realistic consideration of what is best for her well-being as well as her child's must be dealt with. Depending on the child's age, the situation, the illness, or the medications being consumed, weaning may be a judicious but difficult decision.

RETURNING TO WORK OR SCHOOL

The mother who is planning to combine mothering and outside employment or school may have unique and individualized needs that must be considered when preparations are being made for the separation. For the mother who is breastfeeding, returning to employment outside the home does not mean she cannot or should not continue her breastfeeding relationship. Two very important and necessary preparations for the lactating mother include making sure she is able to express her breastmilk whether it be manually or with a breast pump, and making sure the infant will accept the chosen feeding method—by a bottle, cup, spoon, or other means—when she misses the breastfeeding time.

The breastfeeding mother should begin expressing her breastmilk for freezer storage before returning to work. This way she can begin building a supply for when she returns to work or is away from the infant during a feeding time. Not only will early expression allow the mother to become comfortable with expressing her milk, but it allows some experimentation so she can determine which method works best for her. It also takes some of the stress and worry away, knowing that she already has some breastmilk in reserve for her infant's nourishment.

The following are some of the multiple alternatives for nourishing the infant when the mother returns to work or school:

1. The mother may be able to arrange her schedule so that she can visit the infant for nursing during break and meal times.
2. The mother may be able to arrange for the infant to be brought to her for feedings during scheduled breaks.
3. The mother may choose to pump her breasts at work, and provide that expressed milk for the next day's feeding.
4. The mother may choose to supplement with formula when away from the infant, breastfeeding before going to work, when returning home from work, and whenever out with the infant.

The mother needs to make preparations to have someone else offer the feedings to the infant if the first two options listed are not possible. If she plans to do this, she will need to know that the infant can and will accept being fed by someone else. While there are various ways of offering feedings, most child-care facilities prefer bottles, depending on the age of the child. The only way to prepare for this is to begin offering the infant supplemental bottles prior to returning to work. Bottles and artificial teats should be discouraged for the first three to four weeks after birth, if at all possible, to help avoid the problem of nipple confusion and not interfere with breastfeeding while the mother is establishing her milk supply.

When the time arrives for the mother to begin preparing for separation from her infant, by allowing an occasional bottlefeeding, she may encounter fewer difficulties. Some mothers may encounter an infant who rejects the bottle. Although this is extremely frustrating, the infant will usually stop resisting. The following are a few tips that may assist with this transition:

1. Begin offering the bottle at least two weeks prior to the separation. This allows time for experimentation and to see what the infant will agree to if he or she objects in the beginning.

2. Have someone other than the mother offer the bottle to the infant. Many times the infant refuses to take the bottle when she or he knows the mother is near for breastfeeding. Often the mother has to leave the room altogether.

3. Try different types of artificial teats. Try different shapes, different size holes, and different materials (silicone, rubber) from which the teats are made.

4. Warm the artificial teats under warm running tap water. Some infants may find a cold teat unappealing.

5. Wrap the infant in something that belongs to the mother—a blouse, pajamas, or something else that smells like mother may entice him or her to accept a bottle.

6. Try offering a bottle when she or he is sleepy.

7. Constant motion such as rocking, or riding in a carseat, may calm the infant, enticing him or her to take a bottle.

If the mother will miss one or more feedings while at work or school, it is imperative for her to be knowledgeable concerning breastmilk expression and storage. Regular expression when separated from the infant helps prevent the breasts from becoming overly full and uncomfortable, which can lead to engorgement, plugged ducts, and mastitis, as well as reducing the chance of abundant leaking, and eventually a decrease in the mother's milk supply. The amount of pumping time needed will depend on the number of hours the mother is away and the infant's age.

The mother will need to explore the variety of expression methods available and find the one that she is comfortable with and that works best for her. There is a wide variety of expression methods including manual expression, manual pumping, battery-operated pumping, and electric pumping (automatic cycling, double pumping systems). See Module 2, *The Process of Breastfeeding,* Chapter 3, for a discussion of pumps and pumping.

It is advisable for the mother to discuss her plans to express her breastmilk with her employer. Longer breaks and meals may be able to be negotiated. Appropriate and convenient areas for her when she needs to express her milk should be identified. The mother also needs to have a place to store her breastmilk after it is expressed. If at all possible, these things should be discussed before returning to work or school.

Women should realize that more time may be needed for pumping the breasts than might be expected. Pumping for 15 to 30 minutes may be appropriate for her, but she also needs to take into account the amount of time it will take her to get to her designated pumping area, put the pump together, pump, disassemble and clean the pump, store the milk, and return to her area of work. Although this may not be too time-consuming, mothers should take note of the responsibilities other than the actual expression when planning for time away from a job or class.

CARE PLAN FOR MOTHERS

When developing a plan of care for the lactating mother returning to work or school, Harakal (1988) suggests that the following items should be included in discussions and preparations to help ensure that all relevant information and recommendations are considered:

1. How she plans to provide nourishment for her infant when they are separated during a feeding
2. What she plans to use for feeding her infant
3. Choices of milk expression methods
4. Where she will be able to express her milk
5. Where she plans to store her expressed milk
6. Type of container to store the expressed milk in
7. Storage time guidelines
8. How to transport her expressed milk
9. Length of time expressed milk can be stored in refrigerator and freezer
10. Preparation of stored expressed milk for infant (i.e., thawing)
11. Discussion of breastfeeding and supplemental feeding methods with day-care workers:
    a. Breastfeed the infant just before leaving him or her at day care and as soon as possible after returning from work or school.
    b. Instruct day-care workers not to feed the infant within one hour of the mother's return so she or he will want to breastfeed.
    c. If formula is needed to supplement the breastmilk left for the infant, give it early in the day because it takes longer to digest than breastmilk.
12. What warning symptoms of problems to watch for (i.e., plugged ducts, mastitis, and so on).

Just as there is a movement toward baby-friendly hospitals, there is a movement toward establishing mother-friendly workplaces. To fully integrate breastfeeding into a culture, a mother must be supported in her breastfeeding efforts while separated from her infant. See Module 1, *The Support of Breastfeeding*, Chapter 1, for more information on working and breastfeeding.

POST-TEST

For questions 1 to 6, choose the best answer using the following key:

A. Tandem nursing
B. Nursing multiples
C. Breastfeeding while pregnant
D. The breastfeeding adolescent
E. None of the above

1. Sore nipples are often reported as a result of hormonal changes.

2. _____ is breastfeeding two or more children of different ages.

3. Breastfeeding positions, such as the cradle and/or football hold and the parallel hold, are often used.

4. _____, according to E. H. Erikson, is experiencing the psychosocial crisis of anatomy vs. shame and doubt.

5. _____ may fear being teased by her peers or others if she breastfeeds.

6. _____, according to Erikson, is experiencing the psychosocial crisis of identity vs. role confusion.

For questions 7 to 10, choose the best answer.

7. Ms. Smith calls you in tears to discuss weaning her 8-week-old infant because she must return to work.

   A. You encourage her to wean as soon as possible.
   B. You give her the information asked for without inquiring about why she feels she must wean her infant at this time.
   C. You discuss alternatives to weaning such as pumping and supplementing the infant with her expressed milk.
   D. You tell her to please call you back later because you're too busy to discuss anything right now.

8. During your scheduled appointment with Ms. Jones, you discuss her plan of care for when she returns to work because she plans to pump her breasts and use that milk to feed her infant when they are away from each other. The care plan includes:

   A. storage of her breastmilk.
   B. transportation of her breastmilk.
   C. methods of milk extraction.
   D. warning symptoms related to her health to watch for.
   E. All of the above.

9. The mother who is pregnant and breastfeeding should consider weaning

   A. if she has a history of difficult pregnancies (uterine pain, bleeding, drastic weight loss).
   B. in all cases, to avoid depriving the unborn child of required nutrients.
   C. if she has a history of giving birth to an infant less than 40 weeks gestational age.
   D. None of the above.

10. In reference to the adolescent mother,
    A. it is physically impossible for a teen mother to adequately nourish her infant by breastfeeding.
    B. it is physically possible for a teen mother to successfully breastfeed her infant.
    C. the quality and quantity of breastmilk produced by the teen mother is inadequate to completely support the needs of her infant.
    D. Both A and C.

For questions 11 to 20, choose the best answer using the following key:

A. True   B. False

11. Studies have been done that show if breastfeeding continues during pregnancy, the unborn child will not be deprived of required nutrients if the mother is healthy and eating a healthy, well balanced diet.

12. Sore nipples are often reported by breastfeeding women who are pregnant, as a result of improper positioning of their other child at the breast.

13. As pregnancy nears term, there is a change in the composition of the breastmilk of the woman breastfeeding while pregnant, and as the production of colostrum for the new infant begins.

14. If the pregnant mother is nursing her child near the end of her pregnancy, the child will receive the colostrum, depriving the newborn infant of it.

15. Breastfeeding after conception is not contraindicated.

16. A decreased milk supply may be noticed in the pregnant woman who is breastfeeding in the last 4 to 5 months of her pregnancy, caused by the hormones being produced to maintain the pregnancy.

17. As pregnancy nears term, there is a change in the composition of the breastmilk of the woman breastfeeding while pregnant, and as the production of colostrum for the new infant begins. This change in flavor may cause the nursing child to lose interest in breastfeeding.

18. A mother who gives birth to twins should be strongly encouraged to breastfeed them individually for the first 4 to 6 weeks to promote bonding.

19. Cups, spoons, and droppers are alternatives to the artificial teat when supplementing the infant.

20. The pregnant mother who is continuing to breastfeed need not watch her dietary intake as long as she is taking a vitamin supplement.

SECTION C

Relactation or Induced Lactation

Jan B. Simpson, RN, BSN, IBCLC

LEARNING OBJECTIVES

At the completion of this section, the learner will be able to do the following:

1. Provide guidance and instruction for the mother wishing to relactate.
2. Provide guidance and instruction for the mother wishing to induce lactation.

OUTLINE

I. Relactation

    A. Management suggestions for relactation

    B. Use of drugs for relactation

    C. Other relactation therapies

II. Induced Lactation

    A. Management suggestions for induced lactation

    B. Use of drugs to induce lactation

PRE-TEST

For questions 1 to 4, choose the best answer from the following key:
    A. Relactation
    B. Induced lactation

1. _____ describes the woman who has given birth and initiated lactation but after a period of weaning chooses to stimulate lactation again.

2. _____ is when a nulliparous woman chooses to breastfeed her adopted child.

3. _____ describes the woman who has given birth but never breastfed who later chooses to stimulate lactation.

4. _____ is when a nulliparous woman begins the process of lactation.

For questions 5 to 15, choose the best answer.

5. Relactation may occur in a number of circumstances.
   A. The infant is allergic to formula preparations.
   B. The nulliparous woman chooses to breastfeed her adopted infant.
   C. There is a long-term separation of the mother and infant.
   D. All but B.
   E. All but C.

6. The process of relactation depends on the
   A. mother's commitment.
   B. mother's determination.
   C. infant's willingness to suck at the breast.
   D. All of the above.

7. Relactation generally occurs
   A. after a period of combined pumping and breastfeeding.
   B. after a six-month period of pumping prior to introducing the infant to the breast.
   C. after a six-week period of pumping prior to introducing the infant to the breast.
   D. after a six-day period of pumping prior to introducing the infant to the breast.

8. _____ is needed by the mother who is planning to relactate.
   A. Encouragement and support
   B. Information about exactly what is involved and required
   C. A person to care for children and all household responsibilities
   D. Only A and B.

9. The most effective means of breast stimulation is
   A. using an automatic, electric breast pump.
   B. manual expression.
   C. breastfeeding every 2 to 3 hours for 20 to 30 minutes during the day, with stretches of no longer than 4 to 5 hours at night.
   D. breastfeeding 5 times a day for approximately 100 minutes total time.

10. The length of time it will take for the mother to relactate fully is
    A. approximately six weeks.
    B. impossible to determine because it is an individual process.
    C. approximately the same length of time as it has been since breastfeeding stopped.
    D. Only A and B.
    E. Only B and C.

11. _____ should be avoided during relactation.
    A. Day and night comfort nursing
    B. Breastfeeding on demand, at least every 2 to 3 hours during the day, with a 4- to 5-hour stretch at night
    C. Breastfeeding combined with pumping
    D. None of the above.

12. The amount of breastmilk the woman is able to produce through induced lactation is
    A. unpredictable.
    B. approximately 30 cc per breast.
    C. determined by the size of her breasts and the age of the infant.
    D. Both A and C.

13. The nulliparous woman who adopts a child
    A. will always be able to totally nourish her infant by breastfeeding.
    B. may not always be able to totally nourish her infant by breastfeeding.
    C. will never be able to totally or partially nourish her infant by breastfeeding.
    D. will be able to comfort nurse only, providing total supplementation for nourishment.

14. The nulliparous woman who adopts a child and plans to induce lactation
    A. may have to include a supplement.
    B. will not experience milk-ejection reflexes.
    C. may be able to fully lactate and produce enough milk to totally nourish her infant.
    D. All of the above.

15. A suggested guideline for determining the amount of nourishment (breastmilk or formula) an infant needs in a 24-hour period is
    A. weight in pounds × 2.5 = amount in ounces.
    B. weight in kilograms × 2.5 = amount in ounces.
    C. weight in pounds × .25 = amount in ounces.
    D. weight in kilograms × .25 = amount in ounces.

For questions 16 to 20, choose the best answer from the following key:
    A. True   B. False

16. You will know the mother's milk supply is increasing when the amount of supplement used decreases and the infant continues to gain in weight.

17. When the adoptive mother has induced lactation, she should keep a record of the duration and frequency of breastfeeding, the amount of supplement taken and the method by which it was given, the number of wet and soiled diapers, and the infant's behavior.

18. Oxytocin is a hormone that is found naturally in the breastmilk of breastfeeding mothers.

19. Metoclopramide is a drug that is used in the treatment of digestive disorders, but has also been shown to cause a marked increase in the production of serum prolactin, which in turn improves milk production.

20. Use of metoclopramide for the purposes of relactation is currently approved by the U.S. Food and Drug Administration.

Relactation

When a mother who has given birth chooses to stimulate lactation later or after a period of weaning, or decides to breastfeed after having never breastfed, the term for it is *relactation*. Relactation may be necessary because of a number of circumstances:

- The infant is allergic to formula preparations
- Long-term separation of the mother and infant
- Premature weaning from the breast
- Birth of a premature or sick infant who must be cared for in the hospital setting for an extended period of time

The process of relactation depends on a number of things, including the mother's commitment and determination and the infant's willingness to cooperate and suck at the breast. Relactation generally occurs after a period of combined pumping and breastfeeding. An exact prediction of the length of time it will take for the mother to relactate is impossible to determine because it is an individual process. Some mothers who have relactated found that it often took approximately the same length of time to relactate fully as it had been since they stopped breastfeeding (Mohrbacher & Stock, 1991; Sutherland & Auerbach, 1985). This does not necessarily hold true for all mothers.

MANAGEMENT SUGGESTIONS FOR RELACTATION

For the mother who is planning to relactate, encouragement, support, and proper instruction are extremely important. The mother should make an informed decision regarding relactation by learning what is involved before she begins. She needs to have a realistic understanding of what relactation will require of her. Suggestions on ways she may help build her milk supply and suggestions for taking care of her own needs are necessary; they include the following:

1. Discuss the principle of supply and demand. The more the infant effectively breastfeeds and is removing milk from the mother's breasts, the more milk she will produce. Frequent breastfeeding must be encouraged. The most effective means of breast stimulation is breastfeeding every 2 to 3 hours for 20 to 30 minutes during the day, with stretches of 4 to 5 hours at night.
2. Day and night comfort nursing should be encouraged.
3. If the infant is not feeding frequently at the breast, or additional stimulation is needed, milk expression should be discussed. Many mothers have found that the use of an electric breast pump with a double pump setup is most beneficial because it provides the most effective nipple stimulation.
4. Discuss milk-expression techniques and ways to help enhance her milk-ejection reflex.
5. The mother should maintain her strength and energy level by following a nutritious diet with adequate fluid intake, and getting ample rest.

6. Some women notice a slight decrease in their milk supply during menstruation (Mohrbacher & Stock, 1991).

7. Discuss good nipple care.

8. Relactation should be discussed with and followed up on by the mother's and infant's physician.

While the mother is working on relactation, it is extremely important to continue to nourish the infant by offering supplements, decreasing the amount of supplement given as the mother's milk supply increases. This should be done slowly and cautiously, with the infant's weight and growth being monitored frequently by his or her physician. Scales, such as the BabyWeigh™ scale by Medela, may be very useful to the relactating mother. These scales are now available for rental through Medela Rental Stations and can assist the mother and health-care team determine more accurately the infant's intake.

One effective means of providing supplemental nourishment is by using a nursing supplementer device, which allows the infant to receive nourishment while sucking the mother's breast. This helps to eliminate nipple confusion, while providing the mother with the stimulation required to relactate.

The LC who works with a mother who is relactating should strongly encourage her to maintain a record to monitor her infant's growth during a time in which her milk supply may or may not be meeting all of the baby's nutritional requirements. This record should include the frequency and duration of breastfeeding sessions, the number of wet and soiled diapers, the infant's behavior while breastfeeding, the type and amount of supplement given, and the method of supplementation. The relactating mother should also be encouraged to maintain a record of her own diet and fluid intake. It is important to assess the mother's support systems and self-confidence, and to offer her encouragement, support, and information.

USE OF DRUGS FOR RELACTATION

Lactation can be affected by any drug that has an impact on the production or secretion of the hormone prolactin, or release of the hormone oxytocin. Use of medications to stimulate the mother's milk production are controversial and should be discussed with the mother's physician. The following paragraphs discuss two drugs that can often be used during relactation.

Metoclopramide (Reglan), a dopamine antagonist, is a drug that is used in the treatment of digestive disorders, but has also been shown to cause a marked increase in the production of serum prolactin, which in turn improves milk production. Studies done by Sousa (1975) show that metoclopramide can greatly assist in the reestablishment of lactation. Use of this drug for the purpose of relactation has faced some controversy because, currently, it is not approved for this use by the U.S. Food and Drug Administration. More studies need to be done to prove that this drug is a safe, effective drug therapy for the reestablishment of lactation. Some physicians refuse to prescribe this form of therapy for fear of the effect on the infant. Other physicians have used this drug therapy with no negative results from the infant's standpoint, and have found it helps to reestablish lactation (Lauwers & Woessner, 1990; Lawrence, 1989; Neville & Neifert, 1983).

Oxytocin is a hormone that is found naturally in the serum of breastfeeding mothers, but it is also available in a synthetic form—syntocinon, pitocin—that can be used to stimulate uterine contractions, or enhance the milk-ejection reflex (MER). The MER has been seen promptly after the intake of oxytocin by either the intranasal route or the intramuscular route. Oxytocin in the form of a nasal spray has been found to be most effective if used by the nursing mother two to three minutes before breastfeeding begins. To date, no ill effect has been shown in the infant; however, the use of drugs to stimulate the production of milk or stimulate the MER remains controversial (Lawrence, 1989; Neville & Neifert, 1983). The availability of this medication has become a problem since the acquisition of the manufacturer by Sandoz Corporation.

OTHER RELACTATION THERAPIES

Other recommended methods to increase milk volume include the use of Brewer's yeast and herbal teas such as Fenugreek and Mother's milk teas. Very little is known about their efficacy from a research standpoint, with testimonials as the main justification given for recommending these products. Vorherr does report that theophylline (an ingredient in tea) increases pituitary prolactin secretion, although excessive tea intake is believed to inhibit MER (1978). For many health-care professionals, until more information is available about the positive benefits and whether they outweigh some of the risks, these therapies are considered controversial.

Induced Lactation

Induced lactation is lactation by a nulliparous woman who purposely begins the process of lactation. This process is often chosen by a woman who wishes to breastfeed her adopted child. The decision to try to induce lactation should be discussed with and followed up on by the mother's and infant's physicians. As always, the infant's health and vitality are of number-one importance.

Inducing lactation, without the biological preparation of pregnancy and birth, takes a long time and the induced milk supply is often minimal. Sufficient growth of lactiferous ducts and alveoli for the production of breastmilk needs to occur. This level of growth in the woman who wants to nurse an adopted child does not equal the level of growth that occurs in the pregnant woman over a 40-week gestational period (Anderson, 1986).

The amount of breastmilk a woman is able to produce through induced lactation is unpredictable, and she may not be able to totally nourish her infant at the breast. Most adoptive mothers will have to include a supplement. A few women may be unable to induce lactation at all.

MANAGEMENT SUGGESTIONS FOR INDUCED LACTATION

If the woman is aware of when her adopted infant will be arriving and has ample time to prepare, she may choose to begin the process of induced lactation four to six weeks in advance by pumping her breasts (Mohrbacher & Stock, 1991). Others do not recommend use of breast pumps for induced lactation to prepare for adopting an infant because the mother's attention tends to be more focused on the milk than the bonding. Sutherland and Auerbach (1985) point out that expression with the specific purpose of developing a milk supply in advance is not appropriate because of the uncertainty of the infant's arrival date. If the mother chooses to pump in advance, she needs to be reminded that this is not a guarantee for establishing a milk supply (Anderson, 1986).

If the adoptive mother does have the luxury of advance notice, and chooses to begin preparing for the infant's arrival, she may begin to pump her breasts several times a day for approximately five minutes on each breast, increasing the time slowly to prevent any discomfort. Suction strength should be kept low (Anderson, 1986). By the time the infant arrives, she should be pumping at least every 2 to 3 hours for about 10 to 15 minutes, mimicking the infant's breastfeeding pattern. Pumping the breasts on a regular schedule may assist in the development of alveoli and ductile tissue in the breast, possibly leading to milk production (Anderson, 1986).

When the infant arrives, the mother should let the infant's suck provide the stimulation to the breasts, using a nursing supplementer device as needed (see Module 2, *The Process of Breastfeeding,* Chapter 3, for information on the nursing supplementer devices). Most adopted infants need to be supplemented completely on arrival and at least partially supplemented throughout the breastfeeding experience (Anderson, 1986). If the mother opts for another method of supplementation, encourage her to avoid artificial teats, possibly using a dropper, cup, or spoon. This will help avoid nipple confusion and aid in proper sucking of the breast. If the mother is not using a nursing supplementation device, she should always allow the infant to breastfeed before offering any supplemental nourishment.

A suggested guideline for determining the amount of nourishment (in ounces) an infant needs in 24 hours is to multiply the infant's weight in pounds by 2.5 (Anderson, 1986). If the mother is producing very little milk, the calculated amount can be divided into 8 to 12 feedings and fed through a nursing supplementer device (see Figure 3C–1). As the milk supply increases, the amount of supplement can be decreased.

The mother will know her milk supply is increasing when the amount of supplement the infant takes decreases and he or she continues to increase in weight (Anderson, 1986). The infant may be noted to breastfeed more slowly, and milk may dribble out of the mouth while sucking at the breast. If the infant seems satisfied and full, stop offering the supplementation for that feeding. If there is supplement left over after several feedings in a row, cut down on the amount being offered. If the infant continues to appear satisfied with a reduced amount, continue to slowly and gradually decrease the amount of supplement offered.

The infant's growth and other health issues should be monitored frequently and closely by the pediatrician. A scale to weigh the infant is especially helpful for this mother. A record should be kept of the duration and frequency of nursings, the amount of supplement taken and method by which it was given, the number of wet and soiled diapers, the infant's weight, and the infant's behavior.

Figure 3C–1

Use of a nursing supplementer device for induced lactation.

Source: Spangler, A (1995), *Breastfeeding, A Parent's Guide*, p. 65. Illustration by Abby Drue, Inc. Copyright © 1995 by Amy Kathryn Spangler. Reprinted with permission.

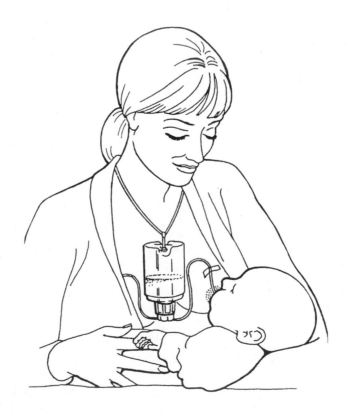

USE OF DRUGS TO INDUCE LACTATION

In induced lactation, the mother has not produced the increased hormonal (estrogen and progesterone) levels that stimulate the proliferation of the alveolar and ductal systems. Therefore, the approach used to induce lactation may need to include drugs that stimulate alveolar and ductal system proliferation. Unfortunately, efforts to stimulate this hormonal response have not been recommended because of concern over milk hormone content and the possible effect on the infant via the milk.

Brown (1973, 1977) has reported that 25 mg to 100 mg of chlorpromazine three times a day for a week to 10 days was successful in inducing lactation in refugee camps in India and Vietnam. The women in these studies also took herbal medicines commonly used in Eastern cultures to stimulate lactation and there was no control group, making the results difficult to interpret. Chlorpromazine is a tranquilizer and is listed by the AAP as a drug. The effect of its use on nursing infants is unknown but may be of concern (AAP, 1994). Using chlorpromazine to induce lactation is not a common clinical practice.

See the previous discussion of drugs used to stimulate relactation.

POST-TEST

For questions 1 to 10, choose the best answer.

1. Oxytocin
   A. is a hormone that is found naturally in the serum of breastfeeding mothers.
   B. is a hormone that is found naturally in the milk of breastfeeding mothers.
   C. can be found in a synthetic form called pitocin.
   D. Only A and C.

2. Metoclopramide
   A. is a dopamine antagonist.
   B. is a drug used in the treatment of digestive disorders.
   C. has been shown to cause a marked increase in the production of serum prolactin, which in turn improves milk production.
   D. is all of the above.

3. The milk-ejection reflex has been seen
   A. after four to six hours of taking a synthetic oxytocin preparation.
   B. promptly after the intake of a synthetic oxytocin preparation by either intranasal route or the intramuscular route.
   C. promptly after the intake of metoclopramide by either intranasal route or the intramuscular route.
   D. None of the above.

4. Reglan
   A. studies have shown that it can greatly assist in the reestablishment of lactation.
   B. currently is not approved by the FDA for use during relactation.
   C. has been used by physicians with no negative results from the infant's standpoint, with a positive reestablishment of lactation.
   D. Only A and C.
   E. All of the above.

5. Syntocinon/pitocin
   A. stimulates the milk-ejection reflex.
   B. has been shown to cause a marked increase in the production of serum prolactin, which in turn improves milk production.
   C. also is a drug used in the treatment of digestive disorders.
   D. None of the above.

6. The nulliparous woman who adopts an infant
   A. will always be able to nourish the infant totally with her breastmilk.
   B. will never have to include a supplement as a part of nourishment.
   C. will never be able to induce lactation at all.
   D. None of the above.

7. A suggested guideline for determining the amount of nourishment an infant needs in a 24-hour period is weight in _____ times _____ equals the amount of breastmilk or formula in ounces.
   A. pounds; 2.5
   B. pounds; 0.25
   C. kilograms; 2.5
   D. kilograms; 0.25

8. During relactation
   A. day and night comfort breastfeedings should be encouraged.
   B. day comfort breastfeedings only should be encouraged because the relactating mother requires extra amounts of rest.
   C. comfort nursings should not be encouraged.
   D. the infant should be put on a nursing schedule so the mother can also put herself on a pumping schedule.

9. The most effective means of breast stimulation
   A. is using an automatic electric breast pump.
   B. is manual expression.
   C. is breastfeeding every 2 to 3 hours for 20 to 30 minutes during the day, with stretches of 4 to 5 hours at night.
   D. is breastfeeding 5 times per day for approximately 100 minutes.

10. The amount of breastmilk a woman is able to produce through induced lactation is
    A. unpredictable.
    B. approximately 30 cc per breast per feeding.
    C. dependent on the infant's age and the woman's breast size.
    D. Both A and C.

For questions 11 to 20, choose the best answer from the following key:
   A. True   B. False

11. There needs to be sufficient growth of lactiferous ducts and alveoli for the production of breastmilk in the woman who is inducing lactation.

12. The level of growth of lactiferous ducts and alveoli in the woman who is adoptive nursing by induced lactation equals the level of growth that occurs in the pregnant woman over a 40-week gestational period.

13. When the adopted infant arrives, the mother who has induced lactation should let the infant's suck provide the stimulation of the breast she receives, using a nursing supplementer device as needed.

14. Most adopted infants are completely supplemented on arrival and at least partially supplemented throughout the breastfeeding experience.

15. Induced lactation applies to any woman who has given birth and later chooses to stimulate lactation after having never breastfed.

16. Relactation refers to a woman who has given birth and later chooses to stimulate lactation after a period of weaning.

17. Induced lactation refers to the multiparous woman who chooses to stimulate lactation after a period of weaning.

18. Pumping the breasts on a regular schedule prior to the adopted infant's arrival may assist in the development of alveoli and ductile tissue in the breast, possibly leading to milk production.

19. Oxytocin is a hormone that is found naturally in the breastmilk of breastfeeding mothers.

20. Relactation generally occurs after a period of combined pumping and breastfeeding.

References

Acolet, D, Sleath, K, Whitelaw, A (1989). Oxygenation, heart rate and temperature in very low birthweight infants during skin-to-skin contact with their mothers. *Acta Paediatrica Scandinavica*, 78(2):189-93.

Affonso, DD, Wahlberg, V, Persson, B (1989). Exploration of mothers' reactions to the kangaroo method of prematurity care. *Neonatal Network*, 7(6):43-51.

Anderson, GC (1990). Kangaroo care and breastfeeding for preterm infants. *Intensive Care Unlimited*, March/April: 1-3.

Anderson, GC (1991). Current knowledge about skin-to-skin (kangaroo) care for preterm infants. *J Perinatolog*, 11(3):216-18.

Anderson, K (1986). *Nursing Your Adopted Baby*. La Leche League International (LLLI) Publication No. 55. Franklin Park, IL: LLLI.

Armand, M, Hamosh, M, Mehta, NR, et al. (1993). Gastric lipolysis in premature infants, effects on diet: human milk or formula. *FASEB J*, 7:A201.

Ashraf, F, Jalil, S, Zaman, S, et al. (1991). Breastfeeding and protection against neonatal sepsis in a high-risk population. *Arch Dis Child*, 66:488-90.

Atinmo, T, Omololu, A (1982). Trace element content of breast milk of mothers of preterm infants in Nigeria. *Early Hum Dev*, 6:309-13.

Atkinson, SA, Anderson, GH, Bryan, MH (1980). Human milk: comparison of the nitrogen composition in milk from mothers of premature and full-term infants. *Am J Clin Nutr*, 33:811-15.

Atkinson, SA, Bryan, MH, Anderson, GH (1978). Human milk: difference in nitrogen concentration in milk from mothers of term and premature infants. *J Pediatr*, 93(1): 67-69.

Atkinson, SA, Fraser, D, Lonnerdal, B (1989). Manganese intakes and excretion in premature infants fed mother's milk or formula. *FASEB J*, 3:A1246, Abstract #5930.

Atkinson, SA, Radde, IC, Chance, GW, et al. (1980). Macro-mineral content of milk obtained during early lactation from mothers of premature infants. *Early Hum Dev*, 4:5-14.

Atkinson, SA, et al. (1978). Human milk: difference in nitrogen concentrations in milk from mothers of term and premature infants. *J Pediatri*, 93:67-9

Barlow, B, et al. (1974). An experimental study of acute necrotizing enterocolitis: the importance of breastmilk. *J Pediatr Surg*, 9:587.

Barness, LA (Ed.) (1993). *Pediatric Nutrition Handbook* (pp. 157, 160-61). Elk Grove Village, IL: AAP.

Bennett, D (1988, March 26). *Cleft lip: Considerations and techniques*. Fifth International Symposium on Maxillofacial Surgery, Denver.

Bernbaum, JC, Pereira, GR, Watkins, JB, et al. (1983). Non-nutritive sucking during gavage feeding enhances growth and maturation in premature infants. *Pediatrics*, 71:41-45.

Bhatia, J, Rassin, DK (1988). Human milk supplementation. *AJDC*, 142:445-47.

Bishop NJ, Dahlenburg, SL, Fewtrell, MS, Morley, R, Lucas, A (1996). Early diet of preterm infants and bone mineralization at age five years. *Acta Paediatr*, 85:230-36.

Bitman, J, Wood, DL, Hamosh, M, et al. (1983). Comparison of the lipid composition of breastmilk from mothers of term and preterm infants. *Am J Clin Nutr*, 38: 300-12.

Bitman, J, Wood, DL, Mehta, NR, et al. (1984). Comparison of the phospholipid composition of breastmilk from mothers of term and preterm infants. *Am J Clin Nutr*, 40:1103-19.

Bixler, D (1981). Genetics and clefting. *Cleft Palate J*, 18: 10-18.

Bocar, D (1993). The Breastfeeding Educator Program. Oklahoma City: Lactation Consultant Services.

Brown, RE (1973). Breastfeeding in modern times. *Am J Clin Nutr*, 26:556.

Brown, RE (1977). Relactation: an overview. *Pediatrics*, 60:116.

Bunting, RW (1957). *Oral Hygiene.* Philadelphia: Lea & Febiger.

Burdi, AR, Lawton, TJ, Grosslight, J (1988). Prenatal pattern emergence in early human facial development. *Cleft Palate J,* 25:8-15.

Clum, D, Primomo, J (1996). Use of a silicone nipple shield with premature infants. *J Hum Lact,* 12(4):287-90.

Countryman, S (1984). *Breastfeeding Your Premature Baby.* La Leche League International (LLLI), Publication No. 13. Franklin Park, IL: LLLI.

Cunningham, A (1977). Morbidity in breastfed and artificially fed infants. *J Pediatr,* 90:29-35.

Danner, S, Cerutti, E (1990a). *Nursing Your Premature Baby.* Rochester, NY: Childbirth Graphics.

Danner, S, Cerutti, E (1990b). *Nursing Your Neurologically Impaired Baby.* Rochester, NY: Childbirth Graphics.

Danner, S, Cerutti, E (1990c). *Nursing Your Baby with Down Syndrome.* Rochester, NY: Childbirth Graphics.

Danner, S, Cerutti, E (1990d). *Nursing Your Baby with a Cleft Palate or Cleft Lip.* Rochester, NY: Childbirth Graphics.

Danner, S, Clay, BW (1986). *Breastfeeding the Infant with a Cleft Lip/Palate.* Unit 10 in Lactation Consultant Series, La Leche League International/Avery Publishing Group.

de Leeuw, R (1988). The kangaroo-method in the care of preterm infants (study 1, 2, and 3). Videotape and data presented at the Eleventh European Congress of Perinatal Medicine, Rome, Italy.

deMonterice, D, Meier, PP, Engstrom, JL, Crichton, CL, Mangurten, HH (1992). Concurrent validity of a new instrument for measuring nutritive sucking in preterm infants. *Nurs Res,* 41(6):342-46.

Ehrenkranz, RA, Ackerman, BA, Nelli, CM (1984). Calcium, phosphorus, zinc and copper content of preterm human milk. *Ped Res,* 18(2):195A, Abstract #597.

Erikson, EH (1963). *Childhood and Society,* 2nd ed. New York: W. W. Norton.

Ernst, JA, Rickard, KA, Neal, PR, et al. (1989). Lack of improved growth outcome related to nonnutritive sucking in very low birthweight premature infants fed a controlled nutrient intake: a randomized prospective study. *Pediatrics,* 83:706-16.

Ferguson, MWJ (1991). The oralfacial region. In: Wigglesworth, JS, Singer, DB (Eds.), *Textbook of Fetal and Perinatal Pathology* (pp. 843-80). London: Blackwell.

Field, T, Ignatoff, E, Stringer, S, et al. (1982). Nonnutritive sucking during feedings: effects on preterm neonates in an intensive care unit. *Pediatrics,* 70:381-84.

Ford, JR, et al. (1983). Comparison of the B vitamin composition of milk from mothers of preterm and term babies. *Arch Dis Child,* 58:367-72.

Gale, SM, Read, LC, George-Nascimento, C, Wallace, JC, Ballard, FJ (1989). Is dietary epidermal growth factor absorbed by premature human infants? *Biol Neonate,* 55:104-10.

Garner, LD, Davis, BW (1983). The team approach to cleft lip and palate. In: McDonald, RE, Avery, DR (Eds.), *Dentistry for the Child and Adolescent,* 4th ed., pp. 687-98. St. Louis: Mosby.

Good, J (1991). *Breastfeeding the Baby with Down Syndrome.* La Leche League International (LLLI) Publication No. 23. Franklin Park, IL: LLLI.

Greene, HL, Hambidge, KM, Schanler, R, Tsang, RC (1988). Guidelines for the use of vitamins, trace elements, calcium, magnesium and phosphorus in infants and children receiving total parenteral nutrition. *Am J Clin Nutr,* 48:1324-42.

Gromada, KK (1991). *Mothering Multiples: Breastfeeding and Caring for Twins.* Franklin Park, IL: La Leche League International.

Gross, SJ (1983). Growth and biochemical response of preterm infants fed human milk or modified infant formula. *N Engl J Med,* 308(5):237-41.

Gross, SJ, David, RJ, Bauman, L, Tomarelli, RM (1980). Nutritional composition of milk produced by mothers delivering preterm. *J Pediatr,* 96(4):641-44.

Gunn, AJ, Gunn, TR, Rabone, DL, et al. (1996). Growth hormone increases breastmilk volumes in mothers of preterm infants. *Pediatrics,* 98(2):279-82.

Hamosh, M, Bitman, J, Liao, TH, et al. (1989). Gastric lipolysis and fat absorption in preterm infants: effect of MCT or LCT containing formulas. *Pediatrics,* 83:86-92.

Hamosh, M, Mehta, NR, Fink, CS, et al. (1991). Fat absorption in premature infants: medium chain triglycerides and long chain triglycerides are absorbed from formula at similar rates. *J Pediatr Gastroenterol Nutr,* 13: 143-49.

Harakal, R (1988). Care plan for employed breastfeeding mothers. *J Hum Lact,* 4(2):68-78.

Hay, WW (1991). *Neonatal Nutrition and Metabolism.* St. Louis: Mosby.

Hayward, JR (1984). Cleft lip and cleft palate. In: Kruger, GO (Ed.), *Textbook of Oral and Maxillofacial Surgery,* 6th ed. (p. 457). St. Louis: Mosby.

Heinonen, OP, Slone, D, Shapiro, S (1977). *Birth Defects and Drugs During Pregnancy.* Littleton, MA: Publishing Sciences Group.

Hopkinson, JM, et al. (1988). Milk production by mothers of premature infants. *Pediatrics,* 81:815-20.

Huggins, K (1990). *The Nursing Mother's Companion.* Boston: Harvard Common Press.

Innis, SM (Ed.) (1992). Lipids in infant nutrition. Symposium. *J Pediatr,* 120:S51-S186.

Kaluger, G, Kaluger, MF (1979) *Human Development: The Span of Life,* 2nd ed. Upper Saddle River, NJ: Prentice-Hall.

King, NM, Wei, SHY (1988). The management of children with cleft lip and palate. In: Wei, SHY (Ed.), *Pediatric Dentistry Total Patient Care.* Philadelphia: Lea & Febiger.

Kruger, GO (1984). *Textbook of Oral and Maxillofacial Surgery,* 6th ed. St. Louis: Mosby.

Lauwers, J, Woessner, C (1990). *Counseling the Nursing Mother,* 2nd ed. Garden City Park, NY: Avery Publishing Co.

Lawrence, R (1989). *Breastfeeding: A Guide for the Medical Profession,* 3rd ed. St. Louis: Mosby.

Lemons, JA, Moyle, L, Hall, D, Simmons, M (1982). Differences in the composition of preterm and term human milk during early lactation. *Pediatr Res*, 16:113-17.

Lizarraga, JL, Maehr, JC, Wingard, DL, Felice, ME (1992). Psychosocial and emotional factors associated with infant feeding intentions of adolescent mothers. *J Adolescent Health*, 13(8):676-81.

Lucas, A, Cole, TJ (1990). Breast milk and neonatal necrotising enterocolitis. *Lancet*, 336:1519-23.

Lucas, A, Hudson, G (1984). Preterm milk as a source of protein for low birthweight infants. *Arch Dis Child*, 59:831-36.

Lucas, A, Morley, R, Cole, TJ, et al. (1990). Early diet in preterm babies and developmental status at 18 months. *Lancet*, 335:1477-81.

Lucas, A, Morley, R, Cole, TJ, Lister, G, Leeson-Payne, C (1992). Breast milk and subsequent intelligence quotient in children born preterm. *Lancet*, 339:261-64.

Ludington-Hoe, SM, Anderson, GC, Hadeed, A (1989). Synchrony in maternal and premature infant temperature during skin-to-skin contact. Poster presented at the American Nurses' Association, Council of Nurse Researchers Conference, Chicago.

Ludington-Hoe, SM, Hadeed, A, Anderson, GC (1990). Energy conservation during kangaroo care. *Heart Lung*, 19:445-51.

Ludington-Hoe, SM, Hadeed, A, Anderson, GC (1991). Randomized trial of cardio-respiratory, thermal, and state effects of kangaroo care for preterm infants. Paper presented at the biennial meetings of the Society for Research in Child Development, Seattle.

Marsh, JL, Vannier, MW (1988). Computer-assisted imaging in the diagnosis, management, and study of dysmorphic patients. In: Vig, KD, Burdi, AR (Eds.), *Craniofacial Morphogenesis and Dysmorphogenesis*, pp. 109-26. Ann Arbor: University of Michigan Press.

Massachusetts General Hospital (MGH), Children's Services (1988). *Pediatric Parenteral Nutrition Manual*. Boston: MGH.

McBride, MC, Danner, SC (1987). Sucking disorders in neurologically impaired infants: Assessment and facilitation of breastfeeding. *Clin Perinatol*, 14(1):109-30.

McGowan, JS, Marsh, RR, Fowler, SM, Levy, SE, Stallings, VA (1991). Developmental patterns of normal nutritive sucking in infants. *Dev Med Child Neurol*, 33:891-97.

Mead, LJ, Chuffo, R, Lawlor-Klean, P, Meier, PP (1992). Breastfeeding success with preterm quadruplets. *JOGNN*, 21(3):221-27.

Measel, CP, Anderson, GC (1979). Nonnutritive sucking during tube feedings: effect on clincial course in premature infants. *JOGNN*, 8:265-72.

Medcoff-Cooper, B (1991). Changes in nutritive sucking patterns with increasing gestational age. *Nurs Res*, 40:245-47.

Medcoff-Cooper, B, Verklan, T, Carlson, S (1993). The development of sucking patterns and physiologic correlates in very-low-birthweight infants. *Nurs Res*, 42:100-104.

Medical College of Georgia (MCG) (1994). *Nutrition Protocols for High Risk Infants*. Department of Pediatrics, Section of Neonatology, Augusta, GA.

Meier, P (1988). Bottle and breastfeeding effects on transcutaneous oxygen pressure and temperature in preterm infants. *Nurs Res*, 37:36-41.

Meier, P, Anderson, GC (1987). Responses of small preterm infants to bottle and breast-feeding. *MCN*, 12:97-105.

Meier, P, Engstrom, JL, Crichton, CL, Clark, DR, Williams, MM, Mangurten, HH (1994). A new scale for in-home test-weighing for mothers of preterm and high risk infants. *J Hum Lact*, 10:163-68.

Meier, P, Lysakowski, TY, Engstrom, JL, Kavanaugh, KL, Mangurten, HH (1990). The accuracy of test-weighing for preterm infants. *J Pediatr Gastroenterol Nutr*, 10:62-65.

Meier, P, Mangurten, HH (1993). Breastfeeding and the preterm infant. In: Riordan, J, Auerbach, KG (Eds.), *Breastfeeding and Human Lactation*, pp. 253-278. Boston: Jones and Bartlett.

Mendelson, RA, Anderson, GH, Bryan, MH (1982). Zinc, copper and iron content of milk from mothers of preterm and full-term infants. *Early Human Dev*, 6:145-51.

Micheli, JL, Schutz, Y (1993). Protein. In: Tsang, RC, Lucas, A, Uauy, R, Zlotkin, S (1993). *Nutritional Needs of the Preterm Infant*, pp. 29-46. Baltimore: Williams & Wilkins.

Mohrbacher, N, Stock, J (1991). *The Breastfeeding Answer Book*. Franklin Park, IL: LLLI.

Moran, JR, Vaughan, R, Stroop, S, et al. (1983). Concentrations and total daily output of micronutrients in breast milk of mothers delivering preterm: a longitudinal study. *J Ped Gastroenterol Nutr*, 2:629-34.

Morley, R, Cole, TJ, Lucas, PJ, et al. (1988). Mother's choice to provide breast milk and developmental outcome. *Arch Dis Child*, 63:1382-85.

Moscone, SR, Moore, M (1993). Breastfeeding during pregnancy. *J Hum Lact*, 9(2):83-88.

Narayanan, I, Mehta, R, Choudhury, DK, Jain, BK (1991). Sucking on the "emptied" breast: nonnutritive sucking with a difference. *Arch Dis Child*, 66:241-44.

Neifert, MR (1983). Routine management of breastfeeding. In: Neville, M, Neifert, M (Eds.), *Lactation: Physiology, Nutrition, and Breastfeeding* (pp. 273-98). New York: Plenum Press.

Neifert, MR, Seacat, J (1985). Milk yield and prolactin rise with simultaneous breast pumping. Presented at the Ambulatory Pediatric Association, Washington, DC, May 7-10.

Neville, M, Neifert, M (1983). *Lactation: Physiology, Nutrition, and Breastfeeding*. New York: Plenum Press.

Nyqvist, KH, Rubertsson, IC, Ewald, U, Sjöden, PO (1996). Development of the preterm infant breastfeeding behavior scale (PIBBS): a study of nurse–mother agreement. *J Hum Lact*, 12:207-19.

Palmer, MM (1993). Identification and management of the transitional suck pattern in premature inants. *J Perinat Neonat Nurs*, 7:66-75.

Peterson, CE, DaVanzo, J (1992). Why are teenagers in the United States less likely to breastfeed than older women? *Demography*, 29(3):431-50.

Putet, G (1993). Energy. In: Tsang, RC, Lucas, A, Uauy, R, Zlotkin, S (Eds.), *Nutritional Needs of the Preterm Infant*, pp. 15-28. Baltimore: Williams & Wilkins.

Raiha, NCR (1991). New perspectives in the nutrition of very low birthweight infants. In: Domenech, E, Castro, R, Ormazahal, C, Mendez, A, Moran, J (Eds.), *Neonatal Nutrition and Metabolism*. Barcelona: Editiones Cientificas y Technicas.

Robertson, AF, Bhatia, J (1993). Feeding premature infants. *Clin Pediatr*, 32(1):36-44.

Saint, L, Maggiore, P, Hartmann, PE (1986). Yield and nutrient content of milk in eight women breastfeeding twins and one woman breastfeeding triplets. *Br J Nutr*, 56:49-58.

Schanler, R, Oh, W (1980). Composition of breastmilk obtained from mothers of premature infants as compared to breastmilk obtained from donors. *J Pediatr*, 96:679.

Schmidt, E, Wittreich, G (1986). Care of the abnormal newborn: a random controlled trial study of the "Kangaroo method of care for low-birthweight newborns." Paper presented at the Euro-Amro Symposium on Appropriate Technology Following Birth, Trieste, Italy, October.

Shaw, GM, Lammer, EJ, Wasserman, CR, et al. (1995). Risks of orofacial clefts in children born to women using multivitamins containing folic acid periconceptionally. *Lancet*, 346:393-97.

Simonin, C, Ruegg, M, Sidiropoulos, D (1984). Comparison of the fat content and fat globule size distribution of breast milk from mothers delivering term and preterm. *Am J Clin Nutr*, 40:820-26.

Slavkin, H (1979). *Craniofacial Development Biology*, pp. 235-97. Philadelphia: Lea & Febiger.

Slavkin, H (1992). Incidence of cleft lips, palates rising. *JADA*, 123:61-65.

Sloan, NL, Camacho, LWL, Rojas, EP, Stern, C, Maternidad Isidro Ayora Study Team (1994). Kangaroo mother method: randomised controlled trial of an alternative method of care for stabilised low-birthweight infants. *Lancet*, 344:782-85.

Snyder, JB (1995). Variation in Infant Palatal Structure and Breastfeeding. Master's Thesis in partial fulfillment for the degree of Master of Arts in Human Development, Pacific Oaks College, CA. (Available from Latch-On Services, PO Box 492, Indianola, IA 50125-0492.)

Sousa, PR (1975). Metaclopramide and breastfeeding. *Br Med J*, 1:512.

Spangler, A (1994). Can I Breastfeed When I Have a Preterm/Low Birthweight Infant?—Lecture Outline.

Stine, MJ (1990). Breastfeeding the premature newborn: a protocol without bottles. *J Hum Lact*, 6:167-70.

Sutherland, A, Auerbach, K (1985). *Relactation and Induced Lactation*. Unit 1 in Lactation Consultant Series, La Leche League International/Avery Publishing Group.

Timko, SW, Culp, YD, Pindell, JG, Harakal, R (1986). *Breastfeeding the Baby with Down Syndrome*. Unit 9 in Lactation Consultant Series, La Leche League International/Avery Publishing Group.

Tsang, RC (Ed.) (1985). *Vitamin and Mineral Requirements in Preterm Infants*. New York: Marcel Dekker.

Tsang, RC, Lucas, A, Uauy, R, Zlotkin, S (1993). *Nutritional Needs of the Preterm Infant*, pp. 15-46, 209-223. Baltimore: Williams & Wilkins.

Tuomikoski-Koiranen, P (1988). Kenguruhoidosta osana keskoster hoitoa ja tutuh yliopistollisen keskussairaalan (Finnish), unpublished manuscript. (Available in English from Anna Maria Laine, University Central Hospital, Department of Pediatrics, 20520 Turku 52 Finland.)

Uauy, RD, Birch, DG, Birch, EE, et al. (1990). Effect of omega-3 fatty acids on retinal function of very low birth weight neonates. *Pediatr Res*, 28(4):85-92.

Veau, V (1931). Treatment of the unilateral harelip. Eighth International Dental Congress (trans.), pp. 126-31.

Vorherr, H (1978). Human lactation and Breastfeeding. In: Larson, BL (Ed.), *Lactation* (pp. 140-65). New York: Academic Press.

Walker, M, Driscoll, JW (1989). *Breastfeeding Your Premature or Special Care Baby: A Practical Guide for Nursing the Tiny Baby*. Weston, MA: Lactation Associates Publication.

Warkany, J (1971). *Congenital Malformation: Notes and Comments*. Chicago: Year Book Medical Publishers.

Weatherly-White, RC, Kuehn, DP, Mirrett, P, et al. (1987). Early repair and breastfeeding for infants with cleft lip. *Plast Reconst Surg*, 79:879-85.

Whitelaw, A (1986). Skin-to-skin contact in the care of very low birth weight babies. *Mater Child Health*, 7:242-46.

Whitelaw, A, Heisterkamp, G, Sleath, K, et al. (1988). Skin-to-skin contact for very low birthweight ifnants and their mothers: a randomized trial of "kangaroo" care. *Arch Dis Child*, 63:1377-81.

Wilson, JG (1963). *Environment and Birth Defects*. New York: Academic.

Woessner, C, Lauwers, J, Bernard, B (1991). *Breastfeeding Today*, p. 189. Garden City Park, NY: Avery Publishing.

Wong, D (1993). *Essentials of Pediatric Nursing*, 4th ed. St. Louis: Mosby.

ADDITIONAL READINGS

Ahmann, E (1996). *Home Care for the High-Risk Infant*. Gaithersburg, MD: Aspen Publishers.

Als, H, Lester, BM, Tronick, E, Brazelton, TB (1982). Manual for the assessment of preterm infants' behavior (APIB). In: Fitzgerald, HE, Lester, BM, Yogman, MW (Eds.), *Theory and Research in Behavioral Pediatrics*, Vol. 1 (pp. 65-132). New York: Plenum Press.

American Dietetic Association (ADA) Report (1986). Promotion of breastfeeding: technical support paper. *J Amer Diet Assoc*, 11.

Anderson, GH (1985). Human milk feeding. *Pediatr Clin North Am*, 32:333-53.

Campbell, SK (1995). *Physical Therapy for Children*. Philadelphia: W.B. Saunders.

Case-Smith, J, Allen, AS, Pratt, PN (1996). *Occupational Therapy for Children*. St. Louis: Mosby.

Dunwar, AJ (1994). *Occupational Therapy: Principles and Practice*. Baltimore: Williams & Wilkins.

Grady, E (1983). *Nursing My Baby with a Cleft of the Soft Palate*. La Leche League International (LLLI) Publication No. 22. Franklin Park, IL: LLLI.

Gross, SJ, Buckley, RH, Wakil, SS, et al. (1981). Elevated IgA concentration in milk produced by mothers delivered of preterm infants. *J Pediatr*, 99:289-93.

Hack, M, Estabrook, MM, Robertson, SS (1985). Development of sucking rhythm in preterm infants. *Early Hum Dev*, 11:133-40.

Hamosh, M (1992). Human milk composition and function in the infant. *Semin Pediatr Gastroenterol Nutr*, 3:4-8.

Hamosh, M (1994). Digestion in the premature infant: the effects of human milk. *Sem Perinatol*, 18(6):485-94.

Lawrence, R (1984). The Lactating Adolescent, pp. 32-42. 15th Round Table, Ross Laboratories.

Lucas, A (1993). Enteral nutrition. In: Tsang, RC, Lucas, A, Uauy, R, Zlotkin, S (Eds.), *Nutritional Needs of the Preterm Infant*, pp. 209-23. Baltimore: Williams & Wilkins.

Ludington-Hoe, SM, Golant SK (1993). *Kangaroo Care— The Best You Can Do to Help Your Preterm Infant*. New York: Bantam Books.

Nelson, KL (1996). Dysphagia: evaluation and treatment. In: Pedretti, LW (Ed.), *Occupational Therapy: Practice Skills for Physical Dysfunction*, pp. 165-192. St. Louis: Mosby.

Vermeiji-Keers, C (1990). Craniofacial embryology and morphogenesis: normal and abnormal. In: Stricker, M, Van Der Meulen, J, Pahpael, B, Mazzola, R (Eds.), *Craniofacial Malformation*, pp. 27-60. Edinburgh: Churchill Livingston.

Walker, M (1990). *Breastfeeding Premature Babies*. Unit 14 in Lactation Consultant Series, La Leche League International/Avery Publishing Group.

Pre- and Post-Test Answer Keys

Postpartum Transitional Period

Pre-Test	Post-Test
1. C	1. E
2. B	2. C
3. B	3. B
4. D	4. C
5. B	5. D
6. D	6. D
7. D	7. B
8. A	8. A
9. B	9. A
10. C	10. A
11. E	11. A
12. C	12. D
13. C	13. E
14. A	14. A
15. B	15. B
16. C	16. A
17. C	17. A
18. B	18. A
19. B	19. B
20. A	20. C

Growing Up Breastfed

Pre-Test	Post-Test
1. C	1. B
2. B	2. D
3. B	3. A
4. C	4. C
5. C	5. A
6. B	6. A
7. B	7. B
8. B	8. B
9. A	9. A
10. A	10. B
11. B	11. A
12. B	12. A
13. C	13. A
14. A	14. C
15. B	15. D
16. C	16. B
17. B	17. A
18. B	18. B
19. A	19. A
20. B	20. A

Nutrition for the Breastfed Infant

Pre-Test	Post-Test
1. C	1. B
2. D	2. C
3. B	3. D
4. D	4. A
5. B	5. B
6. B	6. B
7. B	7. B
8. A	8. A
9. C	9. D
10. D	10. C
11. B	11. C
12. D	12. C
13. D	13. A
14. C	14. B
15. B	15. C
16. A	16. E
17. B	17. B
18. C	18. B
19. A	19. A
20. C	20. C

Maternal Health Issues

Pre-Test	Post-Test
1. B	1. C
2. D	2. D
3. D	3. C
4. A	4. B
5. A	5. B
6. B	6. B
7. D	7. C
8. A	8. D
9. C	9. A
10. C	10. C
11. A	11. C
12. B	12. C
13. D	13. D
14. E	14. A
15. A	15. C
16. A	16. B
17. B	17. B
18. A	18. B
19. A	19. B
20. A	20. A

Infant Health Issues

Pre-Test	Post-Test
1. D	1. E
2. C	2. A
3. D	3. D
4. D	4. B
5. B	5. B
6. E	6. B
7. B	7. D
8. D	8. C
9. A	9. C
10. C	10. E
11. D	11. B
12. E	12. C
13. B	13. B
14. D	14. E
15. B	15. A
16. C	16. B
17. D	17. C
18. A	18. D
19. D	19. C
20. C	20. B

Breastfeeding Infants with Special Needs

Pre-Test	Post-Test
1. B	1. C
2. A	2. E
3. D	3. B
4. B	4. D
5. C	5. A
6. C	6. D
7. D	7. E
8. A	8. D
9. E	9. D
10. E	10. B
11. E	11. D
12. C	12. A
13. A	13. B
14. B	14. B
15. C	15. B
16. A	16. A
17. B	17. A
18. B	18. A
19. A	19. A
20. A	20. A

Breastfeeding in Special Situations

Pre-Test	Post-Test
1. B	1. C
2. C	2. A
3. B	3. B
4. A	4. E
5. D	5. D
6. C	6. D
7. B	7. C
8. A	8. E
9. E	9. A
10. D	10. B
11. B	11. A
12. B	12. B
13. A	13. A
14. A	14. B
15. B	15. A
16. A	16. A
17. A	17. B
18. A	18. B
19. A	19. A
20. B	20. B

Relactation or Induced Lactation

Pre-Test	Post-Test
1. A	1. D
2. B	2. D
3. A	3. B
4. B	4. E
5. D	5. A
6. D	6. D
7. A	7. A
8. D	8. A
9. C	9. C
10. E	10. A
11. D	11. A
12. A	12. B
13. B	13. A
14. A	14. A
15. A	15. B
16. A	16. A
17. A	17. B
18. B	18. A
19. A	19. B
20. B	20. A

Index

How to Receive Continuing Education Credits

The four individual modules of the *Lactation Specialist Self-Study Series* have been approved for continuing education hours/continuing education recognition points (CERPs)/contact hours from the following organizations:

Commission on Dietetic Registration (CDR): The credentialing agency for the American Dietetic Association.

Georgia Nurses Association (GNA): The Georgia Nurses Association is accredited as an Approver of Continuing Education in Nursing by the American Nurses Credentialing Center Commission on Accreditation.

International Board of Lactation Consultant Examiners (IBLCE): The International Board of Lactation Consultant Examiners is the credentialing agency for the International Lactation Consultant Association.

The individual purchasing the module(s) can apply for continuing education credits/contact hours/CERPs for any **one** or **all** of the four modules in the series. The following chart explains the credits approved by each organization for each of the four modules:

		CDR*	GNA	IBLCE
Module 1	*The Support of Breastfeeding*	15 CE Category II	18	18L Independent
Module 2	*The Process of Breastfeeding*	15 CE Category III	18	18L Independent
Module 3	*The Science of Breastfeeding*	23 CE Category III	27	27L Independent
Module 4	*The Management of Breastfeeding*	15 CE Category III	18	18L Independent

---

*The Commission on Dietetic Registration has approved all four modules for specialist CE approval for Board Certified Specialists in Pediatric Nutrition.

Procedure to Follow to Apply for Credits

Step 1   Remove the application for continuing education, answer sheet and evaluation from the back of the module. Do not lose the application form because it has been specially processed to identify originals packaged with each module and can only be replaced for a $25.00 fee accompanied by the original receipt of purchase. Photocopies of the application form will not be accepted. Only one application is needed to apply for credits from more than one organization. Complete the application for continuing education.

Step 2   Review the objectives for each section prior to reading the section or taking the pre-test. Take the pre-test and fill in your answers on the answer sheet for the section to be studied. You must complete the pre-test to obtain credits, although your score on the pre-test will not influence whether you obtain credits. Please answer the pre-test to the best of your ability because the score on the pre-test will be pooled with the scores of other applicants and used to assist the editors in identifying areas applicants are weak in and will be compared to your post-test to quantify the success of the module in enhancing learning.

After you have taken the pre-test and recorded your answers on the official answer sheet, read and study the section. Finally, complete the post-test and fill in the answers on the official answer sheet. **Only the answers on the post-test will be scored for continuing education**. You must receive a 70% correct on the post-test for each section in the module to obtain credit. If you score less than 70% on any one post-test of the module, you will be sent a list of references pertinent to the section(s) you did not complete successfully and can re-apply for continuing education credits for a discounted fee of $1.00 per continuing education credit. Should this occur, you will be sent another answer sheet to use because photocopies of the answer sheets are not accepted.

Step 3   Complete the module evaluation after reading each section. The module evaluations will be analyzed and the information obtained used to improve and enhance the series. Send the module evaluation(s), official answer sheets(s), and check, money order, or credit card information to ANC, Inc., 4833 McGahee Road, Evans, GA 30809.

Allow three weeks for processing. Rush processing is available for an extra $25.00. Scoring and notification of credits to credentialing agencies will be completed within three business days of receiving your application and the rush processing fee.

Step 4   Upon successful completion of all the post-tests for a module, you will be sent a certificate of completion for each organization that you have requested credit from; your name will be forwarded to the appropriate credentialing organization, if appropriate; and a record will be maintained of your successful completion for five years. Requests for duplicate certificates can be honored for a processing fee of $10.00.

Module 4   The Management of Breastfeeding
APPLICATION FOR CONTINUING EDUCATION CREDITS

Name _____

as it will appear on certificate

Address _____

street, rural route, or post office box

City _____ State/Province _____ Zip code _____

Country _____

Daytime phone no. _____ e-mail _____

area code and number

Please complete the information for the organization(s) from which you are requesting credit:

Commission on Dietetic Registration   CE hours: _____ × $2.00 = _____

Are you a board certified specialist in pediatric nutrition?   Yes ___   No ___

Registration number _____

Georgia Nurses Association   Contact hours: _____ × $2.00 = _____

SSN/SIN _____

International Board of Lactation   CERPs: _____ × $2.00 = _____
Consultant Examiners

SSN/SIN or IBLCE 9-digit ID number _____

Optional rush processing ($25.00 fee) _____

TOTAL _____

Checks, money orders, and credit cards accepted. No purchase orders.

_____ MasterCard   _____ Visa   _____ American Express

Account number _____ Expiration date _____

Name as it appears on the card _____

Checks or money orders should be made out to **Augusta Nutrition Consultants, Inc. (ANC)** and sent with the evaluation and completed answer sheet to 4833 McGahee Road, Evans, GA 30809.

DO **NOT** SEND TO JONES AND BARTLETT PUBLISHERS.

Note: You must submit this **original** form to receive continuing education units. Photocopies cannot be accepted.

Evaluation of
The Management of Breastfeeding

Please comment on the degree of content difficulty, effectiveness of learning method, and objectives for the following topics by putting a checkmark in the circle next to the response that best describes the material.

Postpartum Transitional Period

Content level	○ too high	○ appropriate	○ too low
Effectiveness of learning method	○ excellent/very good	○ good	○ fair/poor
Information	○ useful		○ not useful

Use the following key for the objectives and circle your response:

1 = STRONGLY MET   **2** = MET   **3** = SOMEWHAT MET   **4** = SOMEWHAT NOT MET   **5** = NOT MET

At the completion of this section, the learner will be able to do the following:

1. Identify the sensory reactions and reflex behaviors of the newborn.   1   2   3   4   5

2. Recognize the importance of mother–baby interdependence during the postpartum period.   1   2   3   4   5

3. Discuss the average, quiet, and active babies' responses during the newborn period in relation to breastfeeding.   1   2   3   4   5

4. Describe the four stages of maternal role acquisition and appropriate counseling strategies for each stage.   1   2   3   4   5

Growing Up Breastfed

Content level	○ too high	○ appropriate	○ too low
Effectiveness of learning method	○ excellent/very good	○ good	○ fair/poor
Information	○ useful		○ not useful

Use the following key for the objectives and circle your response:

1 = STRONGLY MET   **2** = MET   **3** = SOMEWHAT MET   **4** = SOMEWHAT NOT MET   **5** = NOT MET

At the completion of this section, the learner will be able to do the following:

1. Recognize the importance of stimulation to emotional growth of mother and baby, and the contributions of breastfeeding to this growth.   1   2   3   4   5

2. Describe developmental milestones in normal child development and their effect on the breastfeeding relationship.   1   2   3   4   5

3. Discuss normal sleep patterns of breastfed infants.   1   2   3   4   5

4. Describe benefits to the infant from prolonged lactation.   1   2   3   4   5

Nutrition for the Breastfed Infant

Content level	○ too high	○ appropriate	○ too low
Effectiveness of learning method	○ excellent/very good	○ good	○ fair/poor
Information	○ useful		○ not useful

Use the following key for the objectives and circle your response:

1 = STRONGLY MET   **2** = MET   **3** = SOMEWHAT MET   **4** = SOMEWHAT NOT MET   **5** = NOT MET

At the completion of this section, the learner will be able to do the following:

1. Give three indications of adequate feedings in breastfed infants.   1 2 3 4 5

2. Give developmental milestones that can guide the introduction and progression of solid foods into the infant's diet.   1 2 3 4 5

3. Explain the recommended sequence for the introduction of solid foods for the breastfed infant.   1 2 3 4 5

4. Cite three contributions of extended breastfeeding to the health and well-being of the toddler.   1 2 3 4 5

5. Cite recommendations for the supplementation of breastfed infants with vitamins and/or minerals.   1 2 3 4 5

Maternal Health Issues

Content level	○ too high	○ appropriate	○ too low
Effectiveness of learning method	○ excellent/very good	○ good	○ fair/poor
Information	○ useful		○ not useful

Use the following key for the objectives and circle your response:

1 = STRONGLY MET   **2** = MET   **3** = SOMEWHAT MET   **4** = SOMEWHAT NOT MET   **5** = NOT MET

At the completion of this section, the learner will be able to do the following:

1. Discuss the influence of maternal cystic fibrosis, multiple sclerosis, phenylketonuria, diabetes, and hyperlipoproteinemia on milk production and milk composition.   1 2 3 4 5

2. Describe how viral and bacterial infections impact feeding.   1 2 3 4 5

3. List the advantages and disadvantages of various contraceptive methods for the lactating woman.   1 2 3 4 5

4. Identify the factors that influence the passage of drugs into human milk and the absorption of drugs by the infants.   1 2 3 4 5

5. Identify drugs that may impair or stimulate lactation.   1 2 3 4 5

6. Identify drugs that are contraindicated during lactation.   1 2 3 4 5

7. Cite the circumstances when breastfeeding is contraindicated.   1 2 3 4 5

Infant Health Issues

Content level	○ too high	○ appropriate	○ too low
Effectiveness of learning method	○ excellent/very good	○ good	○ fair/poor
Information	○ useful		○ not useful

Use the following key for the objectives and circle your response:

1 = STRONGLY MET   **2** = MET   **3** = SOMEWHAT MET   **4** = SOMEWHAT NOT MET   **5** = NOT MET

At the completion of this section, the learner will be able to do the following:

1. Describe techniques for maintaining the infant's thermal regulation. 1 2 3 4 5

2. Discuss the prevention and treatment of newborn hypo-glycemia. 1 2 3 4 5

3. Differentiate among the types of jaundice and discuss care for the breastfeeding infant who has hyperbilirubinemia. 1 2 3 4 5

4. Cite the research on infections in breast- versus bottle-feeding populations. 1 2 3 4 5

5. Recognize symptoms of growth deficit, or failure to thrive, and cite three interventions. 1 2 3 4 5

6. State biochemical guidelines for the assessment of iron-deficiency anemia. 1 2 3 4 5

7. Discuss the factors that contribute to optimal infant oral health care. 1 2 3 4 5

Breastfeeding Infants with Special Needs

Content level	○ too high	○ appropriate	○ too low
Effectiveness of learning method	○ excellent/very good	○ good	○ fair/poor
Information	○ useful		○ not useful

Use the following key for the objectives and circle your response:

1 = STRONGLY MET   **2** = MET   **3** = SOMEWHAT MET   **4** = SOMEWHAT NOT MET   **5** = NOT MET

At the completion of this section, the learner will be able to do the following:

1. Discuss suggestions for the successful initiation and continuation of breastfeeding of the infant who is born prematurely. 1 2 3 4 5

2. Discuss tongue and jaw movements that are disorganized and/or dysfunctional and how these variations and movements impact feeding. 1 2 3 4 5

3. Discuss suggestions for the successful initiation and continuation of breastfeeding of the neurologically impaired infant. 1 2 3 4 5

4. Discuss suggestions for the successful initiation and continuation of breastfeeding of the infant with Down syndrome. 1 2 3 4 5

5. Identify classifications of cleft lip and/or cleft palate.   1 2 3 4 5

6. Discuss suggestions for the successful initiation and/or con-   1 2 3 4 5
   tinuation of breastfeeding of the infant with cleft lip and/or
   cleft palate.

Breastfeeding in Special Situations

Content level	○ too high	○ appropriate	○ too low
Effectiveness of learning method	○ excellent/very good	○ good	○ fair/poor
Information	○ useful		○ not useful

Use the following key for the objectives and circle your response:

1 = STRONGLY MET   **2** = MET   **3** = SOMEWHAT MET   **4** = SOMEWHAT NOT MET   **5** = NOT MET

At the completion of this section, the learner will be able to do the following:

1. Provide information and guidance to the mother who chooses   1 2 3 4 5
   to continue breastfeeding while pregnant.

2. Provide breastfeeding management suggestions for the mother   1 2 3 4 5
   who chooses to tandem nurse.

3. Provide breastfeeding management suggestions for the mother   1 2 3 4 5
   who is nursing multiples.

4. Offer guidance and information to the adolescent who is con-   1 2 3 4 5
   sidering breastfeeding or who is breastfeeding.

5. Identify ways to help the lactating mother who will be sep-   1 2 3 4 5
   arated from her infant for brief or extended lengths of time
   to have a successful breastfeeding relationship.

6. Advise the breastfeeding mother who is returning to work or   1 2 3 4 5
   school about methods for continuing a successful breastfeeding relationship.

Relactation or Induced Lactation

Content level	○ too high	○ appropriate	○ too low
Effectiveness of learning method	○ excellent/very good	○ good	○ fair/poor
Information	○ useful		○ not useful

Use the following key for the objectives and circle your response:

1 = STRONGLY MET   **2** = MET   **3** = SOMEWHAT MET   **4** = SOMEWHAT NOT MET   **5** = NOT MET

At the completion of this section, the learner will be able to do the following:

1. Provide guidance and instruction for the mother wishing to   1 2 3 4 5
   relactate.

2. Provide guidance and instruction for the mother wishing to   1 2 3 4 5
   induce lactation.

Describe how the information presented is applicable to your practice:

Please tell us what you liked the best about the material:

Please tell us what you liked the least about the material:

Please evaluate the time required to complete the module when compared to the continuing education hours offered (check one):

　　　○ more time required than hours awarded

　　　○ approximately the same time required as hours awarded

　　　○ less time required than hours awarded

Additional comments:

Module 4   *The Management of Breastfeeding*
Answer Sheet

Please use a number 2 pencil to mark your responses.

Chapter 1 Section A
Postpartum Transitional Period

	Pre-Test a b c d e	Post-Test a b c d e
1.	O O O O O	1. O O O O O
2.	O O O O O	2. O O O O O
3.	O O O O O	3. O O O O O
4.	O O O O O	4. O O O O O
5.	O O O O O	5. O O O O O
6.	O O O O O	6. O O O O O
7.	O O O O O	7. O O O O O
8.	O O O O O	8. O O O O O
9.	O O O O O	9. O O O O O
10.	O O O O O	10. O O O O O
11.	O O O O O	11. O O O O O
12.	O O O O O	12. O O O O O
13.	O O O O O	13. O O O O O
14.	O O O O O	14. O O O O O
15.	O O O O O	15. O O O O O
16.	O O O O O	16. O O O O O
17.	O O O O O	17. O O O O O
18.	O O O O O	18. O O O O O
19.	O O O O O	19. O O O O O
20.	O O O O O	20. O O O O O

Chapter 1 Section B
Growing Up Breastfed

	Pre-Test a b c d e	Post-Test a b c d e
1.	O O O O O	1. O O O O O
2.	O O O O O	2. O O O O O
3.	O O O O O	3. O O O O O
4.	O O O O O	4. O O O O O
5.	O O O O O	5. O O O O O
6.	O O O O O	6. O O O O O
7.	O O O O O	7. O O O O O
8.	O O O O O	8. O O O O O
9.	O O O O O	9. O O O O O
10.	O O O O O	10. O O O O O
11.	O O O O O	11. O O O O O
12.	O O O O O	12. O O O O O
13.	O O O O O	13. O O O O O
14.	O O O O O	14. O O O O O
15.	O O O O O	15. O O O O O
16.	O O O O O	16. O O O O O
17.	O O O O O	17. O O O O O
18.	O O O O O	18. O O O O O
19.	O O O O O	19. O O O O O
20.	O O O O O	20. O O O O O

Chapter 1 Section C
Nutrition for the Breastfed Infant

	Pre-Test						Post-Test				
	a	b	c	d	e		a	b	c	d	e
1.	O	O	O	O	O	1.	O	O	O	O	O
2.	O	O	O	O	O	2.	O	O	O	O	O
3.	O	O	O	O	O	3.	O	O	O	O	O
4.	O	O	O	O	O	4.	O	O	O	O	O
5.	O	O	O	O	O	5.	O	O	O	O	O
6.	O	O	O	O	O	6.	O	O	O	O	O
7.	O	O	O	O	O	7.	O	O	O	O	O
8.	O	O	O	O	O	8.	O	O	O	O	O
9.	O	O	O	O	O	9.	O	O	O	O	O
10.	O	O	O	O	O	10.	O	O	O	O	O
11.	O	O	O	O	O	11.	O	O	O	O	O
12.	O	O	O	O	O	12.	O	O	O	O	O
13.	O	O	O	O	O	13.	O	O	O	O	O
14.	O	O	O	O	O	14.	O	O	O	O	O
15.	O	O	O	O	O	15.	O	O	O	O	O
16.	O	O	O	O	O	16.	O	O	O	O	O
17.	O	O	O	O	O	17.	O	O	O	O	O
18.	O	O	O	O	O	18.	O	O	O	O	O
19.	O	O	O	O	O	19.	O	O	O	O	O
20.	O	O	O	O	O	20.	O	O	O	O	O

Chapter 2 Section A
Maternal Health Issues

	Pre-Test						Post-Test				
	a	b	c	d	e		a	b	c	d	e
1.	O	O	O	O	O	1.	O	O	O	O	O
2.	O	O	O	O	O	2.	O	O	O	O	O
3.	O	O	O	O	O	3.	O	O	O	O	O
4.	O	O	O	O	O	4.	O	O	O	O	O
5.	O	O	O	O	O	5.	O	O	O	O	O
6.	O	O	O	O	O	6.	O	O	O	O	O
7.	O	O	O	O	O	7.	O	O	O	O	O
8.	O	O	O	O	O	8.	O	O	O	O	O
9.	O	O	O	O	O	9.	O	O	O	O	O
10.	O	O	O	O	O	10.	O	O	O	O	O
11.	O	O	O	O	O	11.	O	O	O	O	O
12.	O	O	O	O	O	12.	O	O	O	O	O
13.	O	O	O	O	O	13.	O	O	O	O	O
14.	O	O	O	O	O	14.	O	O	O	O	O
15.	O	O	O	O	O	15.	O	O	O	O	O
16.	O	O	O	O	O	16.	O	O	O	O	O
17.	O	O	O	O	O	17.	O	O	O	O	O
18.	O	O	O	O	O	18.	O	O	O	O	O
19.	O	O	O	O	O	19.	O	O	O	O	O
20.	O	O	O	O	O	20.	O	O	O	O	O

Chapter 2 Section B
Infant Health Issues

	Pre-Test						Post-Test				
	a	b	c	d	e		a	b	c	d	e
1.	O	O	O	O	O	1.	O	O	O	O	O
2.	O	O	O	O	O	2.	O	O	O	O	O
3.	O	O	O	O	O	3.	O	O	O	O	O
4.	O	O	O	O	O	4.	O	O	O	O	O
5.	O	O	O	O	O	5.	O	O	O	O	O
6.	O	O	O	O	O	6.	O	O	O	O	O
7.	O	O	O	O	O	7.	O	O	O	O	O
8.	O	O	O	O	O	8.	O	O	O	O	O
9.	O	O	O	O	O	9.	O	O	O	O	O
10.	O	O	O	O	O	10.	O	O	O	O	O
11.	O	O	O	O	O	11.	O	O	O	O	O
12.	O	O	O	O	O	12.	O	O	O	O	O
13.	O	O	O	O	O	13.	O	O	O	O	O
14.	O	O	O	O	O	14.	O	O	O	O	O
15.	O	O	O	O	O	15.	O	O	O	O	O
16.	O	O	O	O	O	16.	O	O	O	O	O
17.	O	O	O	O	O	17.	O	O	O	O	O
18.	O	O	O	O	O	18.	O	O	O	O	O
19.	O	O	O	O	O	19.	O	O	O	O	O
20.	O	O	O	O	O	20.	O	O	O	O	O

Chapter 3 Section A
Breastfeeding Infants with Special Needs

	Pre-Test						Post-Test				
	a	b	c	d	e		a	b	c	d	e
1.	O	O	O	O	O	1.	O	O	O	O	O
2.	O	O	O	O	O	2.	O	O	O	O	O
3.	O	O	O	O	O	3.	O	O	O	O	O
4.	O	O	O	O	O	4.	O	O	O	O	O
5.	O	O	O	O	O	5.	O	O	O	O	O
6.	O	O	O	O	O	6.	O	O	O	O	O
7.	O	O	O	O	O	7.	O	O	O	O	O
8.	O	O	O	O	O	8.	O	O	O	O	O
9.	O	O	O	O	O	9.	O	O	O	O	O
10.	O	O	O	O	O	10.	O	O	O	O	O
11.	O	O	O	O	O	11.	O	O	O	O	O
12.	O	O	O	O	O	12.	O	O	O	O	O
13.	O	O	O	O	O	13.	O	O	O	O	O
14.	O	O	O	O	O	14.	O	O	O	O	O
15.	O	O	O	O	O	15.	O	O	O	O	O
16.	O	O	O	O	O	16.	O	O	O	O	O
17.	O	O	O	O	O	17.	O	O	O	O	O
18.	O	O	O	O	O	18.	O	O	O	O	O
19.	O	O	O	O	O	19.	O	O	O	O	O
20.	O	O	O	O	O	20.	O	O	O	O	O

Chapter 3 Section B
Breastfeeding in Special Situations

	Pre-Test						Post-Test				
	a	b	c	d	e		a	b	c	d	e
1.	O	O	O	O	O	1.	O	O	O	O	O
2.	O	O	O	O	O	2.	O	O	O	O	O
3.	O	O	O	O	O	3.	O	O	O	O	O
4.	O	O	O	O	O	4.	O	O	O	O	O
5.	O	O	O	O	O	5.	O	O	O	O	O
6.	O	O	O	O	O	6.	O	O	O	O	O
7.	O	O	O	O	O	7.	O	O	O	O	O
8.	O	O	O	O	O	8.	O	O	O	O	O
9.	O	O	O	O	O	9.	O	O	O	O	O
10.	O	O	O	O	O	10.	O	O	O	O	O
11.	O	O	O	O	O	11.	O	O	O	O	O
12.	O	O	O	O	O	12.	O	O	O	O	O
13.	O	O	O	O	O	13.	O	O	O	O	O
14.	O	O	O	O	O	14.	O	O	O	O	O
15.	O	O	O	O	O	15.	O	O	O	O	O
16.	O	O	O	O	O	16.	O	O	O	O	O
17.	O	O	O	O	O	17.	O	O	O	O	O
18.	O	O	O	O	O	18.	O	O	O	O	O
19.	O	O	O	O	O	19.	O	O	O	O	O
20.	O	O	O	O	O	20.	O	O	O	O	O

Chapter 3 Section C
Relactation or Induced Lactation

	Pre-Test						Post-Test				
	a	b	c	d	e		a	b	c	d	e
1.	O	O	O	O	O	1.	O	O	O	O	O
2.	O	O	O	O	O	2.	O	O	O	O	O
3.	O	O	O	O	O	3.	O	O	O	O	O
4.	O	O	O	O	O	4.	O	O	O	O	O
5.	O	O	O	O	O	5.	O	O	O	O	O
6.	O	O	O	O	O	6.	O	O	O	O	O
7.	O	O	O	O	O	7.	O	O	O	O	O
8.	O	O	O	O	O	8.	O	O	O	O	O
9.	O	O	O	O	O	9.	O	O	O	O	O
10.	O	O	O	O	O	10.	O	O	O	O	O
11.	O	O	O	O	O	11.	O	O	O	O	O
12.	O	O	O	O	O	12.	O	O	O	O	O
13.	O	O	O	O	O	13.	O	O	O	O	O
14.	O	O	O	O	O	14.	O	O	O	O	O
15.	O	O	O	O	O	15.	O	O	O	O	O
16.	O	O	O	O	O	16.	O	O	O	O	O
17.	O	O	O	O	O	17.	O	O	O	O	O
18.	O	O	O	O	O	18.	O	O	O	O	O
19.	O	O	O	O	O	19.	O	O	O	O	O
20.	O	O	O	O	O	20.	O	O	O	O	O